Refractive Surgery: Current Techniques and Management

Refractive Surgery: Current Techniques and Management

Olivia N. Serdarevic, M.D.
Professor of Ophthalmology
University of Paris VI
Hôtel-Dieu
Paris, France
Cornell University Medical College
The New York Hopsital-Cornell Medical Center
The Manhattan Eye, Ear, and Throat Hospital
Beth Israel Medical Center
New York, New York

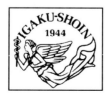

IGAKU-SHOIN   New York   •   Tokyo

Igaku-Shoin Medical Publishers. Inc. gratefully acknowledges
the assistance of Chiron Vision, Nidek, Inc., Technomed Technology,
and VisX, Inc., for their support of this project.

Published and distributed by

IGAKU-SHOIN Medical Publishers, Inc.
One Madison Avenue, New York, New York 10010

IGAKU-SHOIN Ltd.,
5-24-3 Hongo, Bunkyo-ku, Tokyo 113-91.

Library of Congress Cataloging-in-Publication Data

Serdarevic. Olivia N.
    Refractive surgery : current techniques and management / Olivia N.
Serdarevic.
        p.   cm.
    Includes bibliographical references and index.
    ISBN 0-89640-325-4 (New York). — ISBN 4-260-14325-5 (Tokyo)
    1. Refractive keratoplasty.   I. Title.
    [DNLM: 1. Refractive Errors—surgery.   2. Keratotomy. Radial.   WW
300 S482r   1997]
RE336. S47   1997
617.7'55—dc20
DNLM/DLC
for Library of Congress   96-29391
                                                                CIP

ISBN: 0–89640–325–4   (New York)
ISBN: 4-260–14325–5   (Tokyo)

Printed and bound in the U.S.A.
10 9 8 7 6 5 4 3 2 1

Dedication

To my mother and late father
who, with their love, altruism, energy, and brilliance,
taught me
to strive for excellence, balance, and integrity in my endeavors
and gave me the courage
to defend my convictions and pursue my dreams

Foreword

It is a great privilege and an honor to have the opportunity to write a Foreword to the magnificent book edited by Olivia Serdarevic, M.D., entitled *Refractive Surgery: Current Techniques and Management.* Dr Serdarevic, along with several other distinguished individuals, enjoys a reputation as one of the world's outstanding refractive surgeons and a leading pioneer in excimer laser correction of refractive errors of the eye.

In the first chapter of this textbook, Dr. Serdarevic has wisely chosen to present background information concerning the etiology, incidence, prevention, and nonsurgical management of refractive errors. Subsequent chapters deal with radial keratotomy as well as mini-radial keratotomy, and then progress to photorefractive keratectomy for low, moderate, and high myopia. Chapters 5 through 8 are concerned with photorefractive keratectomy, the particular application of this therapy, and most importantly, the management of complications and retreatment procedures. As this brilliant book develops, the subjects of laser in situ keratomileusis, automated lamellar keratoplasty, phakic myopic intraocular lenses, clear lens extraction, intraocular lens power calculations after refractive surgery, as well as the latest approaches and statistics regarding astigmatic keratotomy, photorefractive keratectomy for astigmatism, and keratophakia for hyperopia are comprehensively addressed.

The next section deals with the relationship of photorefractive keratectomy and laser thermal keratoplasty for hyperopia and presbyopia as well as hyperoptic astigmatism. In addition, the complications of laser thermal keratoplasty and other forms of corneal refractive surgery are clearly enunciated, and suggestions for their management are proposed.

The final four chapters of this twenty-four chapter textbook deal with the organization and management of refractive centers, as well as co-management, medical-legal aspects, and the regulatory aspects of refractive surgery. In many respects, the final sections are those portions of the entire refractive surgical spectrum that are least known to ophthalmologists and are a superb addition to this remarkable book.

This textbook, for which Dr. Serdarevic should be congratulated, displays an exceptionally well-defined and brilliant view of the entire subject of the correction of refractive errors of the eye by all currently available surgical approaches. This volume brings together the finest clinical research scientists and ophthalmic intellects, who have described their various surgical approaches and techniques to correct refractive conditions of the eye. Each chapter is comprehensive in nature, exhaustive in scope, and represents the most current thinking. Furthermore, the book has magnificent illustrations throughout the chapters which, combined with information regarding the most recent statistics and surgical trends, eloquently positions this volume as the foremost treatise of its kind. This textbook is unparalleled in the world literature in its comprehensive and outstanding compilation of information regarding the various forms of surgical treatment of refractive errors of the eye.

Francis A. L'Esperance, Jr., M.D.
Professor of Clinical Ophthalmology
Columbia University College of Physicians and Surgeons
New York, New York
USA

Preface

Ophthalmologists have been interested in the surgical correction of refractive errors for over 200 years. The earliest attempts involved manipulation of the crystalline lens in Italy in the late 1700s. However, it is just over the past 10 years that widespread interest and technological advances have led to the development and successful application globally of many refractive procedures.

My personal experience performing and teaching refractive surgery in the United States, Europe, and Asia made me realize the need for a book that would provide comprehensive, authoritative, and up-to-date information about major refractive disorders, current techniques and devices. I have been extremely fortunate to have the outstanding assistance of more than 50 of my American and international colleagues who write about the refractive subjects that have gained them worldwide recognition. The contributors discuss their most recent results and strategies regarding patient selection and management, surgical approaches, and management of complications in an attempt to present a balanced guide to accepted procedures.

It has been very rewarding for me to "grow up" in ophthalmology together with the field of refractive surgery. As a medical student at the Columbia University College of Physicians and Surgeons, I became particularly interested in corneal pathology, morphology, and wound healing during my first research project involving specular microscopy and light effects on the cornea. As a resident at the Columbia Presbyterian E.S. Harkness Eye Institute, I learned, particularly from the extraordinary advice, teaching, and example of Dr. Francis L'Esperance, Jr., to respect Nature's complex design for the human optical system and to search for innovative approaches for treating ocular disorders.

During my residency I was excited by the pioneering work in corneal and intraocular refractive surgery and was eager to work on a procedure that would not destabilize the cornea. I felt that it was inadvisable to pursue procedures such as radial keratotomy for myopia or keratomileusis for high hyperopia that achieve their refractive effects by "stable" destabilization.

I was intrigued in 1983 by the excimer laser after Drs. Trokel and Srinivasan demonstrated in enucleated bovine corneas that the excimer laser could be a very precise cutting device. I am very grateful to Dr. Stephen Trokel for kindling my interest in photoablation and providing the opportunity to work on the excimer laser. While Dr. Trokel was interested in assessing the possibility of replacing steel knives with the excimer laser for radial keratotomy or replacing the cryolathe with the excimer laser for intrastromal procedures, I proceeded to evaluate the laser's potential for surface ablation. My first interest in surface ablation was as a technique for thereapeutic keratectomy. Since it was not possible to create a model of corneal dystrophy in the rabbit, I induced fungal ulcers in an experimental model and performed the first phototherapeutic keratectomy to remove the infected tissue. It has been extremely rewarding to have this work recognized by Dr. Trokel who wrote in 1992, "When it was found (Serdarevic, 1985) that circular ablations on animal corneas healed with remarkable clarity, the way was open to investigation of direct surface-recontouring in human subjects,"[1] and by Dr. L'Esperance who wrote in 1993, "in 1984, Serdarevic and her associates were the first to apply argon fluoride excimer laser radiation to create a therapeutic lamellar keratectomy. . . The fact that the cornea healed with minimal surface irregularities and scarring stimulated further investigation into the use of lamellar keratectomies for therapeutic and refractive procedures."[2]

Improvements in excimer laser systems and techniques over the past decade have permitted this technology to achieve widespread clinical application and acceptance for the correction of refractive errors. Photorefractive keratectomy has been judged to be reasonably safe and effective even by the world's most demanding regulatory agencies. I had the privilege of chairing in March 1994 the Ophthalmic Device Panel Meeting of the United States Food and Drug Administration, where the first two Premarket Applications of two excimer laser companies were presented and recommended for approval subject to some conditions. I hope that in the future regulatory agencies in all countries will ensure reasonable safety to protect public health while allowing evolution of, and timely access to, new devices and techniques. Regulatory agencies should not preclude surgeons from offering the best therapy to their patients. Global standardization of regulatory requirements with international cooperation and collection of data would enable more rapid progress in the field of refractive surgery.

Although international collaboration for regulatory purposes is not yet a reality, refractive surgeons are interacting more and more with colleagues in other countries. It is now widely recognized that excellent medical care and cutting edge technology are available in many countries and continents. Moreover, advances in refractive surgery have been pioneered by ophthalmologists throughout the world.

Just as there is no one country that has the monopoly on development of new refractive techniques and devices, there is no single refractive procedure that is or will be the panacea for the correction of all refractive errors. Although tremendous advances have occurred in refractive surgery in the past few years, many more are needed. Promising new procedures should be evaluated and developed with cautious enthusiasm. New approaches should not be prematurely condemned and rejected before adequate, unbiased evaluation. The development of new experimental models to assess refractive techniques, devices, and adjunct pharmacologic therapy either by computer simulation or by in vitro testing will permit more rapid advances and less need for premature clinical testing. Improved understanding of visual function and control of wound healing will contribute to the safety and efficacy of refractive surgery. It is well known that surgical alteration of the optical system will always compromise some aspect of visual function of anatomy, but the best corneal and intraocular refractive techniques will optimize and maintain optical quality and adequately exploit compensatory mechanisms.

I am extremely grateful for the friendship, collaboration, expertise, and instruction that my American and international colleagues have offered me over the years. Many of them are contributors to this book. I would like to thank all of them for the enormous time and effort that they expended to share their wealth of experience, knowledge, and perspectives with the readers.

I also would like to thank the staff of Igaku-Shoin and particularly Beth Kaufman Barry for asking me to edit this book and understanding the necessity of publishing in a very timely fashion a text on the rapidly evolving field of refractive surgery.

REFERENCES

1. Trokel S: The excimer laser. In Noyori K, Shimizu K, Trokel S: *Ophthalmic Laser Therapy*. Tokyo, Igaku-Shoin Ltd., 1992, p 68.
2. L'Esperance FA Jr: History and development of the excimer laser. In Thompson FB, McDonnell PJ (eds): *Color Atlas and Text of Excimer Laser Surgery: The Cornea*. New York, Igaku-Shoin Medical Publishers, 1993, p 13.

Olivia N. Serdarevic

Contributors

Jorge L. Alio, M.D., Ph.D.
Professor and Chairman
Division of Ophthalmology
University of Alicante School of Medicine
Alicante, Spain

Till Anschütz, M.D.
Department of Ophthalmology
Stadtklinik Baden-Baden
Laserinstitut
Gaggenau, Germany

Maria Clara Arbelaez, M.D.
Founder and Director
Refractive Surgery Department
Ophthalmology Clinic of Cali
Cali, Colombia

Jan Ashton, B.A., C.O.A.
Vice President, Business Development
Vista Laser Centers of the Northwest
New Westiminster, British Columbia
Canada

Kerry K. Assil, M.D.
Medical Director
Sinskey Eye Institute
National Medical Director
Vision Correction Centers
Santa Monica, California

Georges Baïkoff, M.D.
Professor of Ophthalmology
Marseille, France

Stephen F. Brint, M.D., F.A.C.S.
Associate Clinical Professor of Ophthalmology
Tulane University School of Medicine
Eye Surgery Center of Louisiana
New Orleans, Louisiana

Lucio Buratto, M.D.
Director
Centro Ambrosiano di Microchirurgia Oculare
Milan, Italy

Raul D. Castro, M.D.
Director Brazilian Society of Refractive Surgery
Staff Hospital de Olhos de Minas Gerais
Unit of Refractive Surgery
Belo Horizonte, Brazil

Emmanuel Caubet, M.D.
Cannes, France

Philippe J. Cénac, M.D.
Adjunct Professor of Ophthalmology
Centre Hospitalier Princesse Grace
Monaco

Ekktet Chansue, M.D.
Director, Cornea and Refractive Surgery Service
Ramathibodi Hospital Faculty of Medicine
Mahidol University
Bangkok, Thailand

**Sek-Jin Chew, M.D., F.R.C.S.(ED), Ph.D.,
   F.R.C.Ophth, MS, MBBS, FAMS**
Deputy Director and Head of Myopia Unit
Singapore Eye Research Institute
Vice President
Myopia International Research Foundation
Consultant, Singapore National Eye Center
Senior Lecturer, National University of Singapore
Visitng Scientist, The Rockefeller University, New York
Visiting Professor, New York Eye and Ear Infirmary
City University of New York
New York, New York

Joseph Colin, M.D.
Professor and Chairman
Department of Ophthalmology
CHRU Morvan
Brest, France

Daniel Epstein, M.D., Ph.D.
Associate Professor
Department of Ophthalmology
University Hospital
Uppsala, Sweden

Massimo Ferrari, M.D.
Milan, Italy

Coni Sweeney Fisher, M.S., C.O.T.
Director of Development
Eye Surgery Center of Louisiana
New Orleans, Louisiana

**David S. Gartry, M.D., F.R.C.S., F.R.C. Ophth,
   B.Sc. (Hons), D.O., F.C.Optom.**
Consultant Ophthalmic Surgeon
Cornea Service
Moorfields Eye Hospital
London, England

Howard V. Gimbel, M.D., F.R.C.S.C.
University of Calgary
Assistant Clinical Professor
Department of Surgery
Calgary, Alberta, Canada
Associate Clinical Professor
Department of Ophthalmology
Loma Linda University, California
Clinical Professor
Department of Ophthalmology
University of California
San Francisco, California

R. Bruce Grene, M.D.
Chief Executive Officer
Grene Vision Group
Clinical Assistant Professor
Department of Surgery
University of Kansas School of Medicine
Wichita, Kansas

José Güell, M.D. Ph.D.
Associate Professor of Ophthalmology
Autonoma University of Barcelona
Director, Cornea and Refractive Surgery
Vall d'Hebron University Hospital
Director, Cornea and Refractive Surgery
Instituto de Microcirurgia Ocular de Barcelona (I.M.O.)
Barcelona, Spain

Marcia Reis Guimaraes, M.D.
Assistant Professor of Pathology and Ophthalmology
Medical School University of Minas Gerais
Belo Horizonte, Brazil
Director Brazilian Society of Refractive Surgery
Director Hospital de Olhos de Minas Gerais
Belo Horizonte, Brazil

Ricardo Q. Guimaraes, M.D., Ph.D.
President Brazilian Society of Refractive Surgery
Director International Society of Refractive Surgery
Assistant Clinical Professor
University of Minas Gerais
Belo Horizonte, Brazil
Director Hospital de Ilhosa de Minas Gerais
Belo Horizonte, Brazil
Refractive Surgery, Cataract/IOL
Cornea and External Disease Specialist
Belo Horizonte, Brazil

Jack T. Holladay, M.D.
McNeese Professor of Ophthalmology
University of Texas Medical School
Houston, Texas

Mahmoud M. Ismail, M.D.
Associate Professor
Department of Ophthalmology
Instituto Oftalmologico de Alicante
University of Alicante School of Medicine
Alicante, Spain

W. Bruce Jackson, M.D., F.R.C.S.C.
Professor and Chairman
Department of Ophthalmology
University of Ottawa
Director General
University of Ottawa Eye Institute
Ottawa General Hospital
Ottawa, Ontario
Canada

Donald G. Johnson, M.D., F.R.C.S.
Medical Director
London Place Eye Centre, Inc.
Chairman
Vista Technologies, Inc.
New Westminster, British Columbia
Canada

Geoffrey B. Kaye, M.B., Ch.B., F.C.S.(SA), F.R.C.S.C.
Gimbel Eye Centre
Calgary, Alberta
Canada

Jae-Ho Kim, M.D.
Professor and Chairman
Department of Ophthalmology
Catholic University Medical College
Seoul, Korea

Richard L. Lindstrom, M.D.
Clinical Professor of Ophthalmology
University of Minnesota
Medical Director
Phillips Eye Institute Center for Teaching
and Research
Minneapolis, Minnesota

Bernard Mathys, M.D.
Consultant in Refractive Surgery
Department of Ophthalmology
Free University of Brussels
Erasmus Hospital, Brussels
Belgium

Cathy McCarty, Ph.D., M.P.H.
Department of Opthalmology
The University of Melbourne
Melbourne, Australia

Lee T. Nordan, M.D.
Assistant Clinical Professor of Ophthalmology
Jules Stein Eye Institute
UCLA
Los Angeles, California

Juan J. Pérez-Santonja, M.D., Ph.D.
Ophthalmology, Instituto Oftalmologico de Alicante
University of Alicante School of Medicine
Alicante, Spain

Alan E. Reider, Esq.
Arent Fox
Washington, D.C.

Gilles J. Renard, M.D.
Professor and Chairman
Department of Opthalmology
University of Paris VI
Hotel-Dieu
Paris, France

Anne Robinet, M.D.
Department of Ophthalmology
CHRU Morvan
Brest, France

David Robinson
Melbourne University Department of Ophthalmology
East Melbourne, Australia

James J. Salz, M.D.
Clinical Professor of Ophthalmology
University of Southern California
Los Angeles, California

Ronald Stasiuk, M.D., F.R.A.C.O., F.R.A.C.S.
Clinical Associate
Melbourne University Department of Ophthalmology
Ophthalmologist in Charge, Consultant
Bellbird Private Hospital
Director
Blackburn South Eye Clinic
Director
LaserSight Australia
East Melbourne, Australia

Mark D. Stern, M.D.
Former Medical Officer
Division of Ophthalmic Devices
Center for Devices and Radiological Health
Food and Drug Administration
Rockville, Maryland

Kazuo Tsubota, M.D.
Chairman
Department of Ophthalmology
Tokyo Dental College
Associate Professor of Ophthalmology
Tokyo Dental College
Assistant Professor of Ophthalmology
Keio University School of Medicine
Tokyo, Japan

Hugh R. Taylor, M.D., F.R.C.S., F.R.A.C.O.
Professor and Chairman
Department of Ophthalmology
The University of Melbourne
Royal Victorian Eye and Ear Hospital
East Melbourne, Australia

Vance Thompson, M.D.
Associate Professor of Ophthalmology
University of South Dakota School of Medicine
Director of Refractive Surgery
Department of Ophthalmology
Sioux Valley Hospital
Sioux Falls, South Dakota

Ray Jui-Fang Tsai, M.D.
Associate Professor of Ophthalmology
Chairman, Department of Ophthalmology
Director, Eye Research Lab
Chang Gung Memorial Hospital
Chang Gung College of Medicine and Technology
Tao Yuan, Taiwan

Peter Tseng, M.D., F.R.C.S., F.R.C.Ophth.
Head, Department A
Singapore National Eye Centre
Singapore

Rasik B. Vajpayee, M.D.
The University of Melbourne
Royal Victorian Eye and Ear Hospital
East Melbourne, Australia

John A. van Westenbrugge, M.D., F.R.C.S.C.
Gimbel Eye Centre
Calgary, Alberta
Canada

Contents

Refractive Errors: Etiology, Incidence, Prevention, and Nonsurgical Management

Sek-Jin Chew

Peter Tseng

INTRODUCTION

A lot has been written about the optics, nonsurgical management, and basic research on refractive errors. Clinicians have very little time to keep abreast of the latest advances in surgical technique in order to maintain the quality care that these patients demand. Why then should they be persuaded to spend time and effort to read yet another review of a topic that appears to be only indirectly relevant to a clinical practice?

The answer lies partly in the demographics of the patients seeking refractive surgery. Their psychological profile frequently sets them apart from typical ophthalmic patients with sight-threatening diseases. They are often more demanding and perfectionist, and can have unrealistic expectations concerning the outcome of surgery. Equally important, the well-established association between myopia and high educational level or intelligence raises the threshold of these patients to health information saturation. Moreover, the bustling information superhighway affords them cheap and ready access to up-to-date health information and research. In part because of their higher disposable income and intellect, these patients are often far more computer literate than most ophthalmologists (who pride themselves on their use of modern technology yet shun the keyboard in favor of the dictaphone). At home or in the office, 24 hr a day, the concerned patient can access the World-Wide Web on a personal computer to browse the homepages of optometric and ophthalmic institutions and private practices. High-quality, prestigious professional on-line journals vie for their attention with advertising for questionable treatments of various disorders. All these factors produce a very discerning and well-informed patient who comes armed with health information of variable value. As in the management of any other disorder, ophthalmologists must help them sift through that information to arrive at an informed consent for surgery.

In this chapter, we summarize key concepts in our recent understanding of the refractive errors which are useful in helping ophthalmologists to manage patients seeking refractive surgery. We focus only on topics with the most advances in the past 5 years. As Figure 1.1 shows, almost twice as many papers have been written on myopia as on all the other forms of refractive errors combined. Moreover, there has been an unabated rise in the number of new publications on myopia and astigmatism in the last decade compared with hyperopia and presbyopia. Much of this interest in myopia focuses on its surgical treatment, as well as its etiology and development (Fig. 1.2). In contrast, genetic and epidemiological studies have yet to ride the tide of exciting discoveries using molecular genetics and molecular epidemiology. These techniques, such as those used to find the genes responsible for multifactorial traits such as glaucoma or obesity, are necessary for the next breakthrough in myopia etiology and gene therapy.

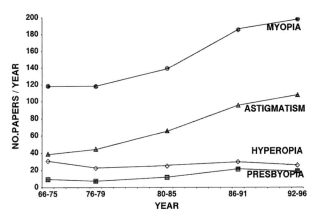

Fig. 1.1. Number of new papers cited each year in Medline on each type of refractive error.

TYPES OF MYOPIA AND ITS CLASSIFICATION

Myopia was well defined almost 150 years ago by Donders and Helmholtz. Donders described the myopic eye as "one in which the dioptric system lies in front of the retina; in other words, parallel rays derived from infinitely remote object units in the myopic eye focus in front of the retina when the eye is at rest."[1] Helmholtz defined the myopic eye as "one for which the far point is a short distance away, sometimes only a few inches from the eye."[2] The far point is the most distant point that is sharply fo-

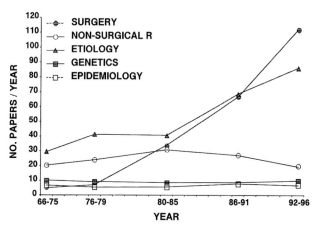

Fig. 1.2. Number of new papers published each year on different aspects of myopia research. Surgical treatment of myopia and studies of its etiology or pathogenesis are mainly responsible for the growing interest in this field.

cused and therefore conjugate with the retina when accommodation is relaxed.

The magnum opus on this subject, Brian Curtin's *The Myopias*, was published in 1985 and still provides the most comprehensive review of the literature.[3] However, with the development of animal models of refractive errors in the last decade, along with more comprehensive epidemiological studies, our concept of the pathogenesis of these errors has undergone radical changes.

A classification of myopia can be based on the degree of myopia, its association with astigmatism, the age of onset, the ocular optical component, or the putative cause.

Severity of Myopia

Curtin and many other authors classify myopia by its severity: low, intermediate, or high.[3] Categorization by degree of myopia unfortunately obscures the fact that low and intermediate refractive errors represent a physiological continuum, and limits the interpretation and comparison of studies conducted using different classification criteria. While high myopias generally represent a distinct pathological or degenerative class, they are now increasingly mixed with progressive physiological myopias, especially in Asia. The only merits of classification by refraction are that this method guides the choice of refractive surgical procedures and provides an arbitrary threshold for the pre- and postoperative screening for related eye problems. The refraction may be supplanted by the use of axial length of vitreous chamber depth, which have a higher correlation with retinal pathology.

Presence of Astigmatism

The combination of astigmatism and myopia occurs frequently. Moreover, higher degrees of myopia are more commonly associated with astigmatism. This classification adds little to our appreciation of the cause or development of the refractive errors.

Refractive Component

Classification by the refractive component invokes terminology such as *axial, refractive, index,* and *lenticular.* The breakdown of the correlation between the various optical components of the eye leads to ametropia. This classification ascribes special responsibility to one component and requires a comparison with population norms for all components. However, its usefulness is limited, as most large-scale studies have now shown that axial myopia predominates among persons with juvenile and adult-onset myopia. Even low degrees of myopia (under −5 D) are primarily due to axial elongation, with normal parameters for corneal and lens powers.[4] This is also the main abnormality found in experimental models of myopia and implicates excessive axial growth (and not simple decorrelation of optical components per se) as the primary pathology in myopia.

Age of Onset

A more useful classification is based on the age of onset of myopia. *School* or *physiological myopia* is the term applied to myopia first detected during the school years. Also called *developmental* or *juvenile myopia*, it is the most common form of myopia and has attracted the greatest attention in clinical studies. Our discussion will therefore center on this entity. In contrast, congenital or neonatal myopia is rare, although it is the subject of close scrutiny using animal models of myopia. Adult-onset myopia is less common than school myopia and is frequently low in severity. This classification is thus useful prognostically, as the age of onset of myopia is closely related to the severity of myopia in adulthood.[5]

Pathogenesis

The most challenging but potentially most promising classification of myopia is by its presumptive etiology, either primary or secondary. This system uses models that are used for the study and management of the glaucomas and demands an exhaustive search for risk factors in every patient. It encompasses such classification schemes as primary versus degenerative, congenital versus acquired, and benign versus malignant myopia. A controversial scheme that is still evolving, it will gradually mature as our meager knowledge of this disorder increases. Additionally, by acknowledging the pathophysiological heterogeneity of the myopias, we will be in a better position in the near future to tailor preventive or therapeutic measures to the specific disturbance which results in excessive axial eye growth.

PREVALENCE OF MYOPIA

Our discussion is restricted to physiological or school myopia. As mentioned above, pathological or degenerative myopia is more severe (often exceeding −10 D) and may begin earlier in childhood. Surgery of this group of patients should be based on far more conservative criteria due to the higher risk of vision loss from chorioretinal degeneration. Even had these patients not developed these complications before surgery, it would be prudent to exclude them, as any subsequent vision loss may too easily be wrongly attributed to the operation.

The prevalence of myopia varies greatly with age, ethnicity, geographic location, and environmental or behavioral factors. The best-referenced statistic is 25% for the prevalence of myopia in the United States in 1983.[6] The same study showed the greater prevalence of myopia with higher educational levels. Recent studies in Asia, such as national studies in Taiwan, show a far higher prevalence of myopia which increases with age: 11.8% at age 6 years, 55.5% at 12 years, 76% at 15 years, and 85% at 18 years[7] (Fig. 1.3).

Generational Changes in Prevalence

Just as new surgical techniques and health care strategies change at almost 6-month intervals, the epidemiology of myopia, surprisingly, is also evolving rapidly. Recent local studies of the prevalence of myopia in the United States suggest an increase

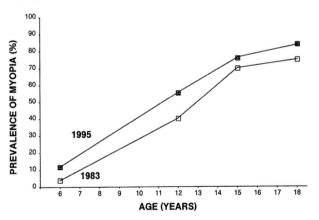

Fig. 1.3. Increasing prevalence of myopia with age in Taiwan. The statistics from 1983 (open squares), when compared with those of a decade later (solid squares), show an increase in prevalence in all age groups.[7a]

from 25% in 1983 to 40% in 1990.[6,8] In Asia, generational changes in the prevalence of myopia appeared coincident with post–World War II increased scholastic activities and with urbanization.[4,9,10] These increases in the frequency and severity of myopia are documented in Taiwan, Japan, Hong Kong, and Singapore, where myopia is endemic. A more alarming observation is the increasing severity of physiological myopia in the present generation of young Chinese adults in Taiwan, where the mean refraction may be as high as -4.00 D in 18-year-olds. Moreover, myopia in excess of -6 D is now seen in an unprecedented 16% of young adults in this country.[7]

These statistics are not only important to health care providers in planning for the burgeoning demands for refractive surgery in Asia over the next decade, but also have important implications for the nonsurgical and postsurgical management of myopes. These concerns include expectations regarding the age of cessation of myopia progression, screening for complications of high myopia, and considerations for adjunctive treatment to retard the pre- and postsurgical progression of myopia.

The changing demography of myopia also sheds light on the risk factors for its onset and progression, many of which are environmentally determined.

RISK FACTORS FOR MYOPIA

Genetic Background

Like many multifactorial traits, such as obesity and hypertension, school myopia is derived from the confluence of selective perturbations in the visual environment acting on a susceptible genetic background. The latter is supported by a higher intrapair concordance in refractive errors for monozygotic twins than for dizygotic twins.[11,12] Parental myopia is also correlated with myopia in their offspring at school age.[13] However, this finding does not necessarily implicate a gene for myopia, as it can be attributed to the inheritance of near-work behavior or the influence of parental behavior on the child's visual world.[14–16] Nonetheless, pedigree analysis indicates that the inheritance of school myopia is not a simple Mendelian trait but rather a complex one.[17]

An environmental influence on myopia has been found in twins. In monozygotic twins with concordant studying and reading habits, this influence is more concordant than in twins with discordant habits. A similar gene–environment effect can be demonstrated by experiments in which visual form deprivation produces myopia reliably in one strain of chickens but not in another strain.[18] As the gene–environment interaction on myopia continues to be explored, modern techniques of molecular biology are now being applied.

Race

As mentioned above, myopia is far more prevalent in Asians than in Caucasians or blacks. These differences may be related to differences in lifestyle, as well as to genetic factors.

Sex

In girls, myopia appears to be more severe and more prevalent than in boys of the same age. In Taiwan, at age 18 the mean myopia in girls is -3.92 D, and in boys it is -2.71 D.[7] However, this sex difference has yet to be linked to genetic, hormonal, or behavioral factors.

Age

The presence and severity of myopia depend to a large extent on the current age of the patient and the age of onset of myopia. While infants are mostly hyperopic, most children become emmetropic by the age of 4 to 6 years. Juvenile myopia commonly develops at about 10 years of age and ceases to progress by late adolescence. From 5% to 10% of children at age 6 are myopic. This proportion increases with age to 80–90% in young adults.[5–7,19–22]

Many studies have also found a high incidence of onset and progression of myopia in adults. Adult-onset myopia may occur in 10–20% of young adults with college or graduate education.[23,24] In the Prospective Evaluation of Radial Keratotomy (PERK) study, myopic adults (mean age of 35 years) without surgery who were followed up for more than 10 years had a mean increase in myopia of -0.67 D.[25] Adult-onset myopia, like juvenile myopia, is axial in nature and may have similar environmental risk factors.[26] These statistics are of clinical relevance in predicting the amount of regression of corrected myopia independent of the method of refractive surgery.

The patient's age is also useful in assessing the risk of the retinal degenerations associated with myopia. While schoolchildren and teenagers with high physiological myopia infrequently exhibit fundus abnormalities, the hallmarks of this disorder become increasingly prevalent with age. Mild scleral crescents and tessellated fundi are common in patients with myopia exceeding −3 D, but staphylomas, posterior pole degeneration, and equatorial degeneration are more frequent in those over the age of 30, especially with longer axial lengths.[27] It is important to perform ultrasound biometry as part of the routine preoperative evaluation of a myope, especially when the cause of any regression is evaluated after refractive surgery.

Body Growth

Myopia is positively associated with height, with myopes being taller than emmetropes and hyperopes.[10,28–30] This information is useful in reminding the clinician to diagnose Marfan's syndrome or a marfanoid syndrome. Interestingly, the association of myopia and height may be linked to the visual environment, as experimental studies suggest. Refraction in birds shows that lower-field myopia is greater in short birds that peck accurately at seeds on the ground (quail and chicken) than in tall birds (cranes) and is totally absent in raptors that seek their prey while airborne.[31] These findings are interpreted as an adaptation to the proximity of the visual environment of greatest ethological significance.

Near Work

Reading, television watching, computer use, video game playing, and other forms of near work constitute the risk factor of greatest interest in the development and progression of school myopia. The prevalence and severity of myopia are indisputably correlated with educational level and intelligence; this implicates either reading or genetic inheritance in the cause of myopia.[19,32,33] That chicks reared in a confined space are more myopic than controls reared in a larger space supports the environmental hypothesis.[34]

More direct evidence in humans comes from the higher prevalence and higher degree of myopia in Orthodox Jewish male students who differ from other Jews mainly in their study habits.[35] Orthodox schooling is characterized by sustained near vision and frequent changes in accommodation due to the swaying habit during study and the variety of print sizes.

Television watching has not been conclusively linked to the development of myopia, although a limited study in young primates found that myopia developed several months after prolonged exposure to television viewing.[36] Similarly, despite great public interest and concern, definitive clinical and experimental studies on video display terminals and myopia development are sorely lacking.

These data led to the theory that myopia is due to excessive accommodation, which in turn spawned mechanistic hypotheses based on the ocular hypertensive effects of sustained convergence, increased ciliary tonus, and consequent scleral stretching.[37,38] However, these considerations are being revised in the light of recent experimental findings that accommodation appears not to play a direct role in myopia at all. Instead, eye growth is an active, visually guided process regulated by the retina and is dependent on the clarity of images and the image plane (see below). Reading material may thus represent a type of visual form deprivation, and emmetropization causes the eye to elongate to help maintain its retinal image in focus on the retina.[39,40] The lack of a reliable and valid measure of near work makes it difficult to draw more substantive epidemiological associations with myopia. This deficiency is being addressed by the development of a standardized Visual Exposure Index by the Myopia International Research Foundation.[16]

Types of Optical Correction

Minus-power spectacle lenses induce myopia and cause axial elongation in primates, as well as in all mammals and birds studied to date.[41–43] Similarly, plus-power spectacle lenses cause infantile hyperopia to be retained and postnatal eye growth to cease almost entirely. These experimental findings support the long-standing concern that spectacle wearing in myopic children contributes to the progression of myopia. Soft contact lenses do not appear to retard the rate of myopia progression, nor do bifocal spectacles.[44,45] Rigid gas-permeable contact lenses may retard axial elongation, although conclusive evidence is still awaited.[46,47]

OCULAR GROWTH AND ITS REGULATION

The newborn's eye is short and hyperopic. It is during the neonatal and early juvenile periods that eye growth exhibits plasticity to environmental influences.[48] In this phase of ocular development, an active, visually guided process of emmetropization occurs in which almost full compensation for infantile refractive error takes place, primarily by regulating axial eye growth.[39,49,50] Corneal and lens changes also assist in this process, but their contributions are modest compared to the changes in vitreous chamber length aimed at attaining emmetropia. In this process, the retina plays the pivotal role in regulating the visual feedback loop that determines scleral growth. This principle is clearly elucidated in animal models of ametropia.[51]

Four experimental paradigms have been used in the last two decades to determine that the visual environment guides ocular growth to emmetropia (reviewed in Ref. 50):

1. *Documenting the normal pattern of ocular development.* In infants and newborn animals the axial length initially is short, so that the retina lies in front of the focal plane of the unaccommodated eye. Subsequent axial elongation moves the photoreceptors into, and not beyond, the focal plane.
2. *Changing the focal plane with minus- and plus-power spectacle lenses.* When animals are raised with the focal plane shifted posteriorly with minus-power lenses, the eyes elongate to approximately match the displaced focal plane. This was strikingly demonstrated in primates when positive or negative lenses caused the eyes of juveniles to grow (or cease growth) appropriately to negate the imposed refractive error.[43] Higher centers in the central nervous system are important, as optic nerve section prevents this type of myopia.
3. *Visual form deprivation.* When information about the location of the focal plane is removed by using diffusers or by eyelid suture, the eyes elongate to become myopic. In chicks, as much as −20 D of myopia can be achieved within a single week of form deprivation. Higher centers in the central nervous system are unimportant in this form of myopia, as optic nerve section does not prevent deprivation myopia.
4. *Reinstating clear vision following visual deprivation.* When developing animal eyes that have become myopic are reexposed to normal vision, their axial elongation can slow, gradually eliminating the myopia. Data from several species suggest that axial length is regulated within the eye itself, involving direct, spatially local communication from the retina to the sclera. It also appears that the regulation of axial elongation involves active control of the scleral extracellular matrix.

If humans have a similar mechanism, then successful emmetropization in children involves an interplay between the possibly inherited set point and gain of this mechanism and its interaction with the visual environment during the formative years. This translates into the familiar nurture–nature complementarity in determining the susceptibility to myopia.[13,14,52] While twin studies implicate genetics, its role is generally considered to be weaker than or permissive for environmental factors.[11,53–56]

VISUAL DISABILITY FROM MYOPIA

For medicolegal reasons, it is imperative to perform a comprehensive evaluation of the patient with high myopia before performing refractive surgery.[27] It is disheartening to have to account for the cause of macular hemorrhage or steroid glaucoma to a disbelieving patient years after a successful operation. In addition to assessing for cataract, motility disturbances, and ametropic or meridional amblyopia, the clinician should pay special attention to the retina disease and to glaucoma.

Retinal Degeneration

The myope is at risk for chorioretinal atrophy, breaks in Bruch's membrane, posterior staphyloma, macular degeneration, peripheral retinal breaks, and retinal detachment. He or she is entitled to at least a dilated fundus examination before surgery, even when the best-corrected visual acuity is normal.

Glaucoma

Open angle glaucoma is more common in myopes than in other patient populations. Unfortunately, it is also more difficult to diagnose glaucoma in high myopes for three reasons:

1. *Perimetry.* Visual field defects such as enlargement of the blind spot may be secondary to the myopic conus, and irregular scotomas may be due to patches of retinal atrophy. Moreover, distortions of visual fields due to high refractive errors occur. An accurate automated perimetry protocol stipules that high myopes must wear contact lenses during the test.

2. *Cup/disc assessment.* Glaucomatous excavation of the disc is difficult to interpret in the presence of a myopic conus. The distance between the lamina cribrosa and retina may be greatly reduced in myopic eyes, and temporally there is a sloping transition from choroid to papilla, leading to a smaller excavation. Nasally, supertraction of scleral and choroidal tissue masks the nerve fiber atrophy of glaucoma, so that cupping of the disc and vessel deviation may not be apparent.

3. *Tonometry.* The reduced ocular rigidity of myopic eyes results in falsely low pressure measurements when the Schiotz indentation tonometer is used. Conversely, applanation tonometry may yield artifactually high intraocular pressure (IOP) in myopes. Flatter corneas, such as those of high myopes, are associated with higher applanation tensions. Fortunately, this accounts for a mere 0.1 mm Hg difference in applanation tonometric values.

Myopia is also a risk factor for the progression of glaucoma.[57] However, another study by the same group paradoxically suggests that once glaucoma is established, the presence of myopia may have a beneficial influence on the course of the disease; that is, myopia is a favorable prognostic factor for glaucoma.

The myope is at higher risk of suffering steroid-induced glaucoma. In a study by Podos, Becker, and Morton, 17 patients with myopia of more than 5 D and no family history of glaucoma were given 0.1% dexamethasone four times a day for 6 weeks in one eye.[58] Fifteen of these patients demonstrated a significant increase in IOP. It is thus the responsibility of the refractive surgeon to determine the IOP

both before surgery and postoperatively at regular intervals.

NONSURGICAL MANAGEMENT OF MYOPIA

Since the advent of spectacles, it has been the goal of ophthalmologists and optometrists to prevent the onset of myopia and to slow its rate of increase. The use of refractive surgery provides an added incentive for seeking methods to retard the progression of myopia. Limiting myopia to low degrees reduces the risk of postoperative regression and improves long-term satisfaction with treatment. Moreover, if the risk of pathological myopia can be reduced by such measures, the population suited for refractive surgery would ultimately be increased. This consideration is especially pertinent in Asia, where high myopia is prevalent.

Unfortunately, as is evident from the plethora of treatments, no single regimen has been substantially rewarded with unequivocal success. Therefore, the American Academy of Ophthalmology does not endorse any particular mode of therapy.[59] However, it is important to review these nonsurgical treatments in the light of recent discoveries about the mechanism of myopia development and as adjunctive treatments for the patient awaiting or recovering from refractive surgery.

The role of the visual environment in determining eye growth has led to a variety of optical techniques to regard the progression of myopia. The development of animal models of myopia[60–62] has also brought an upsurge in interest in myopia prevention and treatment with pharmacological agents. Cycloplegics such as atropine have long been used in children to reduce the rate of progression of myopia. Atropine, in particular, has been reported to be effective in clinical use.[63–66] By impairing accommodation, it was hypothesized to reduce the passive stretching of the globe. Furthermore, it was said to reduce the excessive accommodation of the lens itself. These theories have been strongly challenged by the lack of supporting evidence, as well as by recent observations on the role of the retina as the regulator of ocular growth. Many of these studies with atropine also suffered from a lack of adequate, detailed follow-up examinations and the use of appropriate clinical controls. The retinoscopic refractions were subject to observer bias and were not correlated with changes in axial growth of the eye. As a result, atropine is not widely used. But in the last few years, our pharmacological armament against myopia has been vastly expanded by the effective inhibition of myopic eye growth in animal models using neurochemicals and growth factors such as b Fibroblast Growth Factor (bFGF) in or around the eye.

Eye Exercises and Biofeedback

The Bates System of Eye Exercises was inexplicably popular at the turn of this century.[67] This technique involved repeated testing with the same Snellen chart daily by children in order to obtain what Bates claimed was a sixfold reduction in the prevalence of myopia. The learning effect and the lack of sound epidemiological practice did not faze his supporters. Additionally, without reporting the refraction or visual acuity, Bates went on to claim therapeutic success in a number of animal species. The mechanism was asserted to be changes in accommodation by the activity of extraocular muscles. These facts would be useful in gently debunking an insistent patient's myths about alternative therapies. Nonetheless, one could do worse than reassure patients that such measures are harmless and may be pursued at their leisure (and expense!).

Unaided visual acuity may be transiently and reversibly improved by modulating accommodation with biofeedback. However, none of these methods change the refractive error, much less retard axial elongation in progressive myopia.[68,69]

Optical Correction

Bifocal Spectacles
With the reduction of accommodation as their goal, several studies have unfortunately failed to demonstrate any benefit of bifocals in reducing the progression of school myopia in children.[44] An exception may be in myopes with esophoria. Problems include the difficulty in ensuring that children use only the bifocal segment of spectacles for near work. This may be avoided by the use of progressive add lenses, which, according to an unpublished report on Asian children, appears to hold promise for myopia control.

Contact Lenses
As mentioned earlier, rigid but not soft contact lenses may retard the progression of myopia. Per-

rigin et al. used the Paraperm $O_2{}^+$ silicone acrylate RGP lens in a masked 3-year case-control study.[47] A total of 100 children aged 8 to 13 years were fitted with the lenses, which had a diameter of 9.0 mm and an optical zone of 7.7 mm. The fit was parallel, and good centration was ascertained. Myopia progression was −0.51 D/year (total, 1.53 D) in the age-matched controls and −0.16 D/year (total, −0.48 D) in the contact lens wearers. The total difference after 3 years of −1.05 D was partly due to corneal flattening (0.37 D), and the balance may be ascribed to a reduction in axial length increase. The results are inconclusive due to deficiencies in the study design and in follow-up. These questions are being addressed in a randomized clinical trial currently underway in Singapore.

Orthokeratology

Flattening of the cornea by flat fitting of rigid contact lenses is ineffective in retarding the progression of axial eye growth in myopes. This was conclusively demonstrated in a well-designed, randomized clinical trial sponsored by the National Institutes of Health.[70,71]

Ocular Hypotensives

Ocular growth and development is partly dependent on the expression of the normal IOP.[72,73] The shape and integrity of the eye are contingent on the maintenance of a balance of forces between the outwardly directed IOP and the resistance of the ocular coats. The IOP depends on the active secretory processes by the ciliary processes and the resistance of the outflow pathways. The progressive elevation of IOP during postnatal development in chicks and in humans has been suggested to contribute to the continued expansion of the globe.[74,75]

It has been argued that the increased eye size in myopia is the result of passive stretching of the sclera due to increased IOP from the accumulation of liquid vitreous.[76] The posterior staphyloma and thinned sclera in humans appear to support this hypothesis.[77] Accommodation and convergence in humans have been claimed to constrict the globe, raising the IOP, which then induces scleral creep.[37,78] In the rabbit, −1 D of myopia can be induced by hyperthermia and ocular hypertension.[79] However, the chicken model of experimental form-deprivation myopia depends on active growth of the sclera rather than stretching.[80] Raised IOP has not been found, either in humans or in animal models.[81]

In addition to the controversy concerning the role of IOP in the pathogenesis of myopic eye growth, the techniques of IOP measurement have compounded the uncertainty. Most of the studies were conducted under general anesthesia, which may elevate or lower the IOP, depending on the agent used. Furthermore, the clinical tonometers used in the IOP determinations were often not calibrated for use in animals, in which the corneal curvature and hence compensations for meniscus effects are different. Two types of ocular hypotensives have been investigated for their potential in retarding myopic progression: miotics and beta-adrenergic blockers. These will now be discussed.

Miotics

The use of pilocarpine is described mainly in the Japanese literature. The rationale behind this treatment may be based on a reduction of IOP or an increase in subnormal accommodation. These drugs, which cause accommodative spasm in young children, are no longer used.

Beta-Adrenergic Receptor Blockers and Pseudomyopia

Children with pseudomyopia have been treated with the beta-adrenergic blockers labetalol and timolol in the hope that these drugs may relax the ciliary muscle. A study by Hosaka (oral presentation, 2nd International Conference on Myopia San Francisco, Oct 28–30, 1982) in 1982 showed that labetalol produced an improvement of more than 0.38 D in 75.8% of the eyes treated, with no change or worsening in 24.2%. Either timolol or a placebo produced an improvement in 28% of the subjects. This was a short-term study, and Hosaka did not take into account the long-term effect of the drug's hypotensive action on the IOP.

Beta-Adrenergic Blockers and Myopia

Jensen and Goldschmidt[81a] performed a pilot study on beta blockers in children, using the pressure-reducing effect of 0.25% timolol, based on the assumption that raised pressure in the posterior chamber can increase the axial length. Their main objectives were to determine whether children could tolerate timolol, whether there were serious side effects from the treatment, and whether the IOP would be reduced. The subjects in this pilot study were 10 children (4 girls and 6 boys) between the ages of 7 and 12 years. The inclusion criteria, in addition to the age limits, were (1) strongly progressive myopia (minimum of 1.00 D per year) during the period before entering the trial and (2) a strong disposition to myopia, so that the family was highly motivated to participate in the study.

Each child was examined by a pediatric specialist, and a complete ophthalmologic examination was performed. Oral and written information was given to the parents, describing the project and the possible side effects from treatment with timolol eye drops. The children were treated with 0.25% timolol twice daily, and all of them were examined every third month by both an ophthalmologist and a pediatrician. The treatment was completed after 12 months, and an eye examination was performed and IOP measurements were taken before treatment and 12 months after treatment.

The study showed that children tolerate beta-blocking drugs, administered as eye drops, quite well and that the local side effects are negligible. None of the children complained of weakness during physical exercise. Any periods of tiredness were recorded, but all were attributed by the family to physical exercise, influenza, or other illnesses. The investigators found that progression of myopia diminished during treatment for a few of the subjects and tended to remain so after the treatment was stopped. Treatment had little effect on the IOP, although those children who respond to the eye drops with lower tension tend to show some inhibition in the development of myopia. Jensen and Goldschmidt concluded that further studies were necessary, including a larger sample, a longer observation period, and a control group.

Cycloplegics or Muscarinic Antagonists in the Treatment of Myopia

The previous use of muscarinic inhibitors in the treatment of myopia was based on the hypothesis that excessive or sustained accommodation leads to increased myopia. The close correlation of academic achievement and reading with myopia, as well as reports of high rates of myopia in carpet weavers and microscopists, led to the use of cycloplegia in one of the earliest attempts to reduce its progression.[19,24,32,33,35,82–85] Another reason for the use of muscarinic receptor antagonists, which are often used as cycloplegics, was that myopia resulted from tension in the extraocular muscles during prolonged convergence.[86] Luedde reported success in retarding the progression of myopia by dissociating the eyes for near work using monocular cycloplegia. However, there was no mention of the number of patients treated, their ages, or whether controls were used.

Most studies on retarding the progression of myopia in children have focused on the use of topical atropine as a cycloplegic. In selecting subjects for such treatment, Bedrossian used the criteria that they were 8 to 13 years of age and that their myopia was increasing more than −0.50 D annually.[87,88] One drop of 1% atropine was instilled in the test eye at bedtime each evening; no drug was instilled in the other (control) eye. After 1 year, the treatment was switched to the other eye. In the 75 subjects, the experimental eyes improved by +0.20 D, while the control eyes progressed by −0.85 D. These trends persisted during subsequent years of follow-up: of 236 control eyes, 201 showed increased myopia compared with 12 of 236 treated eyes.[88] Oddly, the rate of myopia increase in the control eyes was relatively low, which may reflect an effect of atropine or of cycloplegia on the other eye. Similarly, Gimbel[89] used 1% atropine bilaterally in 279 subjects aged 5 to 15 years. Controls consisted of 572 other subjects of similar age. Only 97 subjects completed 1 year of treatment, and a mere 16 reached 3 years. Gimbel reported that refraction improved by +0.48 D after 1 month of treatment, with an average yearly reduction of myopia of +0.11 D in the treated group. In contrast, the controls continued to deteriorate at the rate of −0.61 D yearly.

Other, weaker cycloplegics have been used in attempts to reduce the side effects and improve compliance with therapy. Scopolamine (0.25%) was effective in reducing the progression of myopia in three patients with unilateral treatment and in two patients with bilateral treatment.[90] Similarly, tropicamide was tested for its efficacy in preventing the progression of myopia.[91] However, Takano used tropicamide for only 1 month, followed by refraction 1 month after cessation, an insufficient period to evaluate changes in eye growth. In another study using tropicamide, Yamaji et al. reported a reduction in myopia in 70% of 95 first- to sixth-grade children (43 boys, 52 girls) after 3 months of using 1 drop of 0.4% tropicamide every night at bedtime.[92] Eighty-one of these children, most of them still using tropicamide, were followed for another 5

months. Of these, 64% continued to have less myopia, as measured by retinoscopy. A combination of tropicamide and epinephrine was used by Tokoro and Kabe in 15 eyes for 1 to 9 months.[93] One year later, the average change was −0.51 D in the experimental group compared to −0.76 D in the control group. More important and more convincing is the finding that the mean axial length increase was 0.284 mm in the treated eyes and 0.349 mm in the control eyes. No eyes with myopia greater than −4 D were included, but there were more high myopes in the control group than in the experimental group. These higher myopes may be progressing faster, thereby negating the significance of the study results.

In contrast to the above investigators who obtained encouraging results with cycloplegics, Curtin did not report a beneficial effect.[3,94] However, in one study, he used only the less potent inhibitor tropicamide at bedtime.[3] In another study, he used atropine in only 10 subjects and did not produce a statistically significant outcome.[94]

Unilateral Topical Atropine in Retarding the Progression of Myopia

We now present data from a clinical trial in Asians to demonstrate the use of topical atropine in improving vision and refraction in myopes and in reducing the progression of myopia.[95] The high prevalence and extremely rapid progression of myopia in this population provided a more statistically powerful and objective determination of the therapeutic efficacy of atropine while minimizing its long-term toxicity. Atropine was applied unilaterally only to the more myopic eye to improve compliance and avoid the need for bifocals. This technique also reduces anisometropia in an age group in which refractive surgery is not normally employed. To confirm its effect on ocular growth, we performed ultrasonic measurements of the length of the globe in addition to refraction.

Patients between the ages of 4 and 17 years (mean, 10 years) in a general ophthalmology practice, with myopia of −0.50 D or more, were invited to participate in a clinical trial of muscarinic antagonist treatment to improve their vision and reduce the progression of myopia. Subjects who were excluded were those with a manifest squint, amblyopia, astigmatism of more than 1.25 D, any other ocular disease, or a disinclination to use the medicine or to be followed closely. The treatment regimen consisted of unilateral atropine 1% eye drops in the more myopic eye once a day in the morning. They were evaluated after the first 2 weeks for immediate complications and allergies. Subsequently, they were seen every 3 months. This frequency of follow-up provided a sensitive measure of the rapid changes in refraction and eye growth occurring in the Asian myope. No bifocal or reading glasses were used, nor were contact lenses of any type prescribed. The spectacle lens prescriptions were gradually reduced in the treated eyes.

Atropine treatment was stopped for at least 48 hr prior to each visit. Cycloplegic refraction and ultrasound biometry were performed. The cycloplegic regimen for examination consisted of tropicamide 1%, 1 drop, repeated once at 5-min intervals, followed by computerized automated refraction 20 min later. Automated refraction was performed by a masked technician to eliminate observer bias. Of the 47 patients started on atropine therapy, all but 1 were included in the statistical analysis. The excluded patient developed contact allergy to the drops after 1 month of use. None of the patients experienced changes or discomfort in bowel habits, respiration, or pulse rates. Occasional complaints of photophobia were managed by prescribing clip-on sunglasses with ultraviolet light blockers. Of the 46 subjects analyzed, 49 eyes were treated and 43 eyes served as controls. Three subjects received bilateral treatment when anisometropia was effectively treated and the previously less myopic (control) eye became more myopic than the treated eye.

When the refractive errors in both groups were compared after periods ranging from 6 months to 1.5 years, a significantly greater increase in myopia was found in the control eyes than in the treated eyes. Of the control eyes, 18 had less than -1.00 D of progression and 25 had -1 to -7 D of progression (mean, -2.00 D increase; standard deviation [SD], 2.06 D). These findings contrasted with those of the treated group, in which more than 70% of subjects experienced a reduction in refractive error of up to 3 D (mean, $+0.17$ D improvement; SD, 0.97). When the rates of myopic progression were compared, over 70% of control eyes were found to have worsened by -0.10 to -0.50 D/month in contrast to the improvement shown by 40% of treated eyes, in which myopia was reduced by $+0.10$ to

$+1.00$ D/month. Control eyes increased in axial length by 1.18 mm (SD, 1.57 mm), while treated eyes were shorter by 0.017 mm (SD, 0.22 mm). The rates of change in globe length were 0.049 mm/month (SD, 0.038 mm) of elongation in the controls and 0.016 mm/month (SD, 0.05 mm) of shortening in the treated eyes. Using an algorithm of 3 D of refractive change for each millimeter of axial length, we found that the changes in eye size correlated well with those of refractive error.[96,97]

When applied judiciously and with frequent follow-up examinations, atropine effectively reduced the progression of myopia and anisometropia and eliminated the problems of optical correction associated with aniseikonia. The effects were reversible; myopia progressed at its previous rate following the cessation of treatment. This finding may necessitate the chronic use of the eyedrops until at least 16 years of age.[66]

The rate of myopia increase in control eyes was almost an order of magnitude greater than that previously reported.[66] The difference may be attributed to the racial or behavioral predisposition of Chinese to myopia compared to that of Caucasians. Therefore, our results were greater than that of other studies, in which atropine at most reduced the yearly myopic progression by 80% but did not reverse the changes.[64,66]

The reduction in axial length following treatment probably represents an expansion of the choroid, as demonstrated in chick eyes during recovery from myopia. Additionally, atropine blockade of growth stimulation by the retina may permit collagenase-mediated remodeling of the sclera toward an emmetropia eye size.[98–101] The possibility of a true reduction in myopia (as opposed to the inhibition of its progression) supports the need to consider early intervention for this condition.

New Horizons for Drug Therapy

Atropine treatment is attended by the distressing side effects of mydriasis, cycloplegia, and photophobia. Although short-term and long-term studies have revealed few side effects, concerns for retinal phototoxicity are real and warrant careful long-term follow-up. Recently, the mode of action of these drugs has been challenged and offers new hope of reducing the side effects. As discussed above, the retina, rather than the ciliary muscle, plays a pivotal role in the control of normal eye growth and elongation. In animals, ciliary ganglionectomy, lesions of the Edinger Westphal nucleus, and optic nerve section do not prevent form deprivation myopia (reviewed in Ref. 40). Moreover, although the chick only has skeletal muscle in its ciliary body, which is unresponsive to muscarinic receptor blockers, atropine effectively prevents myopia. Experimental myopia in birds and mammals is also inhibited by other muscarinic receptor antagonists which cause minimal cycloplegia or which are applied by retroorbital injection.[102–110] These observations have led to the search for muscarinic receptor subtype-specific antagonists which reduce myopia while sparing the muscarinic receptors in the ciliary body.

Atropine sulfate is a nonselective antagonist of muscarinic receptors, of which there are at least five subtypes. These receptor subtypes show distinctive and specific localizations in the eye, with the m1 subtype being plentiful in the retina but rarer in the ciliary body. Antagonists to the m1 subtype prevent experimental myopia.[102,107,111] Drugs acting on this receptor may thus minimize the side effects of atropine treatment while retaining its myopia-inhibitory benefits.

Similarly, substantive evidence for the role of retinal dopamine and vasoactive intestinal polypeptide (VIP) in regulating eye growth in myopia have led to the use of a number of other neuromodulators to inhibit myopia in animals. Dopamine and its metabolite, 3,4-dihydroxyphenyacetic acid (DOPAC), are reduced in myopic eyes but not in controls.[112] Moreover, dopamine agonists such as apomorphine prevent deprivation myopia.[113]

HYPEROPIA

In contrast to myopia, hyperopia has created far less interest despite its ubiquity. This may be attributed to its tendency to regress rather than progress from infancy and to its lower risk of causing eye disease.

Etiology

Spherical refractive errors form a continuum, ranging from high hyperopia through emmetropia to severe myopia. This progression is not only one of semantics but is also of physiological significance

during postnatal development. Reflecting the effect of emmetropization or its perturbation, a myopic shift of refraction from a greater to a lesser degree of hyperopia can be brought about by the same factors that cause the progression of myopia.[14]

While variations in the degree of neonatal hyperopia may be inherited, it is now clear that the loss of hyperopia in early childhood through emmetropization may be interrupted by environmental factors. In particular, pathology affecting foveal vision in the first 3 years of life causes adult hyperopia. Strabismic amblyopia also results in hyperopia in nonhuman primates.[114] More striking (but not unexpected in light of the above discussions on spectacle lens–induced myopia) is that positive lenses worn early in life can prevent emmetropization in a variety of primates and other species.[43,115,116] These findings argue strongly against the use of optical correction for patients with low hyperopia in childhood.

Eye Disorders Associated with Hyperopia

Infants
Apart from amblyopia, hyperopia is of little concern in childhood. Correction may also be needed for esotropia.

Children
In school-age children, hyperopia has been associated with weaker scholastic performance than myopia and emmetropia.[8,117] Therefore, it has been suggested that even moderate uncorrected hyperopia can be detrimental to a child's cognitive abilities.[118] However, this is less likely to be a directly negative impact of hyperopia on learning ability than a reflection of near-work behavior leading to the development of myopia (and better school results!).

Adults
In adults, hyperopia is notable mainly for its latent form, which becomes symptomatic with presbyopia. However, it should be recognized that the smaller eye in hyperopia carries the risks of angle closure glaucoma and central retinal vein occlusion. The high prevalence of acute and chronic angle closure glaucoma in Asia is associated with the shallow anterior chambers in hyperopic elderly patients. Interestingly, the increasing prevalence of axial

myopia may ultimately replace the risk of angle closure glaucoma with open angle glaucomas in the coming decades.[119]

ASTIGMATISM

The etiology of astigmatism is even more obscure than that of hyperopia. Among the various causes of refractive astigmatism, corneal toricity predominates: lenticular, retinal surface toricity and variability in the angle alpha between the visual axis and optic axis are other causes.

Infants have a high prevalence of astigmatism. In most cases, this is against the rule and decreases in the first 2 years of life.[120] In the preschool and school years, with-the-rule astigmatism is more common.

In Chinese patients, astigmatism has been attributed to the tight lids.[121] This permanent effect may be mechanistically related to transient changes when narrowing the lid aperture by squinting increases astigmatism by 1.25 to 1.50 D, generally in the with-the-rule direction. For corneas with astigmatism of 1.00 D or more, Wilson et al. showed that lifting the eyelids reduced corneal toricity, principally in the horizontal meridian. They concluded that lid pressure produced some with-the-rule astigmatism.[122]

Astigmatism often coexists with myopia and is related to its progression. The relation between astigmatism and myopia was analyzed by Fulton et al. in 298 myopic children.[123] In children under the age of 3 years, myopia progressed in eyes with at least 1 D of cylinder and tended to increase through age 8 years in those with at least 3 D of cylinder. These data suggest that uncorrected astigmatism during a period of visual immaturity influences the course of myopia. Other studies suggest that against-the-rule astigmatism carries a higher risk of myopia than with-the-rule astigmatism. Myopia and astigmatism can be induced experimentally by performing astigmatic keratotomy or by applying cylindrical contact lenses to normal chick eyes.[115,124,125]

Thus, astigmatic errors, which are frequent among infants and young children, appear to predate the onset of myopia and may have a role similar to that of the defocusing that causes myopia in young animals. Screening and the full correction of astigmatism in young children are thus important in ensuring the best possible vision.

CONCLUSION

Myopia and astigmatism are increasingly the products of our times. Because the prevalence and severity of these refractive errors have worsened in recent decades, ophthalmologists must be well trained in refractive surgery to meet this challenge. This need is especially great in Asia, where myopia is endemic and severe. In addition, there are many nonsurgical factors in refractive errors, an appreciation of which will enhance the practice of the surgeon. This knowledge reinforces the role of the surgeon as a provider of comprehensive and continuing care.

We must be familiar with the natural history and risk factors for myopia and its progression. The recognition of physiological myopia as an environmentally determined disturbance of emmetropization is the key to designing treatment strategies for the future. For the present, a safe, successful practice must include a discerning screen for eye problems associated with refractive errors, as well as the ability and willingness to discuss their etiology and mythology accurately with patients who are exceptionally well informed and perceptive. Accurate biometry is necessary both in the baseline evaluation of axial myopia and to distinguish its progression from the regression of therapeutic effects. Finally, consideration may be given to adjunctive medical therapy and optical aids which may limit the progression of myopia in young adults.

Fortunately, the final chapter on myopia and its nonsurgical management has yet to be written. With the rapid advances being made in our knowledge of the physiology and biochemistry of myopia, the refractive surgeon must be familiar with the latest discoveries being made.

REFERENCES

1. Donders FC. *On the Anomalies of Accommodation and Refraction of the Eye.* London: New Sydenham Society; 1864.

2. Helmholtz HV. *Treatise on Physiological Optics*. New York, NY: Optical Society of America; 1924.

3. Curtin BJ. *The Myopias: Basic Science and Clinical Management*. Philadelphia, PA: Harper & Row; 1985.

4. Hosaka A. Population studies—myopia experience in Japan. *Acta Ophthalmol—Suppl.* 1988; 185: 37–40.

5. Chew SJ, Ritch R, Leong YK, et al.: The age of onset of myopia is a predictor of adult myopia severity. In: Shimizu K, ed. *Current Aspects in Ophthalmology*. Amsterdam: Elsevier Science Publishers BV; 1992; 680–685.

6. Sperduto RD, Seigel D, Roberts J, Rowland M. Prevalence of myopia in the United States. *Arch Ophthalmol* 1983;101:405–407.

7. Lin LLK, Shih Y, Tsai C, et al. Epidemiological study of ocular refractions among school-children (aged 6 through 18) in Taiwan. *Invest Ophthalmol Vis Sci* 1996:37;S1002.

7a. Lin LLK, Chen CJ, Hung P, Ko L. Nation-wide survey of myopia among schoolchildren in Taiwan, 1986. *Acta Ophthalmol*—Suppl. 1988;185:29–33.

8. Wang Q, Klein BEK, Klein R, Moss SE. Refractive status in the Beaver Dam eye study. *Invest Ophthalmol Vis Sci.* 1994;35:4344–4347.

9. Alward WL, Bender TR, Demske JA, Hall DB. High prevalence of myopia among young adult Yupik Eskimos. *Can J Ophthalmol.* 1985;20:241–245.

10. Johnson GJ, Matthews A, Perkins ES. Survey of ophthalmic conditions in a Labrador community. I. Refractive errors. *Br J Ophthalmol.* 1979;63: 440–448.

11. Lin LLK, Chen CJ. Twin study on myopia. *Acta Genet Med Gemellol.* 1987;36:535–540.

12. Chen CJ, Cohen BH, Diamond EL. Genetic and environmental effects on the development of myopia in Chinese twin children. *Ophthalmic Paediatr Genet.* 1985;6:353–359.

13. Zadnik K, Satariano WA, Mutti DO, Sholtz RI, Adams AJ. The effect of parental history of myopia on children's eye size. *JAMA.* 1994;271:1323–1327.

14. Chew SJ, Ritch R. Parental history and myopia: Taking the long view. *JAMA.* 1994;272:1255.

15. Wallman J. Parental history and myopia: Taking the long view. *JAMA.* 1994;272:1255–1256.

16. Lam DSC, Fan DSP, Saw SM, Islam M, Chew SJ. Parental history of myopia is not a predictor of eye size in pre-school children. Invest *Ophthalmol Vis Sci.* 1996;37(ARVO suppl):

17. Grice KM, DelBono EA, Haines SJ, Wiggs CL, Gwiazda JE. Genetic analysis of pedigrees affected by juvenile onset myopia. *Invest Ophthalmol Vis Sci.* 1996;37:S1002.

18. Schmid KL, Wildsoet CF. Breed- and gender-dependent differences in eye growth and form deprivation responses in chick. *J Comp Physiol A.* 1996;178:551–561.

19. Chew SJ, Chia SC, Lee LKH. The pattern of myopia in young Singaporean men. *Singapore Med J.* 1988; 29:201–211.

20. Chow YC, Dhillon B, Chew PTK, Chew SJ. Refractive errors in Singapore medical students. *Singapore Med J.* 1990;31:472–473.

21. Au Eong KG, Tay MTH, Lim MK. Race, culture and myopia in 110,236 young Singaporean males. *Singapore Med J.* 1993;34:29–32.

22. Rajan U, Tan FT, Chan TK, Wye-Dvorak J, Chew SJ. Increasing prevalence of myopia in Singapore school children. In: Chew SJ, Weintraub J, eds. *Proceedings of the Fifth International Conference on Myopia.* New York, NY: Myopia International Research Foundation; 1995;41–46.

23. O'Neal MR, Connon TR. Refractive error change at the United States Air Force Academy class of 1985. *Am J Optom Physiol Opt.* 1987;64:344–354.

24. Parssinen TO. Relation between refraction, education, occupation, and age among 26- and 46-year-old Finns. *Am J Optom Physiol Opt.* 1987;64: 136–143.

25. Nizam A, Waring GO III. Stability of refraction during 11 years in eyes with simple myopia. *Invest Ophthalmol Vis Sci.* 1996;37:S1004.

26. Adams AJ. Axial length elongation, not corneal curvature, as a basis of adult onset myopia. *Am J Optom Physiol Opt.* 1986;63:150–151.

27. Tokoro T, Shih Y, Yoshino Y. Correlation between myopic macular chorioretinal atrophy and refractive error, axial length and age. In: Khoo CY, ed. *New Frontiers in Ophthalmology.* Amsterdam: Elsevier Science Publishers BV; 1991;935–938.

28. Goss DA, Cox VD, Herrin-Lawson GA, Nielsen ED, Dolton WA. Refractive error, axial length, and height as a function of age in young myopes. *Optom Vis Sci.* 1990;67:332–338.

29. Teasdale TW, Goldschmidt E. Myopia and its relationship to education, intelligence and height. Preliminary results from an on-going study on Danish draftees. *Acta Ophthalmol—Suppl* 1988; 185:41–43.

30. Gardiner P. Physical growth and the progress of myopia. *Lancet.* 1955;2:952–953.

31. Hodos W, Erichsen JT. Lower-field myopia in birds: an adaptation that keeps the ground in focus. *Vision Res.* 1990;30:653–657.

32. Tay MTH, Au Eong KG, Ng CY, Lim MK. Myopia and educational attainment in 421,116 young Singaporean males. *Singapore Med J.* 1992;21:785–791.

33. Teasdale TW, Fuchs J, Goldschmidt E. Degree of myopia in relation to intelligence and educational level. *Lancet.* 1988;8624:1351–1354.

34. Young FA. Primate myopia. *Am J Optom Arch Am Acad Optom.* 1981;58:560–566.

35. Zylbermann R, Landau D, Berson D. The influence of study habits on myopia in Jewish teenagers. *J Pediatr Ophthalmol Strabismus.* 1993;30:319–322.

36. Shih Y, Chen M, Lin LLK, et al. TV watching and development of myopia in baby monkeys. *Invest Ophthalmol Vis Sci.* 1994;35(ARVO suppl):1802.

37. McCollim RJ. On the nature of myopia and the mechanism of accommodation. *Med Hypotheses.* 1989;28:197–211.

38. Kotulak JC, Morse SE. Is increased accommodation a necessary condition for instrument myopia? *SPIE.* 1994;

39. Wallman J. Retinal control of eye growth and refraction. *Prog Retinal Res.* 1992;12:243–249.

40. Wallman J. How many myopias? In: Christen Y, Doly M, Droy-Lefaix MT, eds. *Vision et adaptation.* Paris: Elsevier; 1995: pp. 103–123.

41. Schaeffel F, Glasser A, Howland HC. Accommodation, refractive error and eye growth in chickens. *Vision Res.* 1988;28:639–657.

42. Ni J, Smith EL III. Effects of chronic optical defocus on the kitten's refractive state. *Vision Res.* 1989;29:929–938.

43. Hung LF, Crawford MLJ, Smith EL III. Spectacle lenses alter eye growth and the refractive status of young monkeys. *Nature Med.* 1995;1:761–765.

44. Grosvenor T, Perrigin DM, Perrigin J, Maslovitz B. Houston myopia control study: a randomized clinical trial. Part II. Final report by the patient care team. *Am J Optom Physiol Opt.* 1987;64:482–498.

45. Bier N, Lowther GE. Myopia control study: effect of different contact lens refractive corrections on the progression of myopia. *Optometry Today.* 1988;28:37–40.

46. Grosvenor T, Perrigin J, Perrigin DM, Quintero S. Use of silicone-acrylate contact lenses for the control of myopia: results after two years of lens wear. *Optom Vis Sci.* 1989;66:41–47.

47. Perrigin J, Perrigin DM, Quintero S, Grosvenor T. Silicone-acrylate contact lenses for myopia control: 3-year results. *Optom Vis Sci.* 1990;67:764–769.

48. Wallman J, Turkel J, Trachtman JN. Extreme myopia produced by modest change in early visual experience. *Science.* 1978;201:1249–1251.

49. Wallman J, McFadden S. Monkey eyes grow into focus. *Nature Med.* 1995;1:737–739.

50. Norton TT, Siegwart JT Jr. Animal models of emmetropization: matching axial length to the focal plane. *J Am Optom Assoc.* 1995;66:405–414.

51. Wallman J. Gottlieb MD, Rajaram V, Fugate-Wentzek LA. Local retinal regions control local eye growth and myopia. *Science.* 1987;237:73–77.

52. Bear JC. Epidemiology and genetics of refractive anomalies. In: Grosvenor T, Flom M, eds. *Refractive Anomalies: Research and Clinical Applications.* Boston, MA: Butterworth-Heinemann; 1990;57–80.

53. Criswell MH, Goss DA. Myopia development in nonhuman primates: a literature review. *Am J Optom Physiol Opt.* 1983;60:250–268.

54. Daubs J. Environmental factors in the epidemiology of malignant myopia. *Am J Optom Physiol Opt.* 1982;59:271–277.

55. Curtin BJ. Physiologic vs pathologic myopia: genetics vs environment. *Ophthalmology.* 1979;86:681–691.

56. Angi MR, Clementi M, Sardei C, Piattelli E, Bisantis C. Heritability of myopic refractive errors in identical and fraternal twins. *Graefes Arch Clin Exp Ophthalmol.* 1993;231:580–585.

57. Perkins ES, Phelps CD. Open angle glaucoma, ocular hypertension, low-tension glaucoma, and refraction. *Arch Ophthalmol.* 1982;100:1464–1467.

58. Podos SM, Becker B, Morton WR. High myopia and primary open-angle glaucoma. *Am J Ophthalmol.* 1966;62:1039–1043.

59. American Academy of Ophthalmology. *Low to Moderate Refractive Errors.* San Francisco, CA: American Academy of Ophthalmology; 1991:1–29.

60. Raviola E, Wiesel TN. An animal model of myopia. *N Engl J Med.* 1985;312:1609–1615.

61. Wiesel TN, Raviola E. Myopia and eye enlargement after neonatal lid fusion in monkeys. *Nature.* 1977;266:66–68.

62. Wiesel TN, Raviola E. Increase in axial length of the macaque monkey eye after corneal opacification. *Invest Ophthalmol Vis Sci.* 1979;18:1232–1236.

63. Dyer JA. Role of cycloplegics in progressive myopia. *Ophthalmology.* 1979;86:692–694.

64. Yen MY, Liu JH, Kao SC, Shiao CH. Comparison

of the effect of atropine and cyclopentolate on myopia. *Ann Ophthalmol.* 1989;21:180–187.

65. Goss DA. Attempts to reduce the rate of increase of myopia in young people—a critical literature review. *Am J Optom Physiol Opt.* 1982;59:828–841.

66. Brodstein RS, Brodstein DE, Olson RJ, Hunt SC, Williams RR. The treatment of myopia with atropine and bifocals: A long-term prospective study. *Ophthalmology.* 1984;91:1373–1378.

67. Bates WH. *The Cure of Imperfect Sight by Treatment Without Glasses.* New York, NY: Central Fixation Pub Co; 1920.

68. Trachtman JN. Biofeedback of accommodation to reduce myopia: A review. *Am J Optom Physiol Opt.* 1987;64:639–643.

69. Gallaway M, Pearl SM, Winkelstein AM, Mitchell S. Biofeedback training of visual acuity and myopia: A pilot study. *Am J Optom Physiol Opt.* 1987;64:62–71.

70. Brand RJ, Polse KA, Schwalbe JS. The Berkeley Orthokeratology, Part I: general conduct of the study. *Am J Optom Physiol Opt.* 1983;60:175–186.

71. Polse KA, Brand RJ, Schwalbe JS, Vastine DW, Keener RJ. The Berkeley Orthokeratology Study, Part II: efficacy and duration. *Am J Optom Physiol Opt.* 1983;60:187–198.

72. Coloumbre AJ. The role of intraocular pressure in the development of the chick eye. *J Exp Zool.* 1956;133;211–225.

73. Neath P, Roche SM, Bee JA. Intraocular pressure-dependent and -independent phases of growth of the embryonic chick eye and cornea. *Invest Ophthalmol Vis Sci.* 1991;32:2483–2491.

74. Touhidi-Baghini S. The relationship between intraocular pressure and experimentally induced myopia in chicks. Master's thesis. New York, NY: City University of New York; 1986:1–50.

75. Kornbleuth W, Aladjemoff L, Magora F, Bed Dor D. Intraocular pressure in children measured under general anesthesia. *Arch Ophthalmol.* 1964; 72:489–490.

76. Seltner RL, Sivak JG. A role for the vitreous humor in experimentally-induced myopia. *Am J Optom Physiol Opt.* 1987;64:953–957.

77. Curtin BJ, Teng CC. Scleral changes in pathological myopia. *Trans Am Acad Ophthalmol Otolaryngol.* 1957;62:777–790.

78. Ku DN, Greene PR., Scleral creep in vitro resulting from cyclic pressure pulses: applications to myopia. *Am J Optom Physiol Opt.* 1981;58:528–535.

79. Tokoro T. Experimental myopia in rabbits. *Invest Ophthalmol Vis Sci.* 1970;9:926–934.

80. Christensen AM, Wallman J. Evidence that increased scleral growth underlies visual deprivation myopia in chicks. *Invest Ophthalmol Vis Sci.* 1991; 32:2143–2150.

81. Wilkinson JL, Hodos W. Intraocular pressure and eye enlargement in chicks. *Curr Eye Res.* 1991;10: 163–168.

81a. Jensen H, Goldschmidt E, Management of Myopia: Pharmaceutical Agents. In: *Refractive Anomalies. Research and Clinical Applications*, edited by Grosvener, T. and Flom, M. Boston: Butterworth-Heinemann, 1991, p. 371–383.

82. Sorsby A. Transmission of refractive errors within Eskimo families. *Am J Optom Arch Am Acad Optom.* 1970;471(3):244–249.

83. Rosner M, Belkin M. Intelligence, education, and myopia in males. *Arch Ophthalmol.* 1987;105: 1508–1511.

84. Grisham JD, Simons HD. Refractive error and the reading process: a literature analysis. *J Am Optom Assoc.* 1986;57:44–55.

85. Simensen B, Thorud LO. Adult-onset myopia and occupation. *Acta Ophthalmol.* 1994;72:469–471.

86. Luedde WH. Monocular cycloplegia for the control of myopia. *Am J Ophthalmol.* 1932;15:603–609.

87. Bedrossian RH. The effect of atropine on myopia. *Ann Ophthalmol.* 1971;3:891–897.

88. Bedrossian RH. The effect of atropine on myopia. *Ophthalmology.* 1979;86;713–719.

89. Gimbel HV. The control of myopia with atropine. *Can J Ophthalmol.* 1973;8:527–532.

90. Gostin SB. Prophylactic management of progressive myopia. *South Med J.* 1962;55:916–920.

91. Takano Y. Treatment of myopia by the instillation of tropicamide. *Jap J Clin Ophthalmol.* 1964;18:45–50.

92. Yamaji R, Yoshihara M, Sakiyama A, Furata I, Ishikawa K. Clinical study on the effect of Mydrin OM on the visual acuity and refraction in myopic children. *Jap J Clin Ophthalmol.* 1964;18:397–405.

93. Tokoro T, Kabe S. Treatment of the myopia and the changes in optical components. Report I. Topical application of neosynephrine and tropicamide. *Acta Soc Ophthalmol Jpn.* 1964;68:1958–1961.

94. Curtin BJ. The management of myopia. *Trans Pa Acad Ophthalmol Otolaryngol.* 1972;25:117–123.

95. Chew SJ, Lind GJ, Marzani D. A direct effect for muscarinic antagonists on the sclera: implications

for the control of myopia. In: Chew SJ, Weintraub J, eds. *Proceedings of the 5th International Conference on Myopia*. New York, NY: Myopia International Research Foundation; 1995;229–230.

96. Duke-Elder S, Abrams D. Ophthalmic optics and refraction. In: Duke-Elder S, ed. *System of Ophthalmology*, vol V. St Louis, MO: CV Mosby; 1970: p 353–371.

97. Sorsby A. The nature of spherical refractive errors. In: *Anonymous Refractive Anomalies of the Eye*. NINDB Monograph No. 5. 1976:

98. Norton TT, Rada JA, Hassell JR. Extracellular matrix changes in the sclera of shrews with induced myopia. *Invest Ophthalmol Vis Sci*. 1992:33(ARVO suppl):1054.

99. Rada JA, Brenza HL. Increased latent gelatinase activity in the sclera of visually deprived chicks. *Invest Ophthalmol Vis Sci*. 1995;36:1555–1565.

100. Guggenheim JA, Crisp MS, Wainwright SD, McBrien NA. Gelatinase activity in tree shrew sclera. *Invest Ophthalmol Vis Sci*. 1995;36(ARVO suppl):760.

101. Guggenheim JA, McBrien NA. Form-deprivation myopia induces activation of scleral matrix metalloproteinase-2 in tree shrew. *Invest Ophthaomol Vis Sci*.; 37:1380–1395.

102. Stone RA, Lin T, Laties AM. Muscarinic antagonist effects on experimental chick myopia. *Exp Eye Res*. 1991;52:755–758.

103. Chew SJ, Beuerman RW. Control of cornea wound healing and myopia by in vivo and in vitro inhibition of scleral and corneal fibroblast proliferation by muscarinic antagonists. *Invest Ophthalmol Vis Sci*. 1993;34:S1320.

104. Rickers M, Schaeffel F, Hagel G, Zrenner E. Dose-dependent effects of intravitreal pirenzepine on deprivation myopia and lens-induced refractive errors in chickens. *Invest Ophthalmol Vis Sci*. 1994; 35(ARVO suppl):1801.

105. McBrien NA, Cottriall CL. Pirenzepine reduces axial elongation and myopia in monocularly deprived tree shrews. *Invest Ophthalmol Vis Sci*. 1993;34(ARVO suppl):1210.

106. Cottriall CL, McBrien NA. The M1 muscarinic antagonist pirenzepine reduces myopia and eye enlargement in tree shrew. *Invest Ophthalmol Vis Sci*. 1996;37:1368–1379.

107. Rickers M, Schaeffel F. Dose-dependent effect of intravitreal pirenzepine on deprivation myopia and lens-induced refractive errors in chickens. *Exp Eye Res*. 1995;61:509–516.

108. McKanna JA, Casagrande VA. Chronic cycloplegia prevents lid-suture myopia in tree shrews. *Invest Ophthalmol Vis Sci*. 1985;26(ARVO suppl):331.

109. McKanna JA, Casagrande VA. Atropine affects lid-suture myopia development. *Doc Ophthalmol Proc Ser*. 1981;28:187–192.

110. Chew SJ, Beuerman RW. Visual form deprivation induces myopia in the infant rabbit, which is reduced by muscarinic antagonists applied directly to the sclera. In: Chew SJ, Weintraub J, eds. *Proceedings of the 5th International Conference on Myopia*. New York, NY: Myopia International Research Foundation; 1995;231–246.

111. Marzani D, Lind GJ, Chew SJ, Wallman J. Muscarinic antagonists act directly to inhibit proteoglycan synthesis in the sclera. *Invest Ophthalmol Vis Sci*. 1994;35:S1801.

112. Stone RA, Lin T, Laties AM, Iuvone PM. Retinal dopamine and form deprivation myopia. *Proc Natl Acad Sci USA*. 1989;86:704–706.

113. Iuvone PM, Tigges M, Stone RA, Lambert S, Laties AM. Effects of apomorphine, a dopamine receptor agonist, on ocular refraction and axial elongation in a primate model of myopia. *Invest Ophthalmol Vis Sci*. 1991;32:1674–1677.

114. Kiorpes L, Wallman J. Does experimentally-induced amblyopia cause hyperopia in monkeys? *Vision Res*. 1995;35:1289–1297.

115. Irving EL, Callender MG, Sivak JG. Inducing myopia, hyperopia, and astigmatism in chicks. *Optom Vis Sci*. 1991;68:364–368.

116. Crewther SG, Nathan J, Kiely PM, Brennan NA, Crewther DP. The effect of defocussing contact lenses on refraction in cynomolgus monkeys. *Clin Vis Sci*. 1988;3:221–228.

117. Gawron VJ. Differences among myopes, emmetropes, and hyperopes. *Am J Optom Physiol Opt*. 1981;58:753–760.

118. Rosner J. Hyperopia. In: Grosvenor T, Flom M, eds. *Refractive Anomalies: Research and Clinical Applications*. Boston, MA: Butterworth-Heinemann; 1991;121–130.

119. Chew SJ, Beuerman RW, Kaufman HE, Ritch R. Marked generational differences in ocular biometric parameters in a Chinese population. *Ophthalmology*. 1992;99(suppl):131.

120. Abrahamsson M, Fabian G, Andersson AK, Sjostrand J. A longitudinal study of a population

based sample of astigmatic children. *Acta Ophthalmol.* 1990;68:428–434.

121. Grey C, Yap M. Influence of lid position on astigmatism. *Am J Optom Physiol Opt.* 1986;63: 966–969.

122. Wilson G, Bell C, Chotai S. The effect of lifting the lids on corneal astigmatism. *Am J Optom Physiol Opt.* 1982;59:670–674.

123. Fulton AB, Hansen RM, Petersen RA. The relation of myopia and astigmatism in developing eyes. *Ophthalmology.* 1982;89:298–302.

124. Callender MG, Sivak JG, Husanini A. Refractive plasticity of the developing chick eye. *Invest Ophthalmol Vis Sci.* 1992;33(ARVO suppl):708.

125. Shih Y, Ho T, Chen M, Lin LLK, Wang P, Hou P. Experimental myopia in chickens induced by corneal astigmatism. *Acta Ophthalmol.* 1994;72: 597–601.

2

Ocular Surface Management in Refractive Surgery

Kazuo Tsubota

IMPORTANCE OF OCULAR SURFACE MANAGEMENT IN REFRACTIVE SURGERY

Most corneal refractive procedures disrupt—and thus require proper wound healing of—the corneal epithelium. Although expected in most patients, this process cannot be taken for granted. Even subtle ocular surface abnormalities, such as subclinical diabetic epitheliopathy, may interfere with epithelial wound healing. In such cases, special attention must be paid after refractive surgery.

Epithelial wound healing has many requirements: a supply of cytokines and growth factors from tears,[1–3] proper blinking,[4] the migration and proliferation of epithelial cells,[5–7] and an intact substrate.[8,9] A disturbance in any of these factors or processes may complicate refractive surgery. Furthermore, it is becoming clear that cytokine communication is not one way, from the keratocytes to the epithelium, but rather two way, including a cytokine supply from the epithelium to the keratocytes.[3] Since keratocyte collagen synthesis is responsible for haze formation and regression of photorefractive keratotomy (PRK), a healthy epithelium is necessary to maintain a clear stroma and the surgical refractive effects. Since the incidence of ocular surface disorders such as dry eye, allergic conjunctivitis, or mild diabetic epitheliopathy is high, meticulous preoperative evaluation is essential.

This chapter begins with a description of normal corneal epithelial wound healing at the cellular level. A practical approach to the preoperative evaluation of the ocular surface is then presented. This is followed by a discussion of how to treat those patients who, for one reason or another, have abnormal wound healing. Finally, management of significant corneal complications, including infection and ulceration, is presented.

CORNEAL EPITHELIAL WOUND HEALING FOLLOWING REFRACTIVE SURGERY

Radial keratotomy (RK) disrupts the corneal epithelium at the incision sites, but the insult is small and reepithelialization usually occurs the next day. Although rare, corneal infection may start at the incision site,[10] and there is some risk of irregular corneal epithelial wound healing, such as epithelial downgrowth. When RK is properly performed, the potential risk to the corneal epithelium is much less than that associated with excimer laser PRK.

In most instances, PRK involves removal of the corneal epithelium with either a blunt spatula or diluted alcohol. The area of epithelium removed depends on the area of the desired ablation, with the former usually slightly larger than the latter (e.g., a 7-mm epithelial diameter for a 6-mm ablation diameter). Since area is proportional to the square of the diameter, a small increase in the diameter of the epithelium removed can have a dramatic effect on the total area (e.g., 95 mm^2 for 5.5 mm but 201 mm^2 for 8 mm). The size of the ablation zone depends on many factors, including the degree of myopia to be corrected and the need to minimize nightime glare, but the surgeon must also consider that larger ablation zones require greater epithelial removal, and hence longer and potentially complicated wound healing.

Following excimer laser treatment, the first phase in wound healing is epithelial migration without proliferation. The surrounding epithelium migrates toward the central ablated zone for the first 6 hr. If the epithelial defect is small enough, as in RK, the whole area can be covered quickly by this mechanism alone. With larger epithelial defects, as in most cases of PRK, there is limited migration from the epithelial periphery, and hence cellular proliferation is necessary to cover the defect.

In the corneal epithelium, only transient amplifying (TA) cells in the basal cell layer and stem cells in the limbal area can proliferate.[6] Ablation disrupts the barrier function of the corneal epithelium, exposing the TA cells to tear components such as epidermal growth factor (EGF). The TA cells along the ablation border form the primary focus of proliferative recovery. At the same time, corneal epithelial stem cells at the limbus react to the wound and begin to provide new TA cells to the central cornea[6] (Fig. 2.1).

In the central cornea, the stromal cells disappear after exposure to the excimer laser, disrupting the supply of such important cytokines as keratocyte growth factor (KGF) and hepatocyte growth factor (HGF)[3] from the stroma to the epithelium. In this situation, cytokine delivery from tears is critical. Reepithelialization of the defect is ordinarily completed within 3–4 days.[11] At this point, the epithelium is still thin and there are spindle-shaped cells in the central area, indicating accelerated movement of the epithelial cells. The barrier function as measured by anterior fluorometry is still high, suggesting that tight junction formation of the corneal epithelium is not fully recovered. The proportion of spindle-shaped cells and the increased fluorescence permeability decrease with time, normalizing at around 1 month after PRK. The disappearance of the spindle-shaped cells reflects proper maintenance of the corneal epithelium by desquamation, differentiation, and migration. The central TA cells allow programmed cell death by desquamating from the superficial epithelium, preventing accelerated centripetal movement of the epithelium. Normalization of the fluorescence permeability signals reestablishment of the tight junctions.

LONG-TERM FOLLOW-UP OF THE CORNEAL EPITHELIUM

Although the mechanism is unknown, the corneal epithelium maintains a thickness of about 80 to 100 μm, divided into five to seven layers. Specular microscopy reveals that superficial epithelial cells have a regular hexagonal shape, with a mean exposed area of 600 ± 100 μm^2. These parameters are maintained by a delicate balance of cell proliferation and cell death. Cell proliferation begins with the TA cells in the basal cell layer, whereas cell death is due to epithelial desquamation. Although desquamation

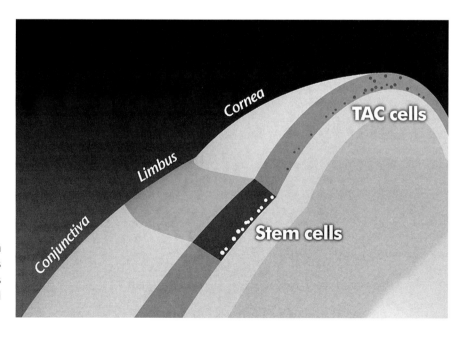

Fig. 2.1. Diagram of corneal stem cells and TA cells. The stem cells are located at the limbus, whereas the TA cells are found in the central cornea.

is thought to be due to the shearing forces of blinking, the most superficial cell layer may also exhibit programmed cell death, or apoptosis. Ordinarily, the superficial cells lose their microvilli and undergo a dense chromatin condensation (as opposed to necrosis). When this balance is disturbed, superficial cell size or epithelial thickness is altered.

After excimer laser treatment, specular microscopy reveals almost normal cell configurations and size in the superficial layer. The elongated cell shape returns to normal within several months.[12] In contrast to the abnormal enlargement of superficial cells seen in users of extended-wear soft contact lenses, which may be due to the blockage of pro-

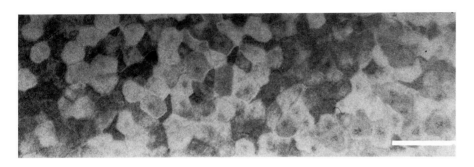

A

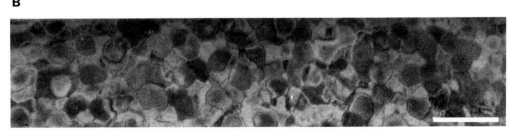

B

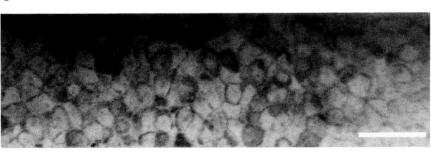

C

D

Fig. 2.2. Specular microscopic view of the corneal epithelium in a normal individual (a), in an extended-wear soft contact lens wearer (b), and in patients following excimer laser treatment (c,d), both female, aged 25 and 33 years, respectively. The specular microscopic view of the corneal epithelium 3 months after laser surgery (c) is similar to that in (a). All bars = 100 μm.

grammed cell death,[13,14] the corneal epithelium is relatively unscathed following PRK[12,15] (Fig. 2.2).

Nevertheless, it is well known that the regression of the PRK effect is due at least in part to abnormal thickening of the corneal epithelium. Greater understanding of cell proliferation and death should improve our management of PRK patients and others in whom epithelial thickness may vary.

PREOPERATIVE MANAGEMENT OF OCULAR SURFACE DISORDERS

The most relevant ocular surface disorders are dry eye, allergic conjunctivitis, and conditions associated with systemic diseases such as diabetes or other autoimmune disorders.

Dry Eye

Preoperative management
Preoperative management of patients with dry eye begins with evaluation of tear dynamics. A routine Schirmer value of at least 10 mm indicates adequate tear production, except in patients with poor tear clearance, in whom tear pooling may show diminished production.[16] For these patients, the preservatives found in ophthalmic solutions may cause epithelial damage, so they are advised to use preservative-free preparations.

Patients with Schirmer test results of less than 10 mm are then assessed for reflex tearing, using the Schirmer test with nasal stimulation.[17] Individuals who cannot produce even reflex tears have lymphocytic infiltration and destruction of the lacrimal glands, typically caused by Sjögren's syndrome (SS) and also associated with dry mouth and elevated autoantibody levels[18] (Table 2.1). In patients with SS dry eye who undergo PRK, wound healing may be impeded by an inadequate supply of growth factors and other cytokines by tears. In contrast,

Table 2.1. Schirmer Tests Results with Non-SS Dry Eye and SS Dry Eye

	Schirmer Test	Schirmer Test with NS
Non-SS Dry Eye	Low	Normal
SS Dry Eye	Low	Low

patients with dry eye who have good reflex tearing should be able to provide the tear components necessary for wound healing after PRK despite their deficient production of basal tears. Our clinical results are consistent with this concept.[19] Patients with dry eye who do not want to undergo the nasal stimulation test may be able to identify their form of dry eye by noting whether they produce tears when crying. If no tears are produced, then they may have the SS form of dry eye, in which case further workup and/or management may be needed if they are to be candidates for PRK.

Postoperative management of patients with non-SS dry eye is essentially the same as routine dry eye management. Patients use preservative-free eye drops, wear protective eyeglasses, and are encouraged to maintain proper blinking. In patients with dry eye, an increased blink rate (40/min on average) is one way to maintain a moist ocular surface.[20,21] Recently, topical anesthesia has been recommended after PRK. Since it is well known that the blink rate decreases dramatically with topical anesthesia, patients with dry eye are particularly vulnerable to desiccation.

Persistent Epithelial Defect Associated with Dry Eye
Slow healing of the corneal epithelium or a persistent epithelial defect should raise the suspicion of dry eye and warrant performance of a Schirmer test if this has not already been done. Patients found to have non-SS dry eye should receive routine dry eye management, whereas those with the SS form should be more aggressively managed. For wounds to heal properly, growth factors and other cytokines must be supplied by tears, especially given the depletion of keratocytes from the ablated area which normally provides these substances. There are two methods for augmenting the supply of those tear components to the ocular surface: punctual occlusion and use of autologous serum eye drops. Currently, there are no exogenous artificial tears which contain cytokines or growth factors.

Punctal occlusion retains existing natural tears in the conjunctival sac. Even patients with SS dry eye can produce small amounts of tears, which can accumulate with punctal occlusion.[22]

Drops derived from autologous serum replace natural tears. Fox et al. reported their clinical efficacy[23] even before tear cytokines were identified. We now know that serum contains most of the components present in tears. In practice, about 100 ml of whole blood is obtained from the patient, and the serum (about 50 ml) is separated by centrifugation (1500 rpm for 5 min). The serum is then frozen in sterile 5-ml containers. Such growth factors as EGF and TGF (transforming growth factor)-β can be maintained for at least 1 month at −20°C. Currently used serum should be refrigerated.

We do not know how many times a day the serum drops are best used. From our experience with ocular surface reconstruction in very severe ocular pemphigoid, the maximal use is every 15 min, or 64 times a day during a 16-hr day.[24] In less severe cases of dry eye, we have found that 5–10 times per day suffices, and we currently recommend that most post-PRK patients with dry eye initially use the drops 10 times a day.

Allergic Conjunctivitis

Since some patients with allergic conjunctivitis never complain of itchiness,[25] a careful ocular surface evaluation by the slit lamp and possibly a systemic workup are necessary to exclude the diagnosis. The most important sign is papillae formation on the upper palpebral conjunctiva, which should be checked in every patient. The presence of any such papillae suggests allergic conjunctivitis. A history of atopic skin disease, asthma, or pruritus in the patient or immediate relatives also raises the suspicion. Serum immunoglobulin E (IgE) levels may also be measured and are typically evaluated in allergic conjunctivitis.

We have found that haze formation and regression are strongly associated with allergic reactions.[26] When we divided the patients into three groups—(1) normal patients, (2) patients with allergic conjunctivitis treated with steroids or antiallergic medication, and (3) patients with allergic conjunctivitis without treatment—only the last group showed significant haze formation and regression of refractive effect following PRK.

The mechanism is unknown, however, in allergic disorders such as asthma and atopic dermatitis; the activated mast cells release cytokines (such as TGF-β and tumor necrosis factor [TNF]-α) and chemical mediators.[27] Activated mast cells promote leukocytes and activate fibroblasts through the released cytokines and/or chemical mediators. Activated fibroblasts increase the development of collagen and other extracellular matrix proteins. Taking this

into consideration, we suspect that PRK patients with allergic conjunctivitis without steroid treatment produce mast cells, which increase fibroblast activation, inducing an increase in collagen. Confirming our belief, the subepithelial haze among our allergic conjunctivitis patients without steroid treatment not only stayed at its peak but actually increased; regression was also apparent.

Patients with allergic conjunctivitis should thus continue to take their medication before and after PRK. Since topical steroids may have long-term side effects, antiallergic drugs such as cromolyn sodium are recommended. Studies are ongoing to determine whether these medications can eventually be tapered or discontinued.

Management of Systemic Conditions, Diabetes Mellitus, and Other Autoimmune Disorders

Although most patients who request refractive surgery are young and healthy, some do have systemic diseases. Such autoimmune conditions as diabetes mellitus, rheumatoid arthritis, and systemic lupus erythematosus are of particular concern because they can affect the ocular surface and interfere with corneal epithelial wound healing.

It is well known that some diabetic patients have delayed wound healing, especially after vitrectomy. The term *diabetic epitheliopathy* refers to any epithelial disorders due to diabetes.[28] In this condition, sorbitol accumulates in the corneal sensory nerves or epithelium, interfering with normal proliferation/maturation and wound healing. Most diabetic patients have no serious postoperative problems, although specular microscopy often reveals enlargement of the superficial epithelial cells following cataract surgery.[29] These patients also generally have some degree of dry eye, but often without complaints, probably because of decreased corneal sensitivity.[30] Meticulous attention should be paid to these patients until the epithelial defect is healed, in addition to the routine epithelial management provided to all patients with dry eye. If epithelial wound healing is compromised, a topical or systemic aldose reductase inhibitor (ARI) is the treatment of choice.[30,31] ARIs inhibit the key enzyme, aldose reductase, in diabetic metabolism and prevent intracellular accumulation of sorbitol. Our limited experience with this approach has yielded satisfactory clinical results. Uncontrolled diabetics may not be good candidates for refractive surgery but may benefit from prophylactic administration of ARI.

Autoimmune disorders can seriously complicate refractive surgery. As we have seen in our clinic, corneal melting may follow surgery, especially in patients with dry eye. All prospective refractive surgery candidates should be questioned about autoimmune disorders. If their disease is active, the procedure should be postponed.

Management of Persistent Epithelial Defect or Corneal Melting

Preoperative evaluation and postoperative management prevent most serious epithelial problems after refractive surgery. Infection is the most severe complication, but it is rare and can be managed by topical or systemic antibiotics. Persistent epithelial defect is another serious development, since it can be a source of corneal infection and haze. The following is a strategy for diagnosing and managing persistent epithelial defect.

The first step is to determine the etiology of the defect. There are seven major causes of compromised reepithelialization: (1) abnormal tear function, (2) dysfunction in proliferation or migration of epithelial cells, (3) substrate problems, (4) inflammation such as allergic conjunctivitis, (5) mechanical stress such as entropion or giant papillary conjunctivitis, (6) neurotrophic components, and (7) topical medications. In order to devise appropriate treatment, it is important to determine which factor or combination of factors is responsible for the persistent epithelial defect.

Abnormal tear function is best treated with punctal occlusion or autologous serum drops, as discussed previously. It may be necessary to occlude the eye with temporary patching or tarsorrhaphy if the patient has decreased blinking or if desiccation is particularly severe.

Dysfunctional epithelial cell proliferation or migration may be caused by diabetes mellitus or defective corneal stem cells. The latter condition, which is sometimes seen in long-term wearers or soft contact lenses, may necessitate stem cell transplantation.

Abnormal substrate, such as the absence of all or part of Bowman's layer following routine PRK, can reduce the smoothness of the ocular surface. Persistent inflammation can inhibit reepithelialization and should be controlled with topical steroids or nonsteroidal anti-inflammatory drugs. The possibility of infection should always be ruled out when steroid use is initiated or increased. Similarly, the desirability of reduced epithelial proliferation must be considered. Mechanical stress should be promptly managed by removing the entropion or using a bandage soft contact lens for protection. There is no definitive treatment for neurotrophic problems, but in our limited experience, autologous serum drops seem to be effective. The side effects of any medications, including topical ones, should always be kept in mind. For example, preservatives may affect the epithelium in patients with poor tear clearance. Very rarely, the etiology of delayed reepithelialization is unknown. In this case, comprehensive management of all possible problems should be undertaken.

CONCLUSION

Most corneal refractive surgery interferes with the health of the ocular surface and depends on proper wound healing of the corneal epithelium. With the increased popularity of such procedures, patients with common ocular surface disorders are presenting for surgical consideration. The proper diagnosis (especially preoperatively) and management of any ocular surface abnormalities are essential to obtain good, stable results of refractive surgery and to prevent complications.

REFERENCES

1. Wilson S. Lacrimal gland epidermal growth factor production and the ocular surface. *Am J Ophthalmol.* 1991;111:763–765.
2. Ohashi Y, Motokura M, Kinoshita Y, et al. Presence of epidermal growth factor in human tears. *Invest Ophthalmol Vis Sci.* 1989;30:1879–1887.
3. Li E, Tseng S. Three patterns of cytokine expression potentially involved in epithelial–fibroblast interactions of human ocular surface. *J Cell Physiol.* 1995;163:61–79.
4. Abelson M, Holly F. A tentative mechanism for inferior punctate keratopathy. *Am J Ophthalmol.* 1977; 83:866–869.

5. Schermer A, Galvin S, Sun T. Differentiation-related expression of a major 64K corneal keratin in vivo and in culture suggests limbal location of corneal epithelial stem cells. *J Cell Biol.* 1986;103:49–62.

6. Sharma A, Coles WH. Kinetics of corneal epithelial maintenance and graft loss. A population balance model. *Invest Ophthalmol Vis Sci.* 1989;30:1962–1971.

7. Tseng S. Concept and application of limbal stem cells. *Eye.* 1989;3:141–157.

8. Tsai R, Tseng S. Effect of stromal inflammation on the outcome of limbal transplantation for corneal surface reconstruction. *Cornea.* 1995;14:439–449.

9. Tsai R, Tseng S. Substrate modulation of cultured rabbit conjunctival epithelial cell differentiation and morphology. *Invest Ophthalmol Vis Sci.* 1988;29:1565–1576.

10. Szerenyi K, McDonnell J, Smith R, Irvine J, McDonnell P. Keratitis as a complication of bilateral, simultaneous radial keratotomy. *Am J Ophthalmol.* 1994;117:462–467.

11. Piebenga L, Matta C, Deitz M, Tauber J, Irvine J, Sabates F. Excimer photorefractive keratectomy for myopia. *Ophthalmology.* 1993;100:1335–1345.

12. Amano S, Shimizu K, Tsubota K. Specular microscopic evaluation of the corneal epithelium after excimer laser photorefractive keratectomy. *Am J Ophthalmol.* 1994;117:381–384.

13. Tsubota K, Toda I, Fujishima H, Yamada M, Sugawara T, Shimazaki J. Extended-wear soft contact lenses induce corneal epithelial changes. *Br J Ophthalmol.* 1994;78:907–911.

14. Tsubota K, Yamada M. Corneal epithelial alterations induced by disposable contact lens wear. *Ophthalmology.* 1992;99:1193–1196.

15. Amano S, Shimizu K, Tsubota K. Corneal epithelial changes after excimer laser photorefractive keratectomy. *Am J Ophthalmol.* 1993;115:441–443.

16. Xu K, Yagi Y, Toda I, Tsubota K. Tear function index: A new measure of dry eye. *Arch Ophthalmol.* 1995;113:84–88.

17. Tsubota K, Xu K, Fujihara T, Katagiri S, Takeuchi T. Decreased reflex tearing is associated with lymphocyte infiltration in lacrimal and salivary glands. *J Rheumatol.* 1996;23:76–82.

18. Lemp M. *Report from the National Institute of Health/Industry Workshop on Clinical Trials in Dry Eye.* 1993.

19. Toda I, Itoh S, Tsubota K. Excimer laser for dry eye patients. *Br J Ophthalmol.* 1996;80:604–609.

20. Tsubota K, Hata S, Okusawa Y, Egami F, Ohtsuki T, Nakamori K. Quantitative videographic analysis of blinking in normal and dry eye patients. *Arch Ophthalmol.* 1996;114:715–720.

21. Tsubota K, Nakamori K. Effects of ocular surface area and blink rate on tear dynamics. *Arch Ophthalmol.* 1995;113:115–158.

22. Ophthalmology editorial: Punctal occlusion for the dry eye. *Ophthalmology.* 1992;99:639–640.

23. Fox R, Chan R, Michelson J, Belmont J, Michelson P. Beneficial effect of artificial tears made with autologous serum in patients with keratoconjunctivitis sicca. *Arthritis Rheum.* 1984;27:459–461.

24. Tsubota K, Satake Y, Ohyama M, et al. Surgical reconstruction of the ocular surface in advanced ocular cicatricial pemphigoid and Stevens-Johnson syndrome. *Am J Ophthalmol.* 1996;122:38–52.

25. Toda I, Shimazaki J, Tsubota K. Dry eye with only decreased tear break-up time is sometimes associated with allergic conjunctivitis. *Ophthalmology.* 1995;102:302–309.

26. Yang H-Y, Bissen-Miyajima H, Toda I, Fujishima H, Shimazaki J, Tsubota K. Allergic conjunctivitis is a risk factor for regression and haze after PRK. International Society of Refractive Surgery, annual meeting, 1995.

27. Gordon JR, Galli SJ. Promotion of mouse fibroblast collagen gene expression by mast cells stimulated via the Fc_ϵ RI. Role for mast cell-derived transforming growth factor β and tumor necrosis factor α. *J Exp Med* 1994;180:2017–2037.

28. Ohashi Y, Matsuda M, Kinoshita S, Manabe R. Aldose reductase inhibitor (CT-112) eyedrops for diabetic corneal epitheliopathy. *Am J Ophthalmol.* 1988;105:233–238.

29. Tsubota K, Chiba K, Shimazaki J. Corneal epithelium in diabetic patients. *Cornea.* 1991;10:156–160.

30. Fujishima H, Shimazaki J, Yagi Y, Tsubota K. Improvement of corneal sensation and tear dynamics in diabetic patients by oral aldose reductase inhibitor, ONO-2235: a preliminary study. *Cornea.* 1996;15:368–372.

31. Hosotani H, Ohashi Y, Yamada M, Tsubota K. Reversal of abnormal corneal epithelial cell morphologic characteristics and reduced corneal sensitivity in diabetic patients by aldose reductase inhibitor, CT-112. *Am J Ophthalmol.* 1995;119:288–294.

3

Radial Keratotomy

James J. Salz
Kerry K. Assil
Joseph Colin

In 1953, Sato et al. reported a study of the use of numerous radial incisions on both the epithelial and endothelial corneal surfaces as a way to flatten the cornea.[1] However, they did not have a full understanding of the complete role of the corneal endothelium. Twenty years later, in 1972, Beliaev and Ilyina demonstrated that placing radial incisions externally and limiting them to the anterior corneal stroma results in flattening of the cornea.[2] Shortly thereafter, radial keratotomy (RK) was adapted as an ophthalmic procedure in the United States.

The original technique of performing RK, as taught by Fyodorov and others, involved a complicated invasive procedure. Regardless of the amount of myopia, the original recommendation involved a 16-incision procedure, with incisions initiated at the limbus and terminated at the optical zone. The amount of correction was titrated only by varying the size of the optical clear zone. For larger amounts of myopia, multiple blade settings based on differences in pachymetry, so-called peripheral redeepening, were advocated in an attempt to stretch the limits of the procedure.

Modern RK has evolved into a much simpler, safer procedure. The Prospective Evaluation of Radial Keratotomy (PERK) study[3] advocated reducing the number of incisions to eight "American-style" incisions, and reports by Salz et al.[4] and Spigelman et al.[5] based on cadaver eye studies[6] introduced the concept of a staged approach to RK by starting with a four-incision operation in many eyes and adding four incisions later if necessary.

Casebeer further popularized the staged approach to RK with a well-defined system of instruments, techniques, and nomograms which were particularly helpful to novice surgeons. Assil introduced the concept of combining the increased effi-

ciency of a centripetal (uphill, Russian-style) incision and the safety of the centrifugal (downhill, American-style) incision with a unique diamond blade design (Genesis). The upper dull portion of the blade acts as a safety bevel, substantially reducing the risk of invading the optical clear zone, an unfortunate complication of the straight Russian technique. Casebeer, Lindstrom, and others also advocate this combined technique with similar blade designs (Duo-Track [Chiron] and Two Step [Mastel, Storz]).

A very recent modification of the radial keratotomy technique involved Lindstrom's concept of mini-RK[7] designed to improve the stability of RK results by reducing the incidence of progressive hyperopic shift and decreasing the potential for rupture of the incisions in the event of blunt trauma. The mini-RK incisions extend from the appropriate optical zone determined by the nomogram, but stop at approximately an outer zone of 8.0 mm rather than just short of the limbus. The details of this approach are covered in Chapter 4.

Although four- and eight-incision RK are quite common, the appropriate combination of mild myopia and astigmatism can be corrected by two-incision RK, an idea first proposed by Enrique Suarez at a meeting of the International Society of Refractive Surgeons (Chicago, November 1993). For example, in a 42-year-old patient with a refractive error of −1.50 × 180 (spherical equivalent −2.25 D), the error can be corrected with a two-incision RK and a 3.75-mm optical clear zone, with the two incisions placed in the steep 90° meridian.

A modern approach to RK consists of two, four, six, or eight incisions performed with a specially designed blade with a safety bevel on the front surface (Genesis, Duo-track, Two Step) using a combined American-Russian technique, with a single blade setting based on ultrasonic pachymetry. The incisions extend from the optical zone, determined by the age-adjusted nomogram for the preoperative spherical equivalent myopia, and terminate at an outer optical zone of approximately 8 mm (mini-RK). One of us (J.S.) has found that the Lindstrom mini-RK nomograms are a useful initial guide to surgical planning. However, surgeons should personalize these nomograms based on their own particular technique and actual results, which may differ from the predicted results in the nomograms. The Lindstrom mini-RK nomograms for two, four, six, and eight incisions can be found in Chapter 4.

SURGICAL TECHNIQUE

Preoperative Planning and Instrumentation

A standardized protocol is recommended to maximize the surgical outcome. Preoperative planning should include ultrasonography, proper equipment (i.e., diamond knives and a microscope), videokeratographic analysis, and incisional nomograms.

Ultrasound
Reliable corneal pachymetry readings are obtained using real-time ultrasound. Paracentral pachymetry done before surgery can supplement intraoperative measurements and establish relative corneal thickness relations. In both the combined and undercut techniques, preoperative and intraoperative pachymetry are used to locate the thinnest area of the cornea. Intraoperative pachymetry conducted at a 3-mm central clear zone (1.5 mm from the surgical centration point) and over the temporal and thinnest paracentral cornea reduces the risk of perforation.

The Diamond Knife
Thinner-width diamond blades are preferred because they produce less resistance during the incision. The angle formed by the radial and enhancement diamond tip should be between 35° and 45° for knives used in the combination (Genesis) technique.[8] Knives with angles greater than 45° encounter more resistance on initial insertion and thus greater difficulty in reaching the desired depth.

The knife design for the combined technique allows the surgeon to begin the incision at the central clear zone, extend it toward the limbus, and reverse direction without invading the clear zone. The front surface, angled at 45°, is the centrifugal cutting component and is sharpened along its entire length. The back surface, which is vertical, is sharpened only for 250 μm from the blade's tip. This helps prevent unwanted invasion of the central clear zone during both the initial insertion and the final centripetal return.

The undercut technique knife differs in having a specially designed footplate that allows the incision to be extended further centrally within the deep stroma without damaging the epithelium or superficial stroma overlying the central clear zone. This diamond blade can be pictured as a triangle with a small square attached to its long vertical side, with the point of the triangle at the bottom of the blade. It has a cutting margin along its entire oblique face, a faceted horizontal (bottom) cutting margin that forms a 300-μm-long base, and a third cutting margin along the distal (back) 250 μm of the vertical margin, which is offset anteriorly 200 μm from the remaining blunt vertical margin of the blade. The remaining horizontal (top) margin of the blade is blunt.[9]

This blade appears to provide more uniform depth throughout the incision, as well as allowing the optical zone to be enlarged. The ability to enlarge the optical zone and have more uniform incision depth may help to reduce astigmatism induced by the procedure.

Footplates
The footplate should maintain the blade at as close to a uniform stromal depth as possible over a broad range of angular deviation. The footplate should minimize the incision-depth variability resulting from surgical movements. Footplates should be relatively broad to provide lateral support. The tips should be curved and polished to reduce resistance against dry epithelium. Importantly, both the diamond blade and the cornea should be visible simultaneously. The spacing of footplates is a significant variable in the determination of incision depth. Wider spacing may cause anterior corneal bowing beneath the knife, resulting in deeper blade penetration, whereas narrow spacing may cause posterior bowing and a more shallow incision.

Diamond Tip Calibration Microscopes
Diamond microscopes with the fewest accessories tend to be more accurate and are more economical

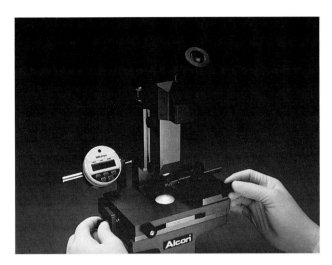

Fig. 3.1. Diamond tip calibration microscope.

(Fig. 3.1). The ideal microscope includes high-quality optics that maximize depth of field and minimize spherical aberration, stages mounted on cross rollers to minimize vibration, and motion detectors to report diamond tip excursion relative to the viewing system.

Computerized Videokeratographic Analysis

Knowledge of the corneal topography is advised and is particularly useful when patients have unusual refractive errors.[10–15] A topographical analysis can help (1) to identify patients with irregular astigmatism, (2) to determine more precisely the axis of astigmatism, (3) to determine the number and symmetry of incisions in patients with asymmetrical astigmatism, (4) to predict the response to astigmatic incisions, (5) to select radial incision sites, (6) to determine the cause and to plan the treatment of patients with decreased visual acuity after keratorefractive surgery, (7) to determine patient staging for secondary procedures, and (8) to provide the surgeon with feedback such as a corneal change map (a topographical map that documents differences in corneal shape before and after surgery).

Incisional Nomograms

Many proposed incisional nomograms have been developed by surgeons over the years. These serve as maps to guide the location and number of incisions used. Standard nomograms account for one or more individual patient variations including age, which is a major variable in the outcome of keratotomy. Centrifugal incision nomograms tend to predict lower degrees of correction compared with centripetal incision nomograms.

Surgical Planning

For the combined surgical technique, the use of a nomogram that allows a surgical outcome with a mean of 0.50 D intended residual myopia is suggested.[16] This combined-technique nomogram includes options for RK with four, six, or eight incisions. The number of incisions is determined by the number required to achieve a central clear zone measuring between 3.5 and 4.0 mm. A four-incision nomogram is advised for cases requiring a central clear zone of 3.5 mm or more, whereas a six- or eight-incision nomogram is recommended for cases of greater myopia.

The presence of significant astigmatism also suggests the use of fewer incisions. Six- or even four-incision nomograms with incision lengths to smaller central clear zones (i.e., <3.5 mm) are preferable to an eight-incision nomogram at a larger clear zone. This facilitates the arcuate or tangential incisions. The six-incision nomogram is preferred in patients with moderate myopia and astigmatism and in older patients.

Astigmatic keratotomy may be deferred until after RK is performed on the myopic spherical equivalents. There are three reasons. First, astigmatism of low magnitude is well tolerated and may not require correction. Second, RK may change the magnitude or axis of astigmatism in patients with mild to moderate astigmatism. Third, performing each surgery alone may be simpler for the surgeon than trying to combine the procedures. It is, however, advisable to perform simultaneous surgeries on patients with significant astigmatism (i.e., >1.75 D). When this occurs, the spherical equivalent is used to determine the extent of radial incisions, and the tangential or arcuate incisions are chosen to eliminate approximately two-thirds of the astigmatism.

Immediate Preoperative Protocol

The sterilized diamond knife should be mounted on the calibrating microscope before the patient is prepared for surgery. Four types of medication are useful in preparing the patient: (1) topical broad-spectrum antibiotics applied 30 min before surgery; (2) 1% pilocarpine to enhance the patient's ability to view the operating microscope undisturbed by the intensity of the light; (3) topical 4% lidocaine given as two successive drops 10 min apart and 0.5% tetracaine, also given as two successive drops with a 10-min break between; and (4) a sedative (e.g., diazepam) that serves as an anxiolytic and muscle relaxant, taken orally 20 min before surgery.

Patient Positioning
A folded towel placed on the operating table beneath the patient's shoulders allows the patient to maintain the chin-up position with less effort. The patient may be covered with a sheet or blanket. Covering the eye not involved in surgery with a patch facilitates fixation on the target.

Preparing the Eye
Periocular povidone-iodine solution is administered, the excess is removed with a sterile gauze pad, and an open eye drape is placed over the patient's face. To avoid corneal desiccation, which can increase friction between the corneal surface and the knife, the patient is asked to blink frequently or to keep the involved eye closed until the surgeon is ready.

The surgeon instills a third drop of lidocaine on the conjunctiva and places the eyelid speculum in a way that exposes the eye without unduly stressing the eyelid.

Visual Axis Determination
A coaxially aligned light reflex corresponds to the center of the corneal optical system, not to the true visual axis. Studies have shown the visual axis to be closely associated with the physiological visual axis.[17] Errors introduced by parallax can be overcome if the patient fixates on the microscope light filament while the surgeon looks through one eyepiece and marks the epithelial surface opposite the surgeon's viewing eye. An alternative technique is to use a coaxial light source mounted on the operating microscope. The administration of a drop of fluid over the corneal axis may enhance a dull corneal light reflex. Using a Sinskey hook, the epithelium over the visual axis is gently indented. If the visual axis is still not clearly marked, a Weck cell applied to the central epithelium will enhance the central epithelial mark.

Central Clear Zone Determination
Using the visual axis as a reference, a central clear zone marker of predetermined diameter is centered.

The central clear zone marker crosshairs should remain aligned with the visual axis epithelial indentation. Because the visual axis site does not usually align with the corneal axis, the central clear zone marker can slip. A quarter-revolution turn to the central clear zone marker before terminating epithelial pressure can ensure a crisply marked epithelium.

Intraoperative Corneal Pachymetry
The pachymeter probe tip is soaked with hydrogen peroxide and dried with an alcohol wipe. The paracentral corneal thickness is measured at the temporal site and at the thinnest paracentral site (determined by preoperative pachymetry). The latter site usually coincides with the paracentral temporal site closest to the anatomical corneal center. If it does not, the knife is set at the measurement of the thinner of the two sites. If the range of paracentral pachymetry values at screening exceeds 75 μm, the refractive range achieved may be less than that predicted by the nomogram. In such cases, the incision is lengthened, either by extending it closer to the limbus or by reducing the central clear zone by 0.25 mm.

Radial Marking and Incision Technique
The thinnest quadrant of the cornea should be incised first because the cornea tends to thin out further throughout the procedure. If the thickest quadrant is incised last, greater tissue penetration is achieved because of this corneal thinning. Using preoperative pachymetry to determine the thinnest quadrant and following this sequence can greatly reduce the incidence of microperforation.[16]

The ideal incision should terminate 1 mm inside the limbus to discourage fibrovascular growth in the RK groove. It should remain consistently within 85% to 95% of the stromal depth and should slightly undermine the clear zone at its central extent.[18] An incision base that does not extend to the central zone can cause some reduction in the resulting refractive effect.

The *centripetal (Russian) incision* gives a deeper incision than the *centrifugal (American) incision*[18] (Fig. 3.2) and has been more popular among surgeons. A third technique, known as the *combined* or *Genesis technique*, has achieved acceptance since its introduction.

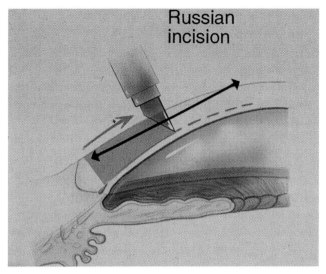
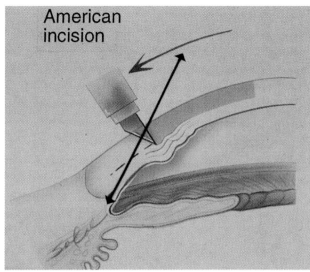

A   **B**

Fig. 3.2. Vector forces in the Russian (centripetal) incision and the American (centrifugal) incision cause significant differences in incision depth. (*A*) In a centripetal incision, the resultant force vector (bold arrow) is relatively parallel to the corneal tissue plane. This results in little displacement of the knife blade relative to the tissue and allows a uniformly deep incision. (*B*) In a centrifugal incision, the diamond blade's angled (downhill) margin performs the incision. The resultant force vectors exerted by the diamond blade, and the equal and opposite forces exerted by the tissue, are oriented at an oblique angle relative to the tissue plane, resulting in a variably shallow incision.

The Combined Technique

Using a specially designed knife, the surgeon can combine the safety features of the centrifugal incision with the efficacy of the centripetal incision.

The surgeon incises along the radial marks, entering at the central clear zone margin. The knife should penetrate the stroma at a slightly oblique angle. After a 2-sec pause, gentle pressure toward the central clear zone further undermines it, and the centrifugal radial incision is made. The centrifugal incision is placed at the beginning of the central clear zone and extended toward the periphery to approximately 1 mm from the limbus. This motion results in a groove that has inconsistent depth but provides a guide to confine the reverse centripetal motion. At the end of the centrifugal motion, the blade is reversed—without being removed from the groove—and returned to the central clear zone (Fig. 3.3). At the end of the incision, the knife is removed from the groove without any pressure on the central clear zone.

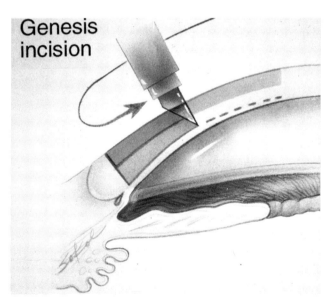

Fig. 3.3. Centripetal component of the combined technique. A centrifugal incision first forms a groove of inconsistent depth. Using this as a guide, a centrifugal incision in the reverse direction creates a second, deeper incision within the initial shallow groove.

The Undercut Technique

A combined-technique nomogram is used, but the optical zone is made 0.25 mm larger in diameter, which decreases the length of the incisions. The optical zone is usually 3.5 to 4.75 μm wide. Larger clear zones are associated with less reliable refractive results.

The undercut technique is performed under topical anesthesia. Six to eight radial incisions are made from the central clear zone toward the limbus and then back toward the center, using the unique undercut knife. The faceted diamond blade used is more bulky than that used in the combined technique and penetrates the cornea more slowly at initial entry. When removing the faceted blade, it is important to life the blade peripherally, which avoids cutting the superficial stroma in the central zone.

Reepithelialization typically occurs by the day after surgery. Patients are given topical antibiotics, topical steroids, and nonsteroidal anti-inflammatory drops. Visual acuity tends to stabilize within 2 weeks.

As with the combined technique, the effectiveness of the undercut technique is highly age dependent. Although this relationship is attributed to corneal biomechanics and wound healing, the actual reason remains unknown. In estimating the greatest expected improvement from RK, a good rule is to add 0.5 D to the patient's age in decades. Preliminary results based on up to a 2-year follow-up period with the undercut technique demonstrate more uniform incisions and a lower incidence of enhancement than the combination technique.

RESULTS OF RK

In reviewing the results of RK, we will briefly summarize the 1- and 10-year results of PERK to gain a historical perspective. We will then analyze three recently published modern approaches to RK: prospective multi-surgeon studies of the Casebeer and Genesis techniques and Lindstrom's results with the mini-RK technique. RK is directly influenced by incision reproducibility. For this reason, the outcome variability for RK decreases sequentially in association with the centrifugal (American), centripetal (Russian), combined (Genesis), undercut, and computer-controlled techniques, respectively.

PERK—One-Year Results

The PERK study was never intended to be the final approach to RK.[3] It was a tightly controlled, carefully monitored study of a relatively simple eight-incision, three-optical zone technique which ignored patients' age in surgical planning. Despite this simple surgical approach, the 1-year results of PERK were generally quite acceptable. Of the 413 eyes studied at 1 year, 78% had an uncorrected visual acuity of 20/40 or better and 60% were corrected to within ± 1 D of emmetropia (Table 3.1). Results according to the amount of preoperative myopia were as follows: low (−2.00 to −3.12 D), 92% 20/40 or better, 84% within 1 D of emmetropia; middle (−3.24 to −4.37 D), 81% 20/40 or better, 62% within 1 D of emmetropia; high (−4.37 to −8.00 D), 63% 20/40 or better, 38% within 1 D of emmetropia. Only 10% of the eyes were overcorrected by +1.00 D or more at 1 year.

PERK—Ten-Year Results

The 1-year PERK study reported the results of a single operation on only one eye of each patient. The 10-year PERK report included the results on both eyes (total, 693 eyes), with a follow-up of 88%.[19] These results also included additional procedures on 89 eyes (about 10%); thus, as a group, the eyes at 10 years actually achieved better uncorrected visual acuity results than they did at 1 year, with 85% now 20/40 or better uncorrected (Table 3.1).

Although the uncorrected visual acuity results were acceptable, only 60% of the eyes were corrected to within ± 1 D of emmetropia. More important, 43% of the eyes experienced a refractive change in a hyperopic direction of 1 D or more between 6 months and 10 years. This hyperopic shift was statistically significantly correlated with optical clear zone size, with the 3.0-mm clear zone eyes experiencing the greatest mean change, 1.12 D, compared to 0.80 D for the 3.50-mm clear zone eyes and 0.62 for the 4.0-mm clear zone eyes. The magnitude of this shift can at times be quite disturbing, with the largest shift reported as +6.37 D.

Casebeer System Results

The prospective study reports on the 1-year results of RK on 546 eyes (−1 to −8 D) operated on by 18 surgeons using the Casebeer system of surgical instruments and surgical technique with primarily

Russian-style incisions[20] (Table 3.1). Repeat operations were performed on 39% of the eyes, and 14% of the eyes had two or more repeat surgeries.

After all the repeat operations, 93% of the eyes achieved an uncorrected visual acuity of 20/40 or better and 54% were 20/20. Postoperative refractions were within ± 1 D of emmetropia in 89% of the eyes, and 68% were within ± 0.5 D. Only 2% of the eyes were overcorrected by more than + 1 D.

Genesis System Results

The Genesis multicenter prospective study reported the results achieved by nine surgeons who operated on 375 eyes with preoperative myopia of between −1 and −9 D[21] (Table 3.1). In all eyes, the incisions were performed with the combined American-Rus-

sian technique discussed earlier. Additional surgery was performed on 27% of the eyes; and only 1% had more than one additional surgery. After all procedures, 95% of the eyes achieved an uncorrected visual acuity of 20/40 or better, 85% were within ± 1 D of emmetropia, and only 1% were overcorrected by 1 D or more.

Three aspects of this study should be of interest to all RK surgeons. The first is the low incidence of decreased best acuity (0.3%) compared with the 1-year PERK data (3.0%), which the authors attributed to more uniform incision depth and the advent of corneal topography. The second aspect involves the issue of globe fixation by the surgeon with forceps or a fixation ring versus fixation by the patient. Eyes fixated by the surgeon had a 23% enhancement rate compared with 43% when the patient

Table 3.1. Comparison of Keratotomy Techniques

Study Design	American Technique PERK Study[23] Prospective	Russian Technique Werblin Study[24] Retrospective	Combined Technique Genesis System[21] Prospective
Radial incision number*	8–16	4–16	2–12
Mean preoperative refraction	−4.1 ± 1.4	Not reported	−3.8 ± 1/6
Mean postoperative refraction	−0.2 ± 1.1†	+0.3 ± 0.6	−0.5 ± 0.6
% of eyes ≥ 20/40 after enhancements	88	99‡	95
% of eyes ≥ 20/40 after one procedure	76	71	75§
% of eyes ± I.0. D of goal	64	Not reported	92
Mean procedure number per eye	1.09	1.48	1.28
% enhancements	12	33	23§
% > 1 enhancement	0	11	1
Maximum number of enhancements	1	7	2
% overcorrection > 1 D	17	Not reported	1
% sutured for consecutive hyperopia	0	3	0
Perforation rate (%)	2.2	Not reported	2.7
% loss of ± 2 lines	3	Not reported	0.3

*Primary procedure maximum incisions numbered 8 in each study.
†Extrapolated data.
‡Residual myopes anticipating further enhancement were excluded.
§In globes with mechanical fixation.

controlled fixation. This suggests that a more uniformly deep incision was achieved with globe fixation.

The third interesting aspect of the study was the incidence of micro-perforation. Surgeons who incised the thinnest portion of the cornea first had a micro-perforation rate of 2.7% compared to 15.5% when the thinnest portion was incised near the end of the surgery.

Mini-RK Results

Lindstrom reported the 6-month results of a retrospective study on 100 eyes with −1.5 to −6.00 D of preoperative myopia utilizing a bidirectional incision approach with the Duo-Track blade in which the outer limit of the incisions was 7.0 to 8.0 mm.[7] After only one procedure, 94% of the eyes achieved an uncorrected visual acuity of 20/40 or better and 92% were within 1 D of emmetropia. After a second procedure in eight eyes (8%), all eyes achieved uncorrected visual acuity of 20/40 or better and were within 1 D of emmetropia. Assil's personal experience with mini-RK incisions suggests an ideal outer diameter slightly in excess of 8 mm (about 8.5 mm).

In summary, all three of these newer approaches to RK have demonstrated results superior to those of the PERK study, with variable degrees of emphasis on additional surgery to achieve these results.

COMPLICATIONS OF RK

Serious complications following RK have been reported. These include endopthalmitis, infectious keratitis, ruptured globe, incisions into the visual axis, severe irregular astigmatism, and cataract.[22] Fortunately, these serious complications are rare, and a properly performed RK is a safe operation. In the 1-year PERK report,[23] there were no serious complications, but there were three cases of delayed bacterial keratitis between 1 and 5 years. By 10 years, two eyes had sustained blunt trauma sufficient to cause vitreous hemorrhages, which cleared without loss of vision or rupture of the globe; three eyes underwent successful cataract surgery; and one eye had successful repair of a retinal detachment.

An excellent indicator of the safety of any refractive surgical procedure is the incidence of loss of best spectacle-corrected visual acuity of two lines or more (many believe that loss of one line is within the normal variation between examinations). In the 10-year PERK study, 23 eyes (2%) lost two lines or more, but 20 of those eyes were still correctable to 20/25 or better and the other three were 20/30. The Casebeer and Genesis studies discussed earlier also reported no serious vision-threatening complications (although the Casebeer study included three eyes with incisions into the optical clear zone) and had a very low incidence (about 0.3% in the Genesis study) of loss of two lines or more of best spectacle-corrected visual acuity.

The unexpected complication of RK that caused great concern was the progressive hyperopic shift of +1 D or more that occurred in 43% of the eyes in the 10-year PERK study. Not all of these patients are unhappy with this shift, since the undercorrected eyes are actually improving. Nevertheless, an operation with this degree of instability is definitely a cause for concern. The survival of RK may well depend on long-term results and the continued stability of newer RK techniques.[24]

MANAGEMENT AND PREVENTION OF COMPLICATIONS

Complications such as microperforation, the effects of astigmatism on the procedure, and progressive hyperopia can be managed with proper planning. Microperforation during surgery requires that the procedure be stopped so that the surgeon can determine whether to continue or to terminate the surgery.[25] Aqueous leakage from a perforation is associated with globe softening and insufficient knife penetration on subsequent incisions, which results in erratic refractive outcomes. The surgeon may decide to terminate the procedure and complete it at another time. A single radial incision provides diffuse central corneal flattening and will not result in severe topographical distortion.

Microperforations can be self-sealing; a Weck cell is used to determine if that is the case. Persistent aqueous leakage indicates that the perforation is more than a microperforation and that treatment is required (usually placement of a nylon suture).

Globe fixation is often desirable, although not always necessary during the primary procedure if a guarded diamond knife is used. If globe fixation is used, it elevates intraocular pressure, which causes the diamond knife to penetrate slightly deeper into the stroma. Retracting the blade 20 μm can counteract this effect.

If patients have less than 1 D of astigmatism, the radial marks are positioned to include the astigmatic meridian because the radial incision will provide preferential flattening along a steep axis. Patients with more than 1 D of astigmatism do not receive a radial incision, so that simultaneous or subsequent astigmatic keratotomy can be performed on that meridian.

Progressive hyperopia after RK is associated with a set of risk factors. These include radial incisions extended to the limbus, multiple enhancement procedures, peripheral redeepening procedures, lack of preoperative cycloplegic refraction (i.e., latent hyperopia), postoperative contact lens wear, and postoperative ocular massage.

ALTERNATIVES TO RADIAL KERATOTOMY FOR CORRECTION OF MYOPIA

Photorefractive keratectomy (PRK) has become globally the major alternative to radial keratotomy. Few comparative studies have been published. Hong and Salz[26] retrospectively compared results at 3 years after RK with those at 3 years after PRK performed with the VisX 20/20 B laser. Both procedures were found to be effective, particularly for low myopia. None of the PRK eyes required retreatments whereas 18% of the RK eyes were retreated. For treatment of myopia up to −3.00 D, 41% of RK eyes and 50% of PRK eyes had uncorrected visual acuity of 20/20. For the same group of patients, 91% of RK eyes and 94% of PRK eyes had uncorrected visual acuity of 20/40 or better. Photorefractive keratectomy, as compared to RK, achieved a higher percentage (86% to 70%) of eyes corrected to within 0.50 D of emmetropia. The details of PRK for myopia are discussed in Chapters 5 through 8.

Laser in situ keratomileusis (LASIK) is another surgical approach that attracts candidates with clinical indications similar to those of RK. Chapter 9 covers the correction of myopia with LASIK.

Reversibility of a refractive procedure increases its safety. Radial keratotomy, PRK, and LASIK are all irreversible procedures for the correction of myopia. Intrastromal corneal ring segments (ICRS) offer a potentially reversible approach. Preservation of positive corneal asphericity is another potential benefit of ICRS.

Nosé and collaborators performed the first ICR implantations with a polymethylmethacryalte (PMMA) 360° ring in blind[27] and sighted[28] eyes in 1991. Clinical studies of ICR and ICRS have been performed in over 500 patients globally but a minimal number of ICR patients and no ICRS patients have more than 2 years of follow-up. Colin (oral presentation, Aegean Cornea III, Samos, 1996) reported on 17 eyes in which ICRS, 0.25 to 0.45 mm in thickness, were inserted for myopia between −1 and −5 D. At 3 months postoperatively, achieved refractions were within 0.5 D, 1.0 D, and 1.5 D in 76%, 88%, and 100% of eyes, respectively. Uncorrected visual acuity was better than or equal to 20/20, 20/25, and 20/40 in 47%, 76%, and 100% of eyes, respectively.

The current clinical ICRS technique involves the insertion of two PMMA arcs of 150°. A typical ICR procedure can be performed in about 10 minutes using topical anesthesia and oral sedation. A diamond blade is used to make a 1.5 mm to 2 mm radial incision in the mid-peripheral cornea at the 12 o'clock position to 2/3 corneal depth. A vacuum centration guide is used, applying suction to the globe. A blunt dissection is made at two-thirds depth in the periphery of the cornea. After suction is removed, the ring segments are slid into place and the incision is closed with two sutures.

Reports of Durrie (oral presentation, European Congress of Cataract and Refractive Surgery, Lisbon, 1994) and Colin (oral presentation, Aegean Cornea III, Samos, 1996) suggest that explantation can be done with preservation of preoperative refraction and corneal shape. Current complications include irregular astigmatism, if the segments are not positioned at the same depth, and halos, if the segments are not well-centered. Abnormal tissue changes include peripheral haze around the lamellar dissection and lamellar deposits along the inside edge of the ring. Long term results are necessary to confirm the biocompatibility of the material in the cornea.

REFERENCES

1. Sato T, Akiyama K, Shibata H. A new surgical approach to myopia. *Am J Ophthalmol.* 1953;36:823–829.
2. Beliaev VS, Ilyina TS. Scleroplasty in the treatment of progressive myopia. *Vestn Oftalmol.* 1972;3:60–63.
3. Waring GO III, Lynn MJ, Gelender H, et al. Results of the Prospective Evaluation of Radial Keratotomy (PERK) study one year after surgery. *Ophthalmology.* 1985;92:177–198.
4. Salz JJ, Villasenor RA, Elander R, et al. Four incision radial keratotomy for low to moderate myopia. *Ophthalmology.* 1986;93:727–738.
5. Spigelman AV, Williams PA, Nichols BD, Lindstrom RL. Four incision radial keratotomy. *J Cataract Refract Surg.* 1988;14:125–128.
6. Salz J, Lee J, Jester JV, et al. Radial keratotomy in fresh human cadaver eyes. *Ophthalmology.* 1981;88:742–746.
7. Lindstrom RL. Minimally invasive radial keratotomy—mini-RK. *J Cataract Refract Surg.* 1995;21:27–34.
8. Assil KK, Kassoff J, Schanzlin DJ, Quantock AJ. A combined incision technique of radial keratotomy: a comparison to centripetal and centrifugal incision techniques in human donor eyes. *Ophthalmology.* 1994;101:746–754.
9. Park R, Quantock AJ, Assil KK. Comparison of the standard combined (bidirectional) radial keratotomy technique with the undercut technique in human donor eyes. *J Refract Surg.* 1996;12:77–84.
10. Assil KK, Schanzlin DJ. Altering corneal topography by incisional keratotomy. In: Assil KK, Schanzlin DJ, eds. *Radial and Astigmatic Keratotomy: A Complete Handbook for the Successful Practice of Incisional Keratotomy Using the Combined Technique.* Thorofare, NJ: Slack; 1994:43–86, 121–132.
11. Assil KK, Sires BS. Altering corneal topography by radial keratotomy. *Ophthalmic Pract.* 1994;12:20–23.
12. Steel D, Jester JV, Salz JJ, et al. Modification of corneal curvature following radial keratotomy in primates. *Ophthalmology.* 1981;88:747–754.
13. Sanders DR, Koch D, eds. *Corneal Topography.* Thorofare, NJ: Slack; 1993:95–122.
14. Schanzlin DJ, Robin JB, eds. *Corneal Topography: Measuring and Modifying the Cornea.* New York, NY: Springer-Verlag; 1992;105–116.
15. McDonnell PJ, Garbus J, Lopez PF, Topographic analysis and visual acuity after radial keratotomy. *Am J Ophthalmol.* 1988;106:692–695.
16. Assil KK, Schanzlin DJ. Radial keratotomy surgical technique and protocol. In: Assil KK, Schanzlin DJ, eds. *Radial and Astigmatic Keratotomy: A Complete Handbook for the Successful Practice of Incisional Keratotomy Using the Combined Technique.* Thorofare, NJ: Slack; 1994;87–110.
17. Waring GO, Casebeer JC, Gordon JF, The Chiron Intraoptics Keratorefractive Study Group. A prospective multicenter clinical trial of the Casebeer systematic approach to incisional refractive surgery for the correction of myopia and astigmatism. *Invest Ophthalmol Vis Sci.* 1993;34(suppl):1243.
18. Melles GRJ, Wijdh RHJ, Cost B, et al. Effect of blade configuration, knife action, and intraocular pressure on keratotomy incision depth and shape. *Cornea.* 1993;12:299–309.
19. Waring GO, Lynn MJ, McDonnell PJ, and the PERK study group. Results of the Prospective Evaluation of Radial Keratotomy (PERK) study ten years after surgery. *Arch Ophthalmol.* 1994;112:1298–1304.
20. Waring GO, Allen R, Berg JC. A prospective multicenter study of refractive keratotomy for myopia and astigmatism. *Ophthalmology.* In press.
21. Verity SM, Talamo JH, Chayet A, et al. The combined technique of radial keratotomy: a prospective multi-centered clinical trial. *Ophthalmology.* 1995;102:1908–1917.
22. Rashid ER, Waring GO. Complications of refractive keratotomy. In: Waring GO, ed. *Refractive Keratotomy for Myopia and Astigmatism.* St Louis, MO: CV Mosby; 1992;863–936.
23. Waring GO III, Lynn MJ, Azhar N, et al. Results of the Prospective Evaluation of Radial Keratotomy (PERK) study at five years after surgery. *Ophthalmology.* 1991;98:11664–1176.
24. Werblin TP, Stafford MG. The Casebeer system for predictable keratorefractive surgery. *Ophthalmology.* 1993;100:1095–1102.
25. Assil KK, Schanzlin DJ. Preventing and managing associated complications of radial keratotomy. In: Assil KK, Schanzlin DJ, eds. *Radial and Astigmatic Keratotomy: A Complete Handbook for the Successful Practice of Incisional Keratotomy Using the Combined Technique.* Thorofare, NJ: Slack, 1994;139–158.
26. Hong JC, Salz JJ. Retrospective comparison of photorefractive keratectomy and radial keratotomy. *J Refract Surg.* 1995;11:477–484.
27. Nosé W, Neves RA, Schanzlin DJ, Belfort R Jr. The Intrastromal Corneal Ring: one-year results of first implants in humans, a preliminary nonfunctional eye study. *Refract Corneal Surg.* 1993;9:452–458.
28. Nosé W, Neves RA, Burris TE, et al. Intrastromal Corneal Ring: 12-month sighted myopic eyes. *J Refract Surg.* 1996;12:20–28.

4

Mini-Radial Keratotomy

Richard L. Lindstrom

Radial keratotomy (RK), a technique which has been gaining momentum for decades, is currently a common surgical procedure for correcting the widespread problem of myopia. With one-fourth of the world's population affected by this condition, if fewer than 1% of myopic individuals chose this surgical alternative, there would have been approximately 500,000 RK patients in 1996 in the United States alone.[1–7]

Despite the popularity of the procedure, classical RK has some significant flaws, not the least of which is the fact that we have no clear idea of what the long-term visual results of the technique will be. A hyperopic shift of 1 D or more occurs in over 40% of eyes during long-term follow-up of RK patients, as indicated by the multicenter Prospective Evaluation of Radial Keratotomy (PERK) study.[8] This continued flattening of the cornea is the Achilles heel of the procedure and is unacceptable. Mini-RK was therefore developed based on the idea that it might be possible to use shorter, less damaging incisions without sacrificing effectiveness (Fig. 4.1).

As the RK nomograms show (Figs. 4.2 to 4.5), the 5.5-mm optical zone is the largest zone with any efficacy. When the optical zone is increased from 6.0 to 7.0 mm or larger in a 4-, 6-, 8-, or even 16-incision RK, my own nomograms, as well as those of others, suggest that the net effect on the patient's refractive error will be nearly zero. As a result, incisions made in the peripheral zone offer very little extra benefit and may actually lead to various side effects, such as diurnal fluctuation and long-term refractive instability with hyperopic drift, by unnecessarily weakening the cornea.[9–13]

The theory behind mini-RK hinged on the idea that since many common side effects of RK result from incisions which permanently weaken the cornea, there might be a point at which it destabilizes.[14–17] If this were true, structural integrity of the cornea might be better maintained with shorter, deeper incisions in which fewer corneal fibers were cut.

A correlation between the degree of hyperopic shift and the length of incisions was indicated by the PERK study. The degree of myopia also came into play, with more myopic patients needing longer incisions to flatten the cornea and becoming more likely to suffer hyperopic drift.[8]

The author began shortening his incisions in response to the drift phenomenon in the early 1990s. Since mid-1991, the mini-RK technique which resulted has been the author's procedure of choice, retaining the benefits of RK for most slightly to moderately myopic patients while significantly reducing the risks.

SURGICAL PLANNING

Mini-RK is suitable for patients in the -1 to -4 D range, who require no more than an eight-incision RK with a 3.0-mm optical zone to achieve full correction or who might benefit from correction of anisometropia. The procedure involves shorter, deeper incisions than those traditionally used. On average, mini-RK incisions are just 1.5 to 2.5 mm in length compared to 4.0 to 5.0 mm for classical RK.

One of the keys to success with the procedure consists of creating a deep, consistent incision stretching from the preferred central optical zone to the 7.0- to 8.0-mm zone. Another key is good surgical planning. The author uses the nomograms shown in Figs. 4.2 to 4.5. If the patient has more

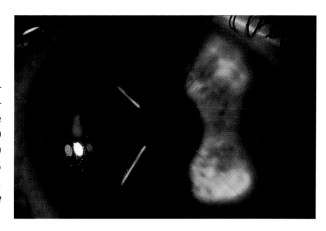

Fig. 4.1. This patient underwent a four-incision mini-RK combined with two 45° arcuate keratotomies for astigmatism 6 months earlier. Note the short length of the oblique radial incisions. Preoperative refraction was −4.50 + 2.00 × 90; postoperative refraction was −0.50 +0.50 × 90. (Reprinted with permission from the January 1995 issue of the *Journal of Cataract and Refractive Surgery* [Vol. 21, No. 1; pp. 30] © *Journal of Cataract and Refractive Surgery.*)

than 1 D of astigmatism, radial and astigmatic keratotomy may be combined, using techniques, previously published.[11]

After selecting appropriate candidates for the mini-RK procedure, these patients are counseled on what to expect, advising them that for safety reasons, usually only one eye will be operated on initially. For patients who intend to have the procedure done in both eyes, the initial operation is done on the nondominant eye and a few weeks later on the dominant one. For those with low myopia who plan to have only one eye operated on, the dominant eye is the one selected.

While the nomograms give us a good idea of what will occur, there is no telling how any individual patient will respond. For the initial nondominant eye, the surgical goal is −0.50 to −1.5 D, depending on the patient's age. In the prepresbyopic or presbyopic patient, a slightly more myopic target is preferable. Patients who have mild residual myopia following the procedure are discouraged from seeking further correction and instead counseled on the positive aspects that this monovision result may have in the long term. In cases where the patient underresponds more dramatically to mini-RK, usually the procedure is repeated 1 week or more postoperatively.

Once the response of the nondominant eye to the mini-RK procedure is known, plans are made to perform the procedure in the dominant eye, with an adjustment in the strength of the procedure based on initial results. For example, a 30-year-old patient who had achieved a 3.0 D result with a four-incision mini-RK instead of the expected 3.5 D refractive correction would be considered to be an 85% responder, and a more powerful procedure would be performed in the second eye. This would take place 1 week or more after completion of the initial surgery.

PERFORMING MINI-RK

To begin the mini-RK procedure, the patient is prepared with 0.5% to 1% povodine-iodine solution and then centered under an operating microscope. After the lids are separated and the lashes isolated with a wire speculum, topical 0.5% proparacaine or the equivalent is applied every 1 to 5 min, for a total of three doses. To lengthen the duration of the anesthesia, just before surgery 0.75% bupivacaine drops are placed in the eye.

Next, as the patient fixates on an appropriate target, the central optical zone marker is centered on the pupil and a second 8.0-mm marker is placed concentrically surrounding the first. Using an ultrasonic pachymeter, the temporal paracentral corneal thickness adjacent to the central optical zone marker is measured. When using a center-to-periphery incision, the diamond micrometer knife is set at 110% of the median temporal paracentral pachymetry. With a periphery-to-center approach or a double-pass approach, the knife is set at 100% of the median paracentral pachymetry.

2 INCISION MRK NOMOGRAM

	SURGICAL OPTION										
AGE	2 x 3.0	2 x 3.25	2 x 3.5	2 x 3.75	2 x 4.0	2 x 4.25	2 x 4.5	2 x 4.75	2 x 5.0	2 x 5.25	2 x 5.5
20	1.60	1.40	1.20	1.08	0.96	0.84	0.72	0.60	0.48	0.36	0.24
21	1.64	1.44	1.23	1.11	0.98	0.86	0.74	0.62	0.49	0.37	0.25
22	1.68	1.47	1.26	1.13	1.01	0.88	0.76	0.63	0.50	0.38	0.25
23	1.72	1.51	1.29	1.16	1.03	0.90	0.77	0.65	0.52	0.39	0.26
24	1.76	1.54	1.32	1.19	1.06	0.92	0.79	0.66	0.53	0.40	0.26
25	1.80	1.58	1.35	1.22	1.08	0.95	0.81	0.68	0.54	0.41	0.27
26	1.84	1.61	1.38	1.24	1.10	0.97	0.83	0.69	0.55	0.41	0.28
27	1.88	1.65	1.41	1.27	1.13	0.99	0.85	0.71	0.56	0.42	0.28
28	1.92	1.68	1.44	1.30	1.15	1.01	0.86	0.72	0.58	0.43	0.29
29	1.96	1.72	1.47	1.32	1.18	1.03	0.88	0.74	0.59	0.44	0.29
30	2.00	1.75	1.50	1.35	1.20	1.05	0.90	0.75	0.60	0.45	0.30
31	2.04	1.79	1.53	1.38	1.22	1.07	0.92	0.77	0.61	0.46	0.31
32	2.08	1.82	1.56	1.40	1.25	1.09	0.94	0.78	0.62	0.47	0.31
33	2.12	1.86	1.59	1.43	1.27	1.11	0.95	0.80	0.64	0.48	0.32
34	2.16	1.89	1.62	1.46	1.30	1.13	0.97	0.81	0.65	0.49	0.32
35	2.20	1.93	1.65	1.49	1.32	1.16	0.99	0.83	0.66	0.50	0.33
36	2.24	1.96	1.68	1.51	1.34	1.18	1.01	0.84	0.67	0.50	0.34
37	2.28	2.00	1.71	1.54	1.37	1.20	1.03	0.86	0.68	0.51	0.34
38	2.32	2.03	1.74	1.57	1.39	1.22	1.04	0.87	0.70	0.52	0.35
39	2.36	2.07	1.77	1.59	1.42	1.24	1.06	0.89	0.71	0.53	0.35
40	2.40	2.10	1.80	1.62	1.44	1.26	1.08	0.90	0.72	0.54	0.36
41	2.44	2.14	1.83	1.65	1.46	1.28	1.10	0.92	0.73	0.55	0.37
42	2.48	2.17	1.86	1.67	1.49	1.30	1.12	0.93	0.74	0.56	0.37
43	2.52	2.21	1.89	1.70	1.51	1.32	1.13	0.95	0.76	0.57	0.38
44	2.56	2.24	1.92	1.73	1.54	1.34	1.15	0.96	0.77	0.58	0.38
45	2.60	2.28	1.95	1.76	1.56	1.37	1.17	0.98	0.78	0.59	0.39
46	2.64	2.31	1.98	1.78	1.58	1.39	1.19	0.99	0.79	0.59	0.40
47	2.68	2.35	2.01	1.81	1.61	1.41	1.21	1.01	0.80	0.60	0.40
48	2.72	2.38	2.04	1.84	1.63	1.43	1.22	1.02	0.82	0.61	0.41
49	2.76	2.42	2.07	1.86	1.66	1.45	1.24	1.04	0.83	0.62	0.41
50	2.80	2.45	2.10	1.89	1.68	1.47	1.26	1.05	0.84	0.63	0.42
51	2.84	2.49	2.13	1.92	1.70	1.49	1.28	1.07	0.85	0.64	0.43
52	2.88	2.52	2.16	1.94	1.73	1.51	1.30	1.08	0.86	0.65	0.43
53	2.92	2.56	2.19	1.97	1.75	1.53	1.31	1.10	0.88	0.66	0.44
54	2.96	2.59	2.22	2.00	1.78	1.55	1.33	1.11	0.89	0.67	0.44
55	3.00	2.63	2.25	2.03	1.80	1.58	1.35	1.13	0.90	0.68	0.45
56	3.04	2.66	2.28	2.05	1.82	1.60	1.37	1.14	0.91	0.68	0.46
57	3.08	2.70	2.31	2.08	1.85	1.62	1.39	1.16	0.92	0.69	0.46
58	3.12	2.73	2.34	2.11	1.87	1.64	1.40	1.17	0.94	0.70	0.47
59	3.16	2.77	2.37	2.13	1.90	1.66	1.42	1.19	0.95	0.71	0.47
60	3.20	2.80	2.40	2.16	1.92	1.68	1.44	1.20	0.96	0.72	0.48
61	3.24	2.84	2.43	2.19	1.94	1.70	1.46	1.22	0.97	0.73	0.49
62	3.28	2.87	2.46	2.21	1.97	1.72	1.48	1.23	0.98	0.74	0.49
63	3.32	2.91	2.49	2.24	1.99	1.74	1.49	1.25	1.00	0.75	0.50
64	3.36	2.94	2.52	2.27	2.02	1.76	1.51	1.26	1.01	0.76	0.50
65	3.40	2.98	2.55	2.30	2.04	1.79	1.53	1.28	1.02	0.77	0.51
66	3.44	3.01	2.58	2.32	2.06	1.81	1.55	1.29	1.03	0.77	0.52
67	3.48	3.05	2.61	2.35	2.09	1.83	1.57	1.31	1.04	0.78	0.52
68	3.52	3.08	2.64	2.38	2.11	1.85	1.58	1.32	1.06	0.79	0.53
69	3.56	3.12	2.67	2.40	2.14	1.87	1.60	1.34	1.07	0.80	0.53
70	3.60	3.15	2.70	2.43	2.16	1.89	1.62	1.35	1.08	0.81	0.54
71	3.64	3.19	2.73	2.46	2.18	1.91	1.64	1.37	1.09	0.82	0.55
72	3.68	3.22	2.76	2.48	2.21	1.93	1.66	1.38	1.10	0.83	0.55
73	3.72	3.26	2.79	2.51	2.23	1.95	1.67	1.40	1.12	0.84	0.56
74	3.76	3.29	2.82	2.54	2.26	1.97	1.69	1.41	1.13	0.85	0.56
75	3.80	3.33	2.85	2.57	2.28	2.00	1.71	1.43	1.14	0.86	0.57
76	3.84	3.36	2.88	2.59	2.30	2.02	1.73	1.44	1.15	0.86	0.58
77	3.88	3.40	2.91	2.62	2.33	2.04	1.75	1.46	1.16	0.87	0.58
78	3.92	3.43	2.94	2.65	2.35	2.06	1.76	1.47	1.18	0.88	0.59
79	3.96	3.47	2.97	2.67	2.38	2.08	1.78	1.49	1.19	0.89	0.59
80	4.00	3.50	3.00	2.70	2.40	2.10	1.80	1.50	1.20	0.90	0.60
AGE	2 x 3.0	2 x 3.25	2 x 3.5	2 x 3.75	2 x 4.0	2 x 4.25	2 x 4.5	2 x 4.75	2 x 5.0	2 x 5.25	2 x 5.5

Find patient age, then move right to find result closest to refractive myopia without going over

Fig. 4.2. Nomogram for two-incision mini-RK.

4 INCISION MRK NOMOGRAM

					SURGICAL OPTION						
AGE	4 x 3.0	4 x 3.25	4 x 3.5	4 x 3.75	4 x 4.0	4 x 4.25	4 X 4.5	4 x 4.75	4 x 5	4 x 5.25	4 x 5.5
20	2.80	2.40	2.00	1.80	1.60	1.40	1.20	1.00	0.80	0.60	0.40
21	2.87	2.46	2.05	1.85	1.64	1.44	1.23	1.03	0.82	0.62	0.41
22	2.94	2.52	2.10	1.89	1.68	1.47	1.26	1.05	0.84	0.63	0.42
23	3.01	2.58	2.15	1.94	1.72	1.51	1.29	1.08	0.86	0.65	0.43
24	3.08	2.64	2.20	1.98	1.76	1.54	1.32	1.10	0.88	0.66	0.44
25	3.15	2.70	2.25	2.03	1.80	1.58	1.35	1.13	0.90	0.68	0.45
26	3.22	2.76	2.30	2.07	1.84	1.61	1.38	1.15	0.92	0.69	0.46
27	3.29	2.82	2.35	2.12	1.88	1.65	1.41	1.18	0.94	0.71	0.47
28	3.36	2.88	2.40	2.16	1.92	1.68	1.44	1.20	0.96	0.72	0.48
29	3.43	2.94	2.45	2.21	1.96	1.72	1.47	1.23	0.98	0.74	0.49
30	3.50	3.00	2.50	2.25	2.00	1.75	1.50	1.25	1.00	0.75	0.50
31	3.57	3.06	2.55	2.30	2.04	1.79	1.53	1.28	1.02	0.77	0.51
32	3.64	3.12	2.60	2.34	2.08	1.82	1.56	1.30	1.04	0.78	0.52
33	3.71	3.18	2.65	2.39	2.12	1.86	1.59	1.33	1.06	0.80	0.53
34	3.78	3.24	2.70	2.43	2.16	1.89	1.62	1.35	1.08	0.81	0.54
35	3.85	3.30	2.75	2.48	2.20	1.93	1.65	1.38	1.10	0.83	0.55
36	3.92	3.36	2.80	2.52	2.24	1.96	1.68	1.40	1.12	0.84	0.56
37	3.99	3.42	2.85	2.57	2.28	2.00	1.71	1.43	1.14	0.86	0.57
38	4.06	3.48	2.90	2.61	2.32	2.03	1.74	1.45	1.16	0.87	0.58
39	4.13	3.54	2.95	2.66	2.36	2.07	1.77	1.48	1.18	0.89	0.59
40	4.20	3.60	3.00	2.70	2.40	2.10	1.80	1.50	1.20	0.90	0.60
41	4.27	3.66	3.05	2.75	2.44	2.14	1.83	1.53	1.22	0.92	0.61
42	4.34	3.72	3.10	2.79	2.48	2.17	1.86	1.55	1.24	0.93	0.62
43	4.41	3.78	3.15	2.84	2.52	2.21	1.89	1.58	1.26	0.95	0.63
44	4.48	3.84	3.20	2.88	2.56	2.24	1.92	1.60	1.28	0.96	0.64
45	4.55	3.90	3.25	2.93	2.60	2.28	1.95	1.63	1.30	0.98	0.65
46	4.62	3.96	3.30	2.97	2.64	2.31	1.98	1.65	1.32	0.99	0.66
47	4.69	4.02	3.35	3.02	2.68	2.35	2.01	1.68	1.34	1.01	0.67
48	4.76	4.08	3.40	3.06	2.72	2.38	2.04	1.70	1.36	1.02	0.68
49	4.83	4.14	3.45	3.11	2.76	2.42	2.07	1.73	1.38	1.04	0.69
50	4.90	4.20	3.50	3.15	2.80	2.45	2.10	1.75	1.40	1.05	0.70
51	4.97	4.26	3.55	3.20	2.84	2.49	2.13	1.78	1.42	1.07	0.71
52	5.04	4.32	3.60	3.24	2.88	2.52	2.16	1.80	1.44	1.08	0.72
53	5.11	4.38	3.65	3.29	2.92	2.56	2.19	1.83	1.46	1.10	0.73
54	5.18	4.44	3.70	3.33	2.96	2.59	2.22	1.85	1.48	1.11	0.74
55	5.25	4.50	3.75	3.38	3.00	2.63	2.25	1.88	1.50	1.13	0.75
56	5.32	4.56	3.80	3.42	3.04	2.66	2.28	1.90	1.52	1.14	0.76
57	5.39	4.62	3.85	3.47	3.08	2.70	2.31	1.93	1.54	1.16	0.77
58	5.46	4.68	3.90	3.51	3.12	2.73	2.34	1.95	1.56	1.17	0.78
59	5.53	4.74	3.95	3.56	3.16	2.77	2.37	1.98	1.58	1.19	0.79
60	5.60	4.80	4.00	3.60	3.20	2.80	2.40	2.00	1.60	1.20	0.80
61	5.67	4.86	4.05	3.65	3.24	2.84	2.43	2.03	1.62	1.22	0.81
62	5.74	4.92	4.10	3.69	3.28	2.87	2.46	2.05	1.64	1.23	0.82
63	5.81	4.98	4.15	3.74	3.32	2.91	2.49	2.08	1.66	1.25	0.83
64	5.88	5.04	4.20	3.78	3.36	2.94	2.52	2.10	1.68	1.26	0.84
65	5.95	5.10	4.25	3.83	3.40	2.98	2.55	2.13	1.70	1.28	0.85
66	6.02	5.16	4.30	3.87	3.44	3.01	2.58	2.15	1.72	1.29	0.86
67	6.09	5.22	4.35	3.92	3.48	3.05	2.61	2.18	1.74	1.31	0.87
68	6.16	5.28	4.40	3.96	3.52	3.08	2.64	2.20	1.76	1.32	0.88
69	6.23	5.34	4.45	4.01	3.56	3.12	2.67	2.23	1.78	1.34	0.89
70	6.30	5.40	4.50	4.05	3.60	3.15	2.70	2.25	1.80	1.35	0.90
71	6.37	5.46	4.55	4.10	3.64	3.19	2.73	2.28	1.82	1.37	0.91
72	6.44	5.52	4.60	4.14	3.68	3.22	2.76	2.30	1.84	1.38	0.92
73	6.51	5.58	4.65	4.19	3.72	3.26	2.79	2.33	1.86	1.40	0.93
74	6.58	5.64	4.70	4.23	3.76	3.29	2.82	2.35	1.88	1.41	0.94
75	6.65	5.70	4.75	4.28	3.80	3.33	2.85	2.38	1.90	1.43	0.95
76	6.72	5.76	4.80	4.32	3.84	3.36	2.88	2.40	1.92	1.44	0.96
77	6.79	5.82	4.85	4.37	3.88	3.40	2.91	2.43	1.94	1.46	0.97
78	6.86	5.88	4.90	4.41	3.92	3.43	2.94	2.45	1.96	1.47	0.98
79	6.93	5.94	4.95	4.46	3.96	3.47	2.97	2.48	1.98	1.49	0.99
80	7.00	6.00	5.00	4.50	4.00	3.50	3.00	2.50	2.00	1.50	1.00
AGE	4 x 3.0	4 x 3.25	4 x 3.5	4 x 3.75	4 x 4.0	4 x 4.25	4 X 4.5	4 x 4.75	4 x 5	4 x 5.25	4 x 5.5

Find patient age, then move right to find result closest to refractive myopia without going over

Fig. 4.3. Nomogram for four-incision mini-RK. (Reprinted with permission from the January 1995 issue of the *Journal of Cataract and Refractive Surgery* [Vol. 21, No. 1; pp. 28] © *Journal of Cataract and Refractive Surgery.*)

6 INCISION MRK NOMOGRAM

	SURGICAL OPTION										
AGE	6 x 3.0	6 x 3.25	6 x 3.5	6 x 3.75	6 x 4.0	6 x 4.25	6 x 4.5	6 x 4.75	6 x 5.0	6 x 5.25	6 x 5.5
20	3.40	2.95	2.50	2.25	2.00	1.75	1.50	1.25	1.00	0.75	0.50
21	3.49	3.02	2.56	2.31	2.05	1.79	1.54	1.28	1.03	0.77	0.51
22	3.57	3.10	2.63	2.36	2.10	1.84	1.58	1.31	1.05	0.79	0.53
23	3.66	3.17	2.69	2.42	2.15	1.88	1.61	1.34	1.08	0.81	0.54
24	3.74	3.25	2.75	2.48	2.20	1.93	1.65	1.38	1.10	0.83	0.55
25	3.83	3.32	2.81	2.53	2.25	1.97	1.69	1.41	1.13	0.84	0.56
26	3.91	3.39	2.88	2.59	2.30	2.01	1.73	1.44	1.15	0.86	0.58
27	4.00	3.47	2.94	2.64	2.35	2.06	1.76	1.47	1.18	0.88	0.59
28	4.08	3.54	3.00	2.70	2.40	2.10	1.80	1.50	1.20	0.90	0.60
29	4.17	3.61	3.06	2.76	2.45	2.14	1.84	1.53	1.23	0.92	0.61
30	4.25	3.69	3.13	2.81	2.50	2.19	1.88	1.56	1.25	0.94	0.63
31	4.34	3.76	3.19	2.87	2.55	2.23	1.91	1.59	1.28	0.96	0.64
32	4.42	3.84	3.25	2.93	2.60	2.28	1.95	1.63	1.30	0.98	0.65
33	4.51	3.91	3.31	2.98	2.65	2.32	1.99	1.66	1.33	0.99	0.66
34	4.59	3.98	3.38	3.04	2.70	2.36	2.03	1.69	1.35	1.01	0.68
35	4.68	4.06	3.44	3.09	2.75	2.41	2.06	1.72	1.38	1.03	0.69
36	4.76	4.13	3.50	3.15	2.80	2.45	2.10	1.75	1.40	1.05	0.70
37	4.85	4.20	3.56	3.21	2.85	2.49	2.14	1.78	1.43	1.07	0.71
38	4.93	4.28	3.63	3.26	2.90	2.54	2.18	1.81	1.45	1.09	0.73
39	5.02	4.35	3.69	3.32	2.95	2.58	2.21	1.84	1.48	1.11	0.74
40	5.10	4.43	3.75	3.38	3.00	2.63	2.25	1.88	1.50	1.13	0.75
41	5.19	4.50	3.81	3.43	3.05	2.67	2.29	1.91	1.53	1.14	0.76
42	5.27	4.57	3.88	3.49	3.10	2.71	2.33	1.94	1.55	1.16	0.78
43	5.36	4.65	3.94	3.54	3.15	2.76	2.36	1.97	1.58	1.18	0.79
44	5.44	4.72	4.00	3.60	3.20	2.80	2.40	2.00	1.60	1.20	0.80
45	5.53	4.79	4.06	3.66	3.25	2.84	2.44	2.03	1.63	1.22	0.81
46	5.61	4.87	4.13	3.71	3.30	2.89	2.48	2.06	1.65	1.24	0.83
47	5.70	4.94	4.19	3.77	3.35	2.93	2.51	2.09	1.68	1.26	0.84
48	5.78	5.02	4.25	3.83	3.40	2.98	2.55	2.13	1.70	1.28	0.85
49	5.87	5.09	4.31	3.88	3.45	3.02	2.59	2.16	1.73	1.29	0.86
50	5.95	5.16	4.38	3.94	3.50	3.06	2.63	2.19	1.75	1.31	0.88
51	6.04	5.24	4.44	3.99	3.55	3.11	2.66	2.22	1.78	1.33	0.89
52	6.12	5.31	4.50	4.05	3.60	3.15	2.70	2.25	1.80	1.35	0.90
53	6.21	5.38	4.56	4.11	3.65	3.19	2.74	2.28	1.83	1.37	0.91
54	6.29	5.46	4.63	4.16	3.70	3.24	2.78	2.31	1.85	1.39	0.93
55	6.38	5.53	4.69	4.22	3.75	3.28	2.81	2.34	1.88	1.41	0.94
56	6.46	5.61	4.75	4.28	3.80	3.33	2.85	2.38	1.90	1.43	0.95
57	6.55	5.68	4.81	4.33	3.85	3.37	2.89	2.41	1.93	1.44	0.96
58	6.63	5.75	4.88	4.39	3.90	3.41	2.93	2.44	1.95	1.46	0.98
59	6.72	5.83	4.94	4.44	3.95	3.46	2.96	2.47	1.98	1.48	0.99
60	6.80	5.90	5.00	4.50	4.00	3.50	3.00	2.50	2.00	1.50	1.00
61	6.89	5.97	5.06	4.56	4.05	3.54	3.04	2.53	2.03	1.52	1.01
62	6.97	6.05	5.13	4.61	4.10	3.59	3.08	2.56	2.05	1.54	1.03
63	7.06	6.12	5.19	4.67	4.15	3.63	3.11	2.59	2.08	1.56	1.04
64	7.14	6.20	5.25	4.73	4.20	3.68	3.15	2.63	2.10	1.58	1.05
65	7.23	6.27	5.31	4.78	4.25	3.72	3.19	2.66	2.13	1.59	1.06
66	7.31	6.34	5.38	4.84	4.30	3.76	3.23	2.69	2.15	1.61	1.08
67	7.40	6.42	5.44	4.89	4.35	3.81	3.26	2.72	2.18	1.63	1.09
68	7.48	6.49	5.50	4.95	4.40	3.85	3.30	2.75	2.20	1.65	1.10
69	7.57	6.56	5.56	5.01	4.45	3.89	3.34	2.78	2.23	1.67	1.11
70	7.65	6.64	5.63	5.06	4.50	3.94	3.38	2.81	2.25	1.69	1.13
71	7.74	6.71	5.69	5.12	4.55	3.98	3.41	2.84	2.28	1.71	1.14
72	7.82	6.79	5.75	5.18	4.60	4.03	3.45	2.88	2.30	1.73	1.15
73	7.91	6.86	5.81	5.23	4.65	4.07	3.49	2.91	2.33	1.74	1.16
74	7.99	6.93	5.88	5.29	4.70	4.11	3.53	2.94	2.35	1.76	1.18
75	8.08	7.01	5.94	5.34	4.75	4.16	3.56	2.97	2.38	1.78	1.19
76	8.16	7.08	6.00	5.40	4.80	4.20	3.60	3.00	2.40	1.80	1.20
77	8.25	7.15	6.06	5.46	4.85	4.24	3.64	3.03	2.43	1.82	1.21
78	8.33	7.23	6.13	5.51	4.90	4.29	3.68	3.06	2.45	1.84	1.23
79	8.42	7.30	6.19	5.57	4.95	4.33	3.71	3.09	2.48	1.86	1.24
80	8.50	7.38	6.25	5.63	5.00	4.38	3.75	3.13	2.50	1.88	1.25
AGE	6 x 3.0	6 x 3.25	6 x 3.5	6 x 3.75	6 x 4.0	6 x 4.25	6 x 4.5	6 x 4.75	6 x 5.0	6 x 5.25	6 x 5.5

Find patient age, then move right to find result closest to refractive myopia without going over

Fig. 4.4. Nomogram for six-incision mini-RK. (Reprinted with permission from the January 1995 issue of the *Journal of Cataract and Refractive Surgery* [Vol. 21, No. 1; pp. 29] © *Journal of Cataract and Refractive Surgery*.)

8 INCISION MRK NOMOGRAM

AGE	8 x 3.0	8 x 3.25	8 x 3.5	8 x 3.75	8 x 4.0	8 x 4.25	8 x 4.5	8 x 4.75	8 x 5.0	8 x 5.25	8 x 5.5
				SURGICAL OPTION							
20	4.00	3.50	3.00	2.70	2.40	2.10	1.80	1.50	1.20	0.90	0.60
21	4.10	3.59	3.08	2.77	2.46	2.15	1.85	1.54	1.23	0.92	0.62
22	4.20	3.68	3.15	2.84	2.52	2.21	1.89	1.58	1.26	0.95	0.63
23	4.30	3.76	3.23	2.90	2.58	2.26	1.94	1.61	1.29	0.97	0.65
24	4.40	3.85	3.30	2.97	2.64	2.31	1.98	1.65	1.32	0.99	0.66
25	4.50	3.94	3.38	3.04	2.70	2.36	2.03	1.69	1.35	1.01	0.68
26	4.60	4.03	3.45	3.11	2.76	2.42	2.07	1.73	1.38	1.04	0.69
27	4.70	4.11	3.53	3.17	2.82	2.47	2.12	1.76	1.41	1.06	0.71
28	4.80	4.20	3.60	3.24	2.88	2.52	2.16	1.80	1.44	1.08	0.72
29	4.90	4.29	3.68	3.31	2.94	2.57	2.21	1.84	1.47	1.10	0.74
30	5.00	4.38	3.75	3.38	3.00	2.63	2.25	1.88	1.50	1.13	0.75
31	5.10	4.46	3.83	3.44	3.06	2.68	2.30	1.91	1.53	1.15	0.77
32	5.20	4.55	3.90	3.51	3.12	2.73	2.34	1.95	1.56	1.17	0.78
33	5.30	4.64	3.98	3.58	3.18	2.78	2.39	1.99	1.59	1.19	0.80
34	5.40	4.73	4.05	3.65	3.24	2.84	2.43	2.03	1.62	1.22	0.81
35	5.50	4.81	4.13	3.71	3.30	2.89	2.48	2.06	1.65	1.24	0.83
36	5.60	4.90	4.20	3.78	3.36	2.94	2.52	2.10	1.68	1.26	0.84
37	5.70	4.99	4.28	3.85	3.42	2.99	2.57	2.14	1.71	1.28	0.86
38	5.80	5.08	4.35	3.92	3.48	3.05	2.61	2.18	1.74	1.31	0.87
39	5.90	5.16	4.43	3.98	3.54	3.10	2.66	2.21	1.77	1.33	0.89
40	6.00	5.25	4.50	4.05	3.60	3.15	2.70	2.25	1.80	1.35	0.90
41	6.10	5.34	4.58	4.12	3.66	3.20	2.75	2.29	1.83	1.37	0.92
42	6.20	5.43	4.65	4.19	3.72	3.26	2.79	2.33	1.86	1.40	0.93
43	6.30	5.51	4.73	4.25	3.78	3.31	2.84	2.36	1.89	1.42	0.95
44	6.40	5.60	4.80	4.32	3.84	3.36	2.88	2.40	1.92	1.44	0.96
45	6.50	5.69	4.88	4.39	3.90	3.41	2.93	2.44	1.95	1.46	0.98
46	6.60	5.78	4.95	4.46	3.96	3.47	2.97	2.48	1.98	1.49	0.99
47	6.70	5.86	5.03	4.52	4.02	3.52	3.02	2.51	2.01	1.51	1.01
48	6.80	5.95	5.10	4.59	4.08	3.57	3.06	2.55	2.04	1.53	1.02
49	6.90	6.04	5.18	4.66	4.14	3.62	3.11	2.59	2.07	1.55	1.04
50	7.00	6.13	5.25	4.73	4.20	3.68	3.15	2.63	2.10	1.58	1.05
51	7.10	6.21	5.33	4.79	4.26	3.73	3.20	2.66	2.13	1.60	1.07
52	7.20	6.30	5.40	4.86	4.32	3.78	3.24	2.70	2.16	1.62	1.08
53	7.30	6.39	5.48	4.93	4.38	3.83	3.29	2.74	2.19	1.64	1.10
54	7.40	6.48	5.55	5.00	4.44	3.89	3.33	2.78	2.22	1.67	1.11
55	7.50	6.56	5.63	5.06	4.50	3.94	3.38	2.81	2.25	1.69	1.13
56	7.60	6.65	5.70	5.13	4.56	3.99	3.42	2.85	2.28	1.71	1.14
57	7.70	6.74	5.78	5.20	4.62	4.04	3.47	2.89	2.31	1.73	1.16
58	7.80	6.83	5.85	5.27	4.68	4.10	3.51	2.93	2.34	1.76	1.17
59	7.90	6.91	5.93	5.33	4.74	4.15	3.56	2.96	2.37	1.78	1.19
60	8.00	7.00	6.00	5.40	4.80	4.20	3.60	3.00	2.40	1.80	1.20
61	8.10	7.09	6.08	5.47	4.86	4.25	3.65	3.04	2.43	1.82	1.22
62	8.20	7.18	6.15	5.54	4.92	4.31	3.69	3.08	2.46	1.85	1.23
63	8.30	7.26	6.23	5.60	4.98	4.36	3.74	3.11	2.49	1.87	1.25
64	8.40	7.35	6.30	5.67	5.04	4.41	3.78	3.15	2.52	1.89	1.26
65	8.50	7.44	6.38	5.74	5.10	4.46	3.83	3.19	2.55	1.91	1.28
66	8.60	7.53	6.45	5.81	5.16	4.52	3.87	3.23	2.58	1.94	1.29
67	8.70	7.61	6.53	5.87	5.22	4.57	3.92	3.26	2.61	1.96	1.31
68	8.80	7.70	6.60	5.94	5.28	4.62	3.96	3.30	2.64	1.98	1.32
69	8.90	7.79	6.68	6.01	5.34	4.67	4.01	3.34	2.67	2.00	1.34
70	9.00	7.88	6.75	6.08	5.40	4.73	4.05	3.38	2.70	2.03	1.35
71	9.10	7.96	6.83	6.14	5.46	4.78	4.10	3.41	2.73	2.05	1.37
72	9.20	8.05	6.90	6.21	5.52	4.83	4.14	3.45	2.76	2.07	1.38
73	9.30	8.14	6.98	6.28	5.58	4.88	4.19	3.49	2.79	2.09	1.40
74	9.40	8.23	7.05	6.35	5.64	4.94	4.23	3.53	2.82	2.12	1.41
75	9.50	8.31	7.13	6.41	5.70	4.99	4.28	3.56	2.85	2.14	1.43
76	9.60	8.40	7.20	6.48	5.76	5.04	4.32	3.60	2.88	2.16	1.44
77	9.70	8.49	7.28	6.55	5.82	5.09	4.37	3.64	2.91	2.18	1.46
78	9.80	8.58	7.35	6.62	5.88	5.15	4.41	3.68	2.94	2.21	1.47
79	9.90	8.66	7.43	6.68	5.94	5.20	4.46	3.71	2.97	2.23	1.49
80	10.00	8.75	7.50	6.75	6.00	5.25	4.50	3.75	3.00	2.25	1.50
AGE	8 x 3.0	8 x 3.25	8 x 3.5	8 x 3.75	8 x 4.0	8 x 4.25	8 x 4.5	8 x 4.75	8 x 5.0	8 x 5.25	8 x 5.5

Find patient age, then move right to find result closest to refractive myopia without going over

Fig. 4.5. Nomogram for eight-incision RK.

After the knife is set, there is a 1-sec pause. Then, using moderate pressure, a continuous incision extending from the inside edge of the central optical zone mark to the outside edge of the 7.0- to 8.0-mark is made. With the American or double-pass technique, the blade is pointed at the center of the lens, with the knife tip set at the inside edge of the central optical zone mark. The knife should be set to pass from the central optical zone to the 8.0-mm optical zone, cutting out both the central optical zone mark and the mark in the periphery.

When cutting from the periphery to the center, the procedure is reversed, with the knife initially set outside the 8.0-mm optical zone marker and extending toward the central mark to be cut out. For the tip of the blade to point toward the center of the lens, it is necessary to rotate the knife slightly at the end of the incision. The author prefers a third option, the double-pass technique, which combines a center-to-periphery and a periphery-to-center cut, because it produces a more consistently deep, short cut and is softer. In cases where mini-RK is combined with astigmatism surgery, it is necessary to make transverse cuts first. These should be made either outside or between the radial incisions (Fig. 4.6).

After completion of the procedure, several drops of antibiotic steroid solution and a nonsteroidal anti-inflammatory agent are placed in the eye. No irrigation of the eye is necessary, and the patient is sent home without a patch and without being treated with cycloplegic agents. Patients must use antibiotic steroid drops for 2 weeks following surgery. At 2 weeks, if the patient is overcorrected by more than +1.0 D, the antibiotic steroid drops are replaced by 5% NaCl and 0.5% pilocarpine, four times daily for 4 to 8 weeks. If the patient is within ±1.0 D, the patient is told to continue taking the remaining antibiotic steroid drops. When the patient is undercorrected by more than −1.0 D, the medication is continued for 4 to 8 weeks postoperatively four times daily.

STUDYING MINI-RK

Mini-RK is an effective procedure, with results that rival those of traditional RK. Efficacy rates are nearly indistinguishable from those attained with full-length incisions. The slightly decreased effec-

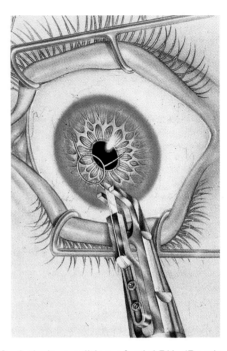

Fig. 4.6. Artist's rendition of mini-RK. (Reprinted with permission from the January 1995 issue of the *Journal of Cataract and Refractive Surgery* [Vol. 21, No. 1; pp. 30] © *Journal of Cataract and Refractive Surgery.*)

tiveness of this procedure, compared to traditional RK, is a fair trade-off for the increase in stability gained by shortening the incision. While the PERK data shows a significant 0.5 hyperopic shift between 6 and 24 months, no measurable long-term instability of the cornea during that period[8] has been observed with mini-RK.

Studies of mini-RK bear out its effectiveness. In a cadaver eye study, eight mini-RK incisions from the 3.0- to the 7.0-mm optical zone proved to be 92% as efficacious as those reaching the 11-mm optical zone. Following the 8-mm mini-RK incision, there was a mean flattening of 7.75 D compared to 8.35 D achieved with a full-length incision.[18]

The potential of mini-RK was also clearly indicated in another study in which patients were evaluated by intraoperative Terry surgical keratometry. Results of this study showed a slim 1% increase in effectiveness with full-length incisions that were twice as long as those used in mini-RK. Following an eight-incision mini-RK procedure, there was a mean flattening of 5.08 D. When this incision was extended into the 11-mm zone, the flattening increased to just 5.13 D.

Table 4.1. Retrospective Review of Mini-RK (*N* = 100) 1996

	Preoperative Vision	Without Reoperation	With Reoperation
Range	−1.5 to −6.0		
20/40 or better	0	94 (94%)	100 (100%)
20/30 or better	0	86 (86%)	94 (94%)
20/25 or better	0	72 (72%)	76 (76%)
20/20 or better	0	64 (64%)	68 (68%)
+/−0.5 D	0	60 (60%)	64 (64%)
+/−1.0 D	0	92 (92%)	98 (98%)
Gain in BCVA (two lines or more)		0	0
Loss in BCVA (two lines or more)		0	0

Visual results with the mini-RK technique are nearly equal to those of RK. In a retrospective study (Table 4.1) involving 100 eyes of 50 patients who underwent four- or eight-incision mini-RK, no patient was overcorrected by more than 1.0 D and 94% of patients had 20/40 or better uncorrected visual acuity. Reoperations were required in eight eyes. With these resulting corrections, 98% of patients were within 1.0 D of emmetropia and 100% had 20/40 or better visual acuity. The one frequent postoperative symptom, starburst, decreased over time. No sight-threatening complications were observed.

GUIDING PRINCIPLES FOR SUCCESS

While mini-RK has proven to be both safe and effective, it is still surgery, and elective surgery at that, and should never be taken lightly. The author's current system of mini-RK hinges on three guiding principles for reducing the potential risk to the patient.

The first principle consists of operating on only one eye at a time. Quite simply, every patient is unique, and there is no telling how he or she will respond to the procedure. If both eyes are operated on simultaneously, we run the unnecessary risk of over- or undercorrection, perhaps subjecting the patient to further surgery. By singling out one eye, we can spare the patient this risk, using the patient's response to the first mini-RK to plan for the second.

If, for example, the patient underresponds to the initial procedure, we can perform a more powerful mini-RK on the second eye and at the same time make any needed enhancements in the first eye.

The second principle involves using a minimum number of incisions, usually two to eight, to achieve the desired result. Determining the number of incisions needed involves weighing the additional risk carried by each new incision. This risk/benefit ratio is lowest with a two- or four-incision mini-RK, which result in approximately 50% and 70%, respectively, of the total flattening achievable by any number of incisions.

Consider the case of a 40-year-old patient. With such a patient, a four-incision mini-RK can be expected to achieve 1.05 D of correction per incision, for a total of 4.20 D of flattening. Four subsequent incisions can be expected to enhance correction by only 0.45 D per incision, for a total of 1.80 D. This amounts to just 43% of the efficacy per incision with 100% of the initial risk. If eight more incisions are added, efficacy drops to a mere 0.075 D per incision, or an overall additional enhancement of just 0.6 D, with the patient still taking on an equal amount of risk per incision.

Bearing this in mind, the author begins with a two- or four-incision RK whenever possible despite the fact that a smaller optical zone must be used than with an eight-incision procedure. Considering the risk/benefit ratio, more than eight incisions are almost never called for. Safety may be further enhanced by placing the incisions in an oblique configuration to decrease the chance of disabling glare.[19]

The third principle—which, unlike the other two, is unique to mini-RK—involves using the shortest possible incisions to reduce the risk while retaining most of the efficacy of RK. By targeting an optimal area in the 3.0- to 8.0-mm optical zone, we can offer the patient greater corneal stability. With the use of shorter incisions, only 50–60% of fibers need be cut, allowing more corneal tissue to remain intact. While prospective trials now underway will require a minimum of 5 years of follow-up to assess clinically the potential benefits of mini-RK, diurnal fluctuation of vision and refractive instability with progressive hyperopic shift will probably be reduced.

In addition to adhering to these three principles, the success of the mini-RK procedure lies in the quality of the incisions. While many surgeons report excellent results with the procedure, others describe problems with significant undercorrection. To enhance efficacy in such cases, the author suggests extending incisions to the 9-mm optical zone. Increases beyond the 9-mm zone should not be needed.

While further study of mini-RK is required, if it holds up to scrutiny, even with the growing acceptance of other procedures such as excimer laser photorefractive keratectomy (PRK) and automated lamellar keratoplasty, there are several long-term possibilities for this procedure. Because of the rapid visual rehabilitation and low morbidity associated with mini-RK, it could remain the procedure of choice for some low to moderate myopes if no significant hyperopic shift occurs and problems with diurnal fluctuation seen with RK are minimized. Mini-RK may also be used to enhance other procedures, such as PRK or LASIK, for correcting residual myopia.

REFERENCES

1. Curtin BJ. *The Myopias: Basic Science and Clinical Management*. Philadelphia, NY: Harper & Row; 1985.
2. Board of Directors of the International Society of Refractive Keratoplasty. Statement on radial keratotomy in 1988. *J Refract Surg*. 1988;4:80–90.
3. Saunders DR, Hofmann RF, Salz JR, eds. *Refractive Corneal Surgery*. Thorofare, NJ: Slack; 1986.
4. Saunders DR, ed. *Radial Keratotomy Surgical Techniques*. Thorofare, NJ: Slack; 1986.
5. Waring GO III. *Refractive Keratotomy Surgical Techniques*. Thorofare, NJ: Slack; 1986.
6. Ophthalmic Procedures Assessment. *Radial Keratotomy for Myopia*. San Francisco, CA: American Academy of Ophthalmology;
7. Waring GO III, Lynn MJ, Nizam A, et al. Results of the Prospective Evaluation of Radial Keratotomy (PERK) study five years after surgery. *Ophthalmology*. 1991;98:1164–1176.
8. Waring GO III, Lynn MJ, McDonnell PJ, et al. Results of the Prospective Evaluation of Radial Keratotomy (PERK) study ten years after surgery. *Arch Ophthalmol*. 1994;112:1298–1308.
9. Simons KB, Linsalata RP. Ruptured globe following blunt trauma after radial keratotomy: a case report. *Ophthalmology*. 1987;94:(suppl):148. Abstract.
10. Binder PS, Waring GO III, Arrowsmith PN, et al. Histopathology of traumatic corneal rupture after radial keratotomy. *Arch Ophthalmol*. 1988;106:1584–1590.
11. Lindstrom RL. The surgical correction of astigmatism: a clinician's perspective. *Refract Corneal Surg*. 1990;6:441–454.
12. Spigelman AV, Williams PA, Nichols BD, et al. Four incision radial keratotomy. *J Cataract Refract Surg*. 1988;14:125–128.
13. Spigelman AV, Williams PA, Lindstrom RL. Further studies of four incision radial keratotomy. *Refract Corneal Surg*. 1989;5:292–295.
14. Ingraham HJ, Guber D, Green WR. Radial keratotomy; clinicopathologic case report. *Arch Ophthalmol*. 1985;103:683–688.
15. Yamaguchi T, Tamaki K, Kaufman HE, et al. Histologic study of a pair of human corneas after anterior radial keratotomy. *Am J Ophthalmol* 1985;100:281–929.
16. Luttrull JK, Jester JV, Smith RE. The effect of radial keratotomy on ocular integrity in an animal model. *Arch Ophthalmol*. 1982;100:319–320.
17. McKnight SJ, Fitz J, Giangiacomo J. Corneal rupture following radial keratotomy in cats subjected to BB gun injury. *Ophthalmic Surg*. 1988;19:165–167.
18. Salz J, Lee JS, Jester JV, et al. Radial keratotomy in fresh human cadaver eyes. *Ophthalmology*. 1981;88:742–746.
19. Chen V, Lindstrom RL. Oblique orientation of incisions in four-incision radial keratotomy. *Ophthalmic Surg*. 1992;23:359.

5

Photorefractive Keratectomy for Low Myopia

Daniel Epstein

Gilles J. Renard

W. Bruce Jackson

Emmanuel Caubet

Philippe J. Cénac

Jae Ho Kim

INTRODUCTION

The interaction between corneal tissue and the excimer laser was first investigated in 1981 by Tabaoda, who studied the response of the epithelium to the argon fluoride (AF) and krypton fluoride (KrF) excimer laser.[1] The word *excimer* is a contraction of the words excited dimers but is a misnomer because the mixed molecular combinations (rare gas-halide) of ArF and KrF are called excimer lasers.

Early interest in ultraviolet lasers for corneal surgery focused on a search for alternatives to steel blades for radial keratotomy (RK). In 1983, Trokel and Srinivasan performed the first argon fluoride (ArF) excimer laser incision/excision.[2] Srinivasan called the interaction between biological tissues and the ArF excimer laser "photoablative decomposition." The ArF excimer laser, which emits radiation at 193 nm in the far-ultraviolet spectrum, photoablates corneal tissue by breaking chemical bonds and ejecting the remnants at supersonic velocity.[3]

Serdarevic performed the first in vivo ArF excimer laser procedure and the first large-area surface ablation of the cornea in 1984.[4] The minimal-scarring healing response observed in that experiment provided the first important indication of the feasibility of excimer laser corneal sculpting for therapeutic and refractive purposes.

Seiler first used the excimer laser in humans to correct astigmatism by linear and arcuate keratectomies in blind eyes (1985) and in sighted eyes (1986).[5] He first performed therapeutic excimer keratectomies in humans in 1986.

L'Esperance performed the first wide-area excimer laser keratectomy in blind and fully sighted eyes in 1987.[6] As this procedure evolved in the following years, it came to be termed *photorefractive keratecomy (PRK).*

Serdarevic first used the excimer laser for corneal trephination in 1987.[7]

Pallikaris first performed laser in situ keratomileusis (LASIK) with the excimer laser in 1990.[8]

Low myopia has proven to be the most fertile refractive soil for successful excimer laser PRK. In the 7 years since large-scale clinical work with sighted human eyes began in 1989–90, hundreds of thousands of eyes have undergone PRK for myopia ranging from −1.00 D to −6.00 D, with generally excellent refractive results.[9–12]

The use of lasers to reshape the anterior corneal curvature to correct refractive errors has become an established clinical procedure. In fact, most countries in which excimer laser systems are available and in which the economic or regulatory environment does not promote nonlaser techniques, PRK is now the treatment of choice to correct low to moderate myopia. Solid state lasers are being developed as other sources of ultraviolet radiation for PRK but are still investigational.

More than a half dozen companies now offer excimer lasers, three of which have been in the market from the start. Different principles have been used in the design of these systems, and the refractive results as well as the postoperative visual rehabilitation vary somewhat according to the system used. Long-term results, covering at least 3 to 4 years of follow-up, are available only from the three initial systems.

This chapter presents the results obtained with different excimer lasers that have been in clinical use on sighted eyes for at least 1 year. The major differences between the systems are outlined, and the current controversies pertaining to post-operative treatment are discussed.

PREOPERATIVE CONSIDERATIONS

Age

Most excimer surgeons require a minimum patient age of about 20 years, the reasoning being that in most cases of low to moderate myopia, refractive stability is generally assured by that age. However, even with that in mind, the refractive surgeon should establish whether a 20-year-old excimer surgery candidate really has attained this stability. Comparing the current refraction with that existing at least a year earlier is generally sufficient to document the presence or absence of refractive stability.

The issue of upper age limits for potential excimer surgery patients has received considerably less attention. As early as the first year of the excimer myopia surgery era, numerous investigators noted that older patients (i.e., over the age of 40–45 years) tended to have a higher risk of residual hyperopia when standard PRK algorithms were used.[9,13] Chatterjee and associates, reporting at the 1996 annual meeting of the Association for Research in Vision and Ophthalmology, stated that when examining the final refractive outcome of 2342 excimer surgery patients, they found that patients 40 to 49 years of age were significantly more hyperopic (mean, +0.14 D) than those below 30 (mean, −0.10 D). They noted a similar significance when comparing patients under 30 with those aged 30 to 39.[14]

Even when the utmost consideration is given to age, adult progression of myopia remains a well-established phenomenon that cannot be foreseen in any given eye. Thus, a patient with stable emmetropia for several years following PRK may develop renewed myopia because of this adult onset of progression.

Contraindications

PRK is contraindicated in the presence of a number of ocular and systemic diseases. Patients with severe dry eye, blepharitis, or neurotrophic keratitis may exhibit delayed epithelial wound healing after PRK. Patients with ocular inflammatory disorders or systemic autoimmune diseases may develop corneal melting after an excimer procedure. Seiler and associates reported a case of severe corneal ulcer in a patient with undiagnosed systemic lupus erythematosus.[15] Assaf and Libert (personal communication, 1996) observed stromal melting and subsequent corneal perforation in a patient with a previously undiagnosed immunological disease (Fig. 5.1). The corneal response may have been aggravated by a week-long use of topical diclofenac against the doctor's orders. Immunological workup suggested an incipient systemic lupus erythematosus.

Patients who are pregnant or who have keratoconus, irregular astigmatism, or contact lens–induced corneal warpage may respond unpredictably to PRK.

Most surgeons also consider the procedure contraindicated in monocular patients. Many refractive centers advise patients with professions that require optimal performance under suboptimal visual conditions (e.g., truck drivers with night shifts, military and commercial pilots) to avoid the procedure.

Approaching or beginning presbyopia is a relative contraindication. Patients (especially those with a myopia of −2.00 D to −3.00 D) should be informed that successful PRK will make them dependent on glasses for reading and other near work. Many refractive surgeons have noted that even after such specific advice is given, most PRK candidates declare that they would rather have good uncorrected distance vision than do without glasses for near work.

Patients with a history of herpetic keratitis appear to be at increased risk of a recurrence after PRK.

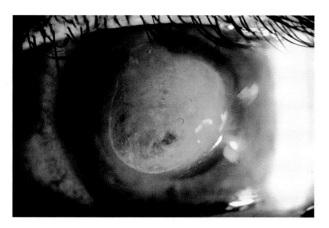

Fig. 5.1. Slit lamp photo of post-PRK eye which developed corneal melting. The patient had previously undiagnosed immunological disease and used topical diclofenac much longer than prescribed. Note the central ulceration/melting and paracentral descemetocele 1 week postoperatively. (Courtesy of J. Assaf, M.D., and J. Libert, M.D., Hôpital Universitaire St. Pierre, Brussels, Belgium.)

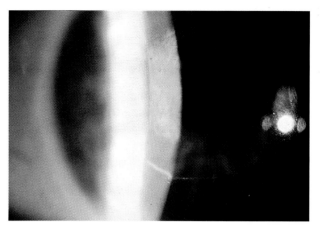

Fig. 5.2. Eye in which PRK was performed after astigmatic keratotomy, with a resulting increase in subepithelial haze. A dense grade 4 haze developed 3 months following PRK that was performed 3 months after astigmatic keratotomy with a pair of arcuate incisions. The contralateral cornea, which had not undergone prior incisional surgery, was clear at all postoperative visits after PRK. (Courtesy of T. David, M.D., Hôtel-Dieu University Hospital, Paris, France.)

Mechanical trauma, ultraviolet radiation, and postoperative topical corticosteroids are all known risk factors for reactivation of herpetic keratitis. McDonnell et al. reported such a reactivation in a patient treated for high postkeratoplasty astigmatism.[16] Subsequently, other reactivation cases after PRK were reported,[17] and this phenomenon has been reproduced in the rabbit model.[18] Accordingly, use of oral acyclovir for 2 weeks after PRK (or after phototherapeutic keratectomy) should be considered when there is a history of ocular herpetic disease.

Performing PRK after incisional refractive surgery remains a controversial issue. Increased subepithelial corneal haze when PRK was used to correct residual myopia after RK has been reported.[19] It has been speculated that keratocytes may remain activated for many years following incisional keratorefractive surgery, thereby provoking a more aggressive wound-healing reaction and more pronounced haze formation after PRK (Serdarevic ON, oral presentation, Annual Meeting of the American Academy of Ophthalmology, New Orleans, 1989) (Fig. 5.2). Lee and collaborators, reporting on 14 eyes which had undergone PRK after an average of 40 months following RK, found haze greater than 2+ and a decrease in best corrected visual acuity in 6% of patients after the excimer procedure. However, 71.4% of patients had an uncorrected visual acuity of 20/25 or better (Table 5.1).[20] David (personal communication) observed a case in which haze intensified when RK was performed after PRK (Fig. 5.3).

Keloid formers, being aggressive wound healers, have often been mentioned as unsuitable for PRK because of the presumed risk of developing significant corneal haze. Epstein (personal communication, 1996) has performed PRK on several known Caucasian keloid formers and did not observe any unusual haze response. Several surgeons have, however, reported a more intense wound-healing response in pigmented individuals (K. Shimizu, 1994, and E. Chansue, 1995, personal communications).

No specific marker has yet been found for use in preoperative assessment to screen patients at risk of aggressive corneal wound healing. Although biochemical testing of tear fluid has been suggested, there is still no test which can be used reliably to predict the post-PRK corneal response of any particular patient.

The preoperative history obtained from any PRK candidate should include systemic medications.

Table 5.1. Clinical Results of PRK for Undercorrected Myopia After RK[20]

Clinical Results	Group I	Group II
No. of Eyes (Patients)	14 (9)	4 (4)
Interval between RK and PRK	40 (12 to 94) months	
Preoperative Values		
Amount of myopia	−3.55 ± 1.45	−7.44 ± 0.90
Keratometry	42.12 ± 2.01	44.93
Postoperative Values		
Visual acuity, uncorrected (corrected)		
20/25 or better	71.4 (100)	0 (75)
20/30 ~ 20/40	14.3 (0)	50 (25)
20/50 ~ 20/200	0 (0)	50 (0)
Amount of myopia	−0.91	−2.50
Keratometry	40.12 ± 2.23	41.56
Complications		
Steroid-induced IIOP	33%	
Decrease in BCVA	6%	
Corneal haze of more than grade 2	6%	
Delayed epithelial wound healing	6%	
Most common subjective symptoms	Glare at night (56%)	

Abbreviations: IIOP = increased intraocular pressure; BCVA = best corrected visual acuity.
(Courtesy of J. H. Kim, M.D., T. W. Hahn, M.D., W. J. Sah, M.D., Catholic University of Korea School of Medicine, Seoul, Korea.)

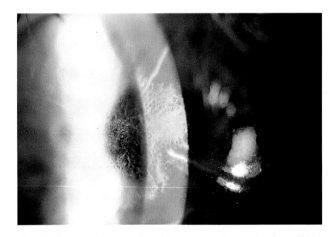

Fig. 5.3. Eye in which RK was performed after PRK, with a resulting increase in subepithelial corneal haze. The cornea was clear at 1 year following PRK and before RK. A dense grade 4 haze developed 6 months following RK. The contralateral cornea, which had no RK, remained clear at 1 year after PRK. (Courtesy of T. David, M.D., Hôtel-Dieu University Hospital, Paris, France.)

Such drugs may influence corneal wound healing. Edmison (personal communication, 1996) observed a case in which a patient on amiodarone developed corneal opacities after PRK (Fig. 5.4).

INTRAOPERATIVE CONSIDERATIONS

Epithelium Removal

Since the corneal epithelium is removed before the PRK procedure, several methods of deepithelialization have been developed. The different approaches to this pre-PRK step have been motivated by a search for the ideal technique that combines the least trauma to the cornea with optimal and stable refractive results.

The most commonly used method is mechanical debridement with a blunt spatula or a sharp blade.[21] Other techniques include chemical removal of the epithelium by synthetic topical anesthetics, cocaine, or alcohol[22] and photoablative deepithelialization. The use of the excimer laser itself for epithelial

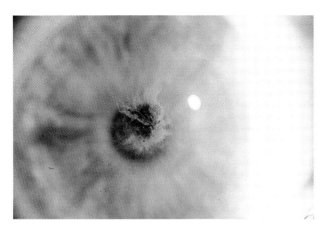

Fig. 5.4. Slit lamp photo of an eye which developed corneal opacities after PRK. The patient had been on amiodarone (200 mg po daily) starting 1 week prior to laser treatment for a preoperative refraction of $-12.75 + 0.50$. Deposits became apparent 3 months following PRK, at which time the best corrected visual acuity (BCVA) was 20/40−. Six months after PRK a whorl-like haze was noted. BCVA decreased to 20/50 at 1 year after PRK, at which time the patient was taken off amiodarone and placed on sotalol. BCVA improved to 20/30 over the following 6 months. (Courtesy of David E. Edmison, M.D., Focus Eye Centre, Ottawa, Ontario, Canada.)

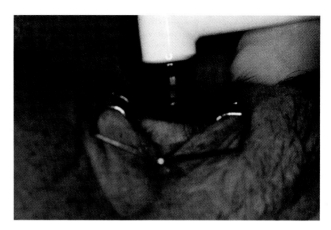

Fig. 5.5. Amoils brush for epithelial removal during PRK. (Courtesy of W. B. Jackson, M.D., University of Ottawa, Ontario, Canada.)

removal (transepithelial PRK) is an unpredictable method, since neither the thickness nor the homogeneity of the epithelium is known. Transepithelial PRK should not be performed with lasers utilizing large-diameter Gaussian beams.

In a retrospective study comparing manual epithelial abrasion with transepithelial ablation in 46 eyes, no significant differences were found with respect to rate of reepithelialization, biomicroscopic assessment of corneal clarity, refractive outcome and uncorrected visual acuity at 6 months, or the incidence of halos and glare.[23]

Some surgeons have developed mechanical devices for removal of the epithelium. These instruments, brush-like in appearance (Fig. 5.5) and function, have the advantage of abrading the epithelium very quickly. They can save the novice PRK surgeon precious seconds and thus decrease the risk of unwanted hydration of the stroma prior to excimer ablation. Usually, after brush action has been completed, a sponge is needed to remove residual epithelial debris. No prospective, masked studies

have been published to document any possible advantage of a brush over manual debridement with regard to long-term refractive outcome.

RESULTS

The efficacy of PRK (and of other refractive procedures) was conventionally measured in terms of two criteria: the percentage of eyes that achieve a postoperative refraction within 1.0 D of emmetropia (or aim) and the percentage of eyes that achieve 20/40 or better uncorrected distance visual acuity. Recently there has been increasing advocacy for tighter criteria, and reports on the percentage of eyes within 0.50 D of aim and the percentage of eyes achieving 20/30 or better uncorrected acuity have become more common.

It is important to keep in mind that these two criteria, often used to define the success rate of a given laser system, do not always provide an accurate reflection of the patient's perception of success. A patient who is practically emmetropic after PRK may have substantial glare problems at night or may require contact lens or spectacle correction for part of the day. Similarly, a patient with a refractive outcome of -2.0 D may consider the procedure successful if preoperative refraction was -9.0 D.

Moreover, since visual acuity and refraction are conventionally tested under optimal conditions in high luminance and with high contrast, loss of contrast vision is usually not detected. A recent study

Table 5.2. Results of Excimer Laser Surgery for Low Myopia

Laser Model	No. of Eyes	Length of Follow-up Period (mo)	Size of Ablation (mm)	Definition of Myopia (D)	Preoperative Myopia (D) and Range
Summit Excimed (David et al) 1995	50	12	5.0	−1 to −6	−3.8 ± 1.54
Summit Omnimed (David et al) 1996	50	1. 6	6.0	1. −1 to −6	1. −4.2 ± 2.0
	35	2. 12		2. −1 to −6	
Summit Excimed (Caubet et al) 1995	148	1. 6	5.0	1. −1 to −6	1. −3.73 ± 1.51
	64	2. 12		2. −1.4 to −6	2. −4.02 ± 1.43
Summit Apex-Plus (Caubet et al) 1996	25	6	6.5	−1.2 to −4.8	−3.32 ± 1.22

by Gauthier and associates.[24] comparing the treated and nontreated eyes of 105 PRK patients tested with high- and low-contrast charts in high and low luminance found that up to 55% of the treated eyes lost two or more lines of best-corrected visual acuity when tested under low contrast and low luminance. While the poorest results were related to optical zone diameters smaller than those in current use, it was clear that significant visual losses, not previously found with standard high-contrast Snellen charts, were detected under these suboptimal viewing conditions.

As the different excimer laser systems on the market have become more sophisticated, and as more advanced algorithms have been developed, refractive outcomes have improved. But in general, results are best in the lower ranges of myopia.[9–11,13,25–31] The results obtained with the various laser systems are reported here in the form of tables to provide the reader with a better overview (Table 5.2). Straightforward comparisons of efficacy are often impossible, since different treatment parameters were used in different clinical studies.

Postoperative Myopia (D) and Range	Percent Attained Refractions (± 0.5 D, 1 D, 2 D)	Percent UCVA ≥20/20 20/25, 20/40	Percent gain 1, 2, >2 Lines BCVA	Percent loss 1, 2, >2 Lines BCVA
	a) 91% 64% cyclo b) 96% 82% cyclo	a) 50% b) 78% c) 94%		c) 2%
	1. a) 78% 68% cyclo b) 94% 92% cyclo 2. a) 82% 78% cyclo b) 96% 92% cyclo	1. a) 52% b) 84% c) 94%	1.	1. c) 6.5%
1. −0.10 ± 0.68	1. a) 78% b) 92%	1. a) 41% b) 57% c) 93%		
2. −0.33 ± 0.46	2. a) 75% b) 93%	2. a) 32% b) 57% c) 89%		
−0.08 ± 0.30	a) 86% b) 100%	a) 83% b) 90% c) 100%		

(continued)

Because PRK success rates must be related to the time interval from surgery, and since it has been established that regression can occur after the procedure,[11,13] several time intervals are included (except for the newest laser [Autonomous]).

The time required for stability of refraction to be achieved postoperatively varies with the depth of ablation (which, in turn, is correlated with the magnitude of attempted myopic correction) and the type of laser used. Studies on patients with optical zone diameters of up to 5.0 mm indicated that post-PRK refraction stabilizes 12 to 18 months after surgery.[11,32] Clinical observations in patients treated with larger (6.0-mm) optical zones suggest that stability of refraction may be attained earlier (Figs. 5.6 to 5.9).

Some investigators have found no change in the contrast sensitivity function after PRK,[33,34] while others have found various degrees of reduction.[10,35,36] It is important to note that a decrease in contrast sensitivity may occur even in eyes that display a clear cornea postoperatively, indicating that this finding is not related to reduced corneal clarity alone. The reported reduction in contrast sensitivity

Table 5.2. Continued

Laser Model	No. of Eyes	Length of Follow-up Period (mo)	Size of Ablation (mm)	Definition of Myopia (D)	Preoperative Myopia (D) and Range
VISX 20/20 B 2.72 (Jackson et al) 1996	1. 20	1. 6	6.0	1. −1 to −6 SE	1. −3.71 ± 1.00 (−5.88 to −2.13)
	2. 19	2. 12		2. −1 to −6 SE	2. −3.29 ± 0.81 (−4.75 to −2.00)
	3. 17	3. 18		3. −1 to −6 SE	3. −3.21 ± 0.70 (−4.50 to −2.00)
VISX 20/20 B Vision Key (Jackson et al) 1996	1. 106	1. 6	6.0	1. −1 to −6 SE	1. −3.94 ± 1.28 (−6.00 to −1.25)
	2. 80	2. 12		2. −1 to −6 SE	2. −4.16 ± 1.27 (−6.00 to −1.25)
	3. 32	3. 18		3. −1 to −6 SE	3. −4.01 ± 1.32 (−5.88 to −1.50)
VISX Star Model C (Jackson et al) 1996	1. 56	1. 6	6.0	1. −1 to −6 SE	1. −4.02 ± 1.30 (−6.00 to −1.25)
	2. 34	2. 12		2. −1 to −6 SE	2. −3.83 ± 1.25 (−6.00 to −1.25)
	3. 8	3. 18		3. −1 to −6 SE	3. −4.13 ± 1.08 (−5.50 to −2.25)

Postoperative Myopia (D) and Range	Percent Attained Refractions (± 0.5 D, 1 D, 2 D)	Percent UCVA ≥20/20 20/25, 20/40	Percent gain 1, 2, >2 Lines BCVA	Percent loss 1, 2, >2 Lines BCVA
1. −0.48 ± 0.39 (−1.00 to +0.25)	1. a) 40.0% b) 85.0% c) 100.0%	1. a) 50.0% b) 80.0% c) 100.0%	1. a) 10.0% b) 0.0% c) 0.0%	1. a) 30.0% b) 5.0% c) 0.0%
2. −0.68 ± 0.42 (−1.25 to 0.00)	2. a) 21.1% b) 63.2% c) 100.0%	2. a) 47.8% b) 82.6% c) 100.0%	2. a) 21.7% b) 0.0% c) 0.0%	2. a) 17.4% b) 0.0% c) 0.0%
3. −0.51 ± 0.43 (−1.25 to 0.00)	3. a) 35.3% b) 76.5% c) 100.0%	3. a) 68.4% b) 94.7% c) 100.0%	3. a) 21.1% b) 0.0% c) 0.0%	3. a) 15.8% b) 0.0% c) 0.0%
1. −0.34 ± 0.47 (−2.38 to +0.63)	1. a) 60.0% b) 89.5% c) 100.0%	1. a) 68.7% b) 87.8% c) 99.1%	1. a) 27.3% b) 3.6% c) 0.0%	1. a) 12.7% b) 1.8% c) 0.0%
2. −0.31 ± 0.40 (−2.00 to +1.38)	2. a) 75.9% b) 96.2% c) 100.0%	2. a) 80.2% b) 93.8% c) 100.0%	2. a) 35.8% b) 7.4% c) 0.0%	2. a) 7.4% b) 1.2% c) 0.0%
3. −0.26 ± 0.39 (−1.25 to +0.25)	3. a) 77.4% b) 93.5% c) 100.0%	3. a) 75.0% b) 87.5% c) 93.8%	3. a) 31.3% b) 9.4% c) 0.0%	3. a) 15.6% b) 3.1% c) 0.0%
1. −0.16 ± 0.51 (−2.25 to +0.75)	1. a) 80.4% b) 94.7% c) 100.0%	1. a) 63.2% b) 80.7% c) 94.7%	1. a) 14.5% b) 0.0% c) 0.0%	1. a) 18.2% b) 3.6% c) 0.0%
2. −0.01 ± 0.33 (−0.50 to +1.38)	2. a) 97.1% b) 97.1% c) 100.0%	2. a) 76.5% b) 88.2% c) 97.1%	2. a) 23.5% b) 2.9% c) 0.0%	2. a) 20.6% b) 0.0% c) 0.0%
3. −0.16 ± 0.30 (−0.75 to 0.00)	3. a) 87.5% b) 100.0% c)	3. a) 75.0% b) 75.0% c) 87.5%	3. a) 25.0% b) 0.0% c) 0.0%	3. a) 25.0% b) 0.0% c) 0.0%

(continued)

Table 5.2. Continued

Laser Model	No. of Eyes	Length of Follow-up Period (mo)	Size of Ablation (mm)	Definition of Myopia (D)	Preoperative Myopia (D) and Range
Aesculap Meditec MEL 50 (Anschütz et al.) 1996	93	12	5.5–6.0	−1 to −6 SE	−4.14 ± 1.00 (−6.00 to −1.25)
Autonomous Technologies (phase IIa) (Pallikaris et al.) 1996	1. 49 2. 26	1. 3 2. 9	6.0	1. −1 to −6 2. −1 to −6	
Autonomous Technologies (phase IIb) (Pallikaris et al.) 1996	25	3	6.0	−1 to −6	
Chiron / Technolas (Schmid et al.) 1996	286	12	6.0	up to −8	−4.03 ± 2.43
Nidek (10 centers worldwide) 1996	118	12	6.0	−1 to −6.5	−3.32 ± 1.30
Schwind (Seiler et al.) 1996	227	12	6.0–6.5	−0.75 to −7	

*20/30.

Postoperative Myopia (D) and Range	Percent Attained Refractions (± 0.5 D, 1 D, 2 D)	Percent UCVA ≥20/20 20/25, 20/40	Percent gain 1, 2, >2 Lines BCVA	Percent loss 1, 2, >2 Lines BCVA
−0.52 ± 0.83 (−1.50 to +1.00)	a) 81% b) 95% c) 100%	a) 72% b) 77% c) 88%		c) 0.8%
	1. a) 42% b) 70% 2. a) 46% b) 61%	1. a) 53% b) 82%* c) 86% 2. a) 52% b) 78%* c) 78%	1. a) 46% b) 8% 2. a) 60% b) 8%	1. a) 10% b) 0% 2. a) 8% b) 0%
	a) 88% b) 92%	a) 72% b) 95%* c) 96%	a) 22% b) 0%	a) 17% b) 0%
−0.53 ± 0.83	a) 47.6% b) 75.2%	a) 67.5% b) 90.6%* c) 97.9%		c) 0%
−0.38 ± 0.70	a) 73.7% b) 89.0%	a) 69.2% b) 82.5% c) 95.0%	a) 18.3% b) 0.9%	a) 9.6% b) 1.7%
	b) 89.3%	a) 58.2% b) c) 98.4%		c) 0.9%

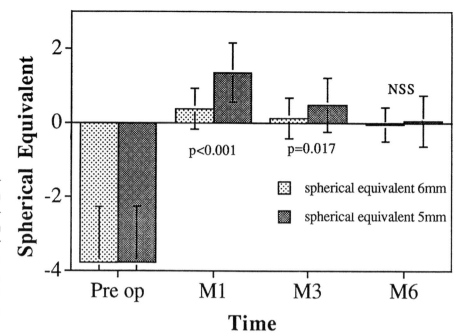

Fig. 5.6. Bar graph show-ing that 6.0-mm ablation zones resulted in signifi-cantly less initial hyperopia (manifest refraction) after PRK than did 5.0-mm zones. (Courtesy of T. David, M.D., Hôtel-Dieu University Hospital, Paris, France.)

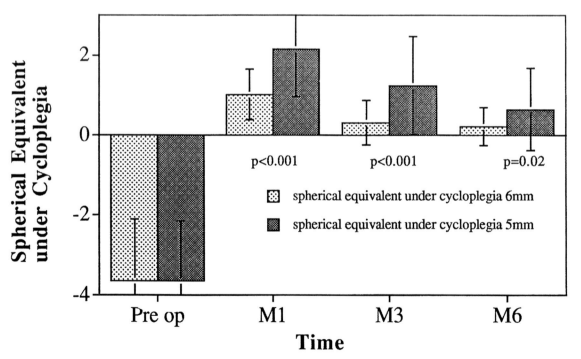

Fig. 5.7. Bar graph showing that 6.0-mm ablation zones resulted in significantly less initial hyperopia (cycloplegic refraction) after PRK than did 5.0-mm zones. (Courtesy of T. David, M.D., Hôtel-Dieu University Hospital, Paris, France.)

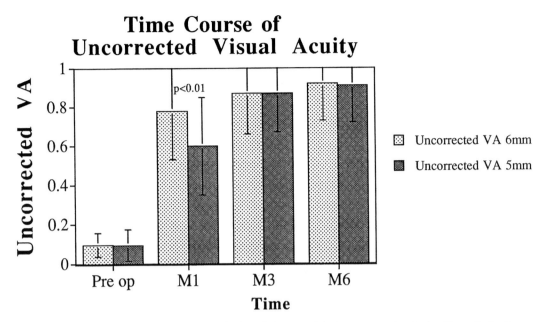

Fig. 5.8. Bar graph showing that patients treated with 6.0-mm ablation zones had significantly better uncorrected visual acuity at 1 month postoperatively than those ablated with 5.0-mm zones. The 6.0-mm treatment thus provided faster visual rehabilitation. (Courtesy of T. David, M.D., Hôtel-Dieu University Hospital, Paris, France.)

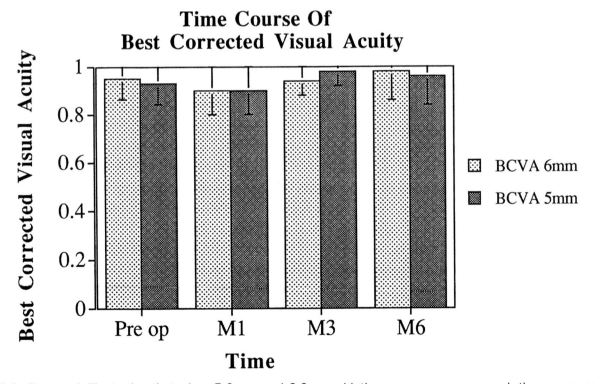

Fig. 5.9. Bar graph illustrating that when 5.0-mm and 6.0-mm ablation zones were compared, there were no significant difference in BCVA during the first 6 months after PRK. (Courtesy of T. David, M.D., Hôtel-Dieu University Hospital, Paris, France.)

may be caused by PRK-induced axial corneal surface changes.[37,38]

Another form of postoperative visual degradation, halos around light sources, is related to optical zone diameter. David and associates (personal communication, 1996) found that when a 5.0-mm ablation zone was used, 18% of the patients complained of halos 6 months postoperatively. After they switched to a 6.0-mm ablation zone, only 2% of patients voiced this complaint. O'Brart and collaborators reported similar observations when comparing 4.0- and 5.0-mm ablation diameters.[39] A more detailed discussion of this phenomenon can be found in Chapter 7.

Potential night-driving problems after small-zone PRK were recently highlighted by Kriegerowski and associates.[40] Visual acuity with low contrast and with glare were examined in 26 eyes 12 to 56 months after uncomplicated PRK (attempted correction −1.00 D to −6.00 D, ablation zone diameter 5.0 mm). The results showed that 19 of the 26 eyes did not meet German night driving requirements.

POSTOPERATIVE REGIMENS

Corticosteroids

The use of topical corticosteroids in the postoperative management of excimer PRK has been controversial since the advent of PRK. But although the potential benefit of corticosteroids remains unresolved, steroid use is routine among the majority of surgeons performing this procedure.

Topical corticosteroids became an integral part of the PRK regimen after initial small-animal studies suggested that they limit postablation subepithelial deposition of new collagen and ground substance.[41] Early clinical observations of the effects of steroids on post-PRK eyes also indicated a beneficial effect on the refractive outcome.[42]

In clinical practice, continued use of topical corticosteroids after excimer PRK has been based mainly on anecdotal observations and retrospective studies.[43] Few controlled prospective studies have examined the value of this therapy. Gartry and associates[44] performed a double-blind, placebo-controlled trial with 113 subjects treated for −3.00 D or −6.00 D. Patients were randomized to either a

3-month course of topical dexamethasone 0.1% or vehicle. At 3 months postoperatively, the dexamethasone-treated eyes had a better mean refractive outcome. However, at 6 and 12 months, there were no statistically significant differences between the groups with respect to refractive outcome or corneal haze intensity.

The relevance of published corticosteroid studies to current clinical practice has been questioned because most of the reports dealt with small ablation zone diameters (4.0 to 5.0 mm), while procedures today commonly are performed with a 6.0-mm diameter. Smaller zones involve a shallower ablation depth, and there may be a depth-specific stromal response to topical corticosteroids. On the other hand, the deeper ablations currently performed could generate a different response to such topical postoperative treatment.

Although the rabbit model shows that topical corticosteroids dramatically reduced the inflammatory response in the superficial stroma after PRK,[45] the relationship between the severity of the post-PRK corneal inflammation and the refractive outcome is yet to be determined.

Despite the uncertainties about the role of topical corticosteroids, there have been repeated and reproducible clinical observations that myopic eyes which regress after routine postoperative corticosteroids are discontinued often respond to a second (and even a third and a fourth) course of corticosteroids by regaining some or all of the initial refractive outcome.[13,46] The mechanism of this reversal of regression is not known.

The potential value of postoperative topical corticosteroids in the routine management of PRK patients remains unresolved. There may be a subset of patients that is very responsive to such therapy, but there is currently no method for identifying such patients preoperatively.

Nonsteroidal Anti-inflammatory Drugs

Nonsteroidal anti-inflammatory agents (NSAIDs) are commonly used to control the postoperative pain which tends to occur immediately after PRK. Where available, they should be used without preservatives.

Diclofenac sodium[47] and other NSAIDs significantly reduce postoperative pain, photophobia, and tearing, as well as burning and stinging sensations.

These agents also substantially decrease the need for oral pain killers after surgery. Indirectly, their use probably also reduces the number of post-PRK sick-leave days, thus bringing down the total cost of the procedure.

NSAIDs, which are believed to influence pain by interfering with certain arachidonic acid metabolites, have been considered as substitutes for topical corticosteroids in the long-term postoperative management of PRK patients.[48] However, there is no evidence that NSAIDs reduce corneal haze or improve the refractive outcome in humans.

NSAIDs with preservatives should be avoided after the first 48 hr following PRK because of the risk of stromal infiltrate formation and melting. Many surgeons advocate using NSAIDs only in combination with topical corticosteroids to avoid stromal infiltrates. Patients should be monitored closely for stromal infiltration. If stromal infiltration occurs, NSAIDs should be discontinued immediately.

Contact Lenses

Therapeutic (soft) contact lenses have been added to the immediate post-PRK regimen because of clinical observations indicating that combining NSAIDs with a contact lens increases pain relief.[47] It has not been shown how contact lenses contribute to the reduction of postoperative pain in such a combination therapy setting, but the mechanism may simply be a more evenly distributed drug release from the lens.

Using an extended-wear soft contact lens on a cornea with a fresh epithelial defect does, however, invite potential complications. There have been numerous reports of culture-negative peripheral corneal infiltrates in patients treated with both contact lens and an NSAID, and patients having microbial keratitis with visual acuity loss have been seen in a number of PRK centers (Epstein D. and Jackson W. B., personal communications, 1995, 1996).

Other Wound-Healing Modulators

In an effort to arrest fibroblast activity and thereby modulate post-PRK corneal wound healing, several known substances have been tested in animal models. Interferon,[49] mitomycin,[50,51] and D-penicillamine[52] are among the drugs tested. There is no re-

producible evidence that any of them modulates the corneal cellular response in a beneficial manner.

EXCIMER LASER SYSTEMS

Excimer laser systems can be classified according to the method of delivering energy to the cornea. There are two basic delivery systems: large-diameter beam and scanning beam.

Large-Diameter Beam Lasers

Fractal Mask Ablation (Schwind) (Trade Name: Keratom)
Computer-generated, randomized patterns are etched onto opaque masks which are imaged in the corneal plane. The mask is rotated continuously during treatment, and the cumulative effect obtained from the rotating pattern provides the desired ablation profile. A constant rate of rotation results in symmetrical profiles. If the rate of rotation is varied, asymmetrical patterns can be produced to correct astigmatism. This design is described as combining the advantages of large-diameter ablation with those of scanning systems.

Summit Technology (Trade Name: Apex Plus)
The computer-controlled iris diaphragm, which masks the stationary, large-diameter beam in a stepwise fashion, has 226 gradations. The ablation zone diameter is 6.5 mm. Ablation depth has been decreased with the aid of an aspheric ablation pattern. Toric ablatable masks enable the simultaneous correction of myopia and astigmatism, replacing an earlier sequential mode of ablation. The maximum diameter for hyperopic corrections is 9.5 mm.

VisX (Trade Name: Star)
The iris diaphragm has up to 240 steps, and a 6.0-mm ablation zone diameter is used. The laser pulse repetition rate has been increased from 5 to 6 Hz, and astigmatism treatment is now automated. Pulses have been redistributed so that more of them are concentrated in the central 2.5 mm (central island pulses). The laser has a smaller cavity than previous models, requiring less gas consumption, no liquid nitrogen, and only three mirrors. The laser's optical pathway resides in a vacuum-sealed tube, a design which is said to boost the longevity of the optics.

Scanning Beam Lasers

Tracker-Assisted Small-Beam Ablation (Autonomous Technologies) (Trade Name: T-PRK)

A scanning system controls a small beam with a spot diameter of approximately 1.0 mm. The system can support ablation zones of up to 10.0 mm in diameter, making possible hyperopic blend zones, for example. The small scanned spot allows the system to correct irregular astigmatism. The eye tracker is based on two-axis tracking mirrors. It is said to have a peak position error of 37 μm (at a target velocity of 100°/sec) and a 50% reduction of peak error within 3.8 msec.

PlanoScan (Chiron/Technolas Laser) (Trade Name: Keracor 117)

An overlapping 2.0-mm beam with variable sequence patterns is used in this scanning spot laser. Preprogrammed beam placement is performed by computer-controlled, movable mirrors. This new system is said to compensate for laser beam inhomogeneity and to provide a smoother ablation surface than that obtained with a multizone technique. The maximum ablation zone diameter is about 8.5 mm for myopia and approximately 9.0 mm for hyperopia.

Meditec (Trade Name: MEL-60)

Each pass of the scanning slit across the cornea occurs vertically. The surgeon controls the procedure by means of a hand-held (nonerodible) mask fixed to a suction ring with which the eye is immobilized. Placement of the mask close to the corneal plane is said to improve centration.

Scanning with a Spin (Nidek) (Trade Name: EC-5000)

The beam simultaneously scans and spins around its axis. The purpose of this two-dimensional beam movement is to reduce the risk of surface irregularities which beam inhomogeneities can cause. By adding the spin element instead of only scanning, the laser compensates for such inhomogeneities by preventing them from repeatedly affecting the same spot on the cornea. This system is said to produce a smoother ablation surface. The system allows for an ablation zone diameter of up to 9.0 mm.

REFERENCES

1. Tabaoda J, Mikesell GW, Reed RD. Response of the corneal epithelium to krypton fluoride excimer laser pulses. *Health Phys.* 1981;40:677.

2. Trokel S, Srinivasan R, Braren B. Excimer laser surgery of the cornea. *Am J Ophthalmol.* 1983;96:710–715.

3. Serdarevic O. Corneal laser surgery. In: L'Esperance FA Jr. *Ophthalmic Lasers.* St. Louis, Mo: The C.V. Mosby Company, 1989.

4. Serdarevic O, Darrell R, Krueger R, Trokel S. Excimer laser therapy for experimental *Candida* keratitis. *Am J Ophthalmol.* 1985;99:534–538.

5. Seiler T, Bende T, Wollensak J, Trokel SL. Excimer laser keratectomy for correction of astigmatism. *Am J Ophthalmol.* 1988;105:117–124.

6. L'Esperance FA Jr, Taylor DM, Warren JW. Human excimer laser keratectomy. Short-term histopathology after refractive surgery. *J Refract Surg.* 1988;4:118.

7. Serdarevic O, Gribomont A, Hanna K. Excimer laser trephination in penetrating keratoplasty: morphological features in wound healing. *Ophthalmology.* 1988;95:493–505.

8. Pallikaris IG, Papatzanaki ME, Stathi EZ, et al. Laser in situ keratomileusis. *Lasers Surg Med.* 1990;10:463–468.

9. Seiler T, Wollensak J. Myopic photorefractive keratectomy with the excimer laser: one-year follow-up. *Ophthalmology.* 1991;98:1156–1163.

10. Gartry DS, Kerr Muir MG, Marshall J. Excimer laser photrefractive keratectmy. 18-month follow-up. *Ophthalmology.* 1992;99:1209–1219.

11. Epstein D, Fagerholm P, Hamberg-Nyström H, Tengroth B. Twenty-four months follow-up of excimer laser photorefractive keratectomy for myopia. *Ophthalmology.* 1994;101:1558–1564.

12. Maguen E, Salz J, Nesburn A, et al. Results of excimer laser photorefractive keratectomy for the correction of myopia. *Ophthalmology.* 1994;101:1548–1557.

13. Tengroth B, Epstein D, Fagerholm P, et al. Excimer laser photorefractive keratectomy for myopia: clinical results in sighted eyes. *Ophthalmology.* 1993;100:739–745.

14. Chatterjee A, Shah S, Doyle SJ. Effect of age on final refractive outcome for 2342 patients following photorefractive keratectomy. *Invest Ophthalmol Vis Sci* (Suppl) 1996;37(suppl):S57. Abstract.

15. Seiler T, Wollensak J. Komplikationen der Laser-keratomileusis mit dem Excimerlaser (193 nm). *Klin Monatsbl Augenheilkd.* 1992;200:648–653.

16. McDonnell PJ, Moreira H, Clapham TN, et al. Photorefractive keratectomy for astigmatism: initial clinical results. *Arch Ophthalmol.* 1991;109:1370–1373.

17. Vrabec MP, Durrie DS, Chase DS. Recurrence of herpes simplex after excimer laser keratectomy. *Am J Ophthalmol.* 1992;114:96–97.

18. Pepose JS, Laycock KA, Miller JK, et al. Reactivation of latent herpes simplex virus by excimer laser photokeratectomy. *Am J Ophthalmol.* 1992;114:45–50.

19. Burnstein Y, Hersh PS. Photorefractive keratectomy following radial keratotomy. *J Refract Surg.* 1996; 12:163–170.

20. Lee YC, Park CK, Sah WJ, et al. Photorefractive keratectomy for undercorrected myopia after radial keratotomy: two-year follow-up. *J Refract Surg.* 1995; 11:S274–S279.

21. Campos M, Herzog L, Wang XW, et al. Corneal surface after deepithelialization using a sharp and a dull instrument. *Ophthalmic Surg.* 1992;23:618–621.

22. Campos M, Raman S, Lee M, McDonnell PJ. Keratocyte loss after different methods of deepithelialization. *Ophthalmology.* 1994;101:890–894.

23. Gimbel HV, DeBroff BM, Beldavs RA, et al. Comparison of laser and manual removal of corneal epithelium for photorefractive keratectomy. *J Refract Surg.* 1995;11:36–41.

24. Gauthier CA, Holden BA, Epstein D, et al. Assessment of high and low contrast visual acuity after photorefractive keratectomy for myopia. *Invest Ophthalmol Vis Sci.* 1996;37:S19. Abstract.

25. McDonald MB, Liu JC, Byrd TJ, et al. Central photorefractive keratectomy for myopia: partially sighted and normally sighted eyes. *Ophthalmology.* 1991; 98:1327–1337.

26. Lavery FL. Photorefractive keratectomy in 472 eyes. *Refract Corneal Surg.* 1993;9:98–100.

27. Piebenga LW, Matta CS, Deitz MR, et al. Excimer photorefractive keratectomy for myopia. *Ophthalmology.* 1993;100:1335–1345.

28. Salz JJ, Maguen E, Nesburn AB, et al. A two-year experience with excimer laser photorefractive keratectomy for myopia. *Ophthalmology.* 1993;100: 873–882.

29. Brancato R, Tavola A, Carones F, et al. Excimer laser photorefractive keratectomy for myopia: results in 1165 eyes. *Refract Corneal Surg.* 1993;9(suppl): 95–104.

30. Kim JH, Hahn TW, Lee YC, et al. Photorefractive keratectomy in 202 myopic eyes: one-year results. *Refract Corneal Surg.* 1993;9(suppl):11–16.

31. Talley AR, Hardten DR, Sher NA, et al. Results one year after using the 193-nm excimer laser for photorefractive keratectomy in mild to moderate myopia. *Am J Ophthalmol.* 1994;118:304–311.

32. Seiler T, Holschbach A, Derse M, et al. Complications of myopic photorefractive keratectomy with the excimer laser. *Ophthalmology.* 1994;101: 153–160.

33. Eiferman RA, O'Neil KP, Forgey DR, Cook YD. Excimer laser photorefractive keratectomy for myopia: six-month results. *Refract Corneal Surg.* 1991;7:344–347.

34. Sher NA, Chen V, Bowers RA, et al. The use of the 193-nm excimer laser for myopic photorefractive keratectomy in sighted eyes: a multicenter study. *Arch Ophthalmol.* 1991;109:1525–1530.

35. Ambrosio G, Cennamo G, De Marco R, et al. Visual function before and after photorefractive keratectomy for myopia. *J Refract Corneal Surg.* 1994;10: 129–136.

36. Butuner Z, Elliott DB, Gimbel HV, et al. Visual function one year after excimer laser photorefractive keratectomy. *J Refract Corneal Surg.* 1994;10:626–630.

37. Seiler T, Genth U, Holschbach A, Derse M. Aspheric photorefractive keratectomy with excimer laser. *Refract Corneal Surg.* 1993;9:166–172.

38. Seiler T, Reckman NW, Maloney RK. Effective spherical aberration of the cornea as a quantitative descriptor in corneal topography. *J Cataract Refract Surg.* 1993;19(suppl):155–165.

39. O'Brart DPS, Gartry DS, Lohmann CP, et al. Excimer laser photorefractive keratectomy for myopia: comparison of 4.0- and 5.0-mm ablation zones. *J Refract Corneal Surg.* 1994;10:87–94.

40. Kriegerowski M, Schlote T, Thiel HJ, et al. Photorefractive keratectomy (PRK) may lead to night driving inability. *Invest Ophthalmol Vis Sci.* 1996;37(suppl):S59. Abstract.

41. Tuft SJ, Zabel RW, Marshall J. Corneal repair following keratectomy: a comparison between conventional surgery and laser photoablation. *Invest Ophthalmol Vis Sci.* 1989;30:1769–1777.

42. Seiler T, Kahle G, Kriegerowski M. Excimer laser (193 nm) myopic keratomileusis in sighted and blind human eyes. *Refract Corneal Surg.* 1990;6:165–173.

43. Fagerholm P, Hamberg-Nyström H, Tengroth B, Epstein D. Effect of postoperative steroids on the

refractive outcome of photorefractive keratectomy for myopia with the Summit excimer laser. *J Cataract Refract Surg.* 1994;20:212–215.

44. Gartry DS, Kerr Muir MG, Marshall J. The effect of topical corticosteroids on refraction and corneal haze following excimer laser treatment of myopia: an update. A prospective, randomised, double-masked study. *Eye.* 1993;7:584–590.

45. Campos M, Abed HM, McDonnell PJ. Topical fluorometholone reduces stromal inflammation after photorefractive keratectomy. *Ophthalmic Surg.* 1993; 24:654–657.

46. Fitzsimmons TD, Fagerholm P, Tengroth B. Steroid treatment of myopic regression: acute refractive and topographic changes in excimer photorefractive keratectomy patients. *Cornea.* 1993;12:358–361.

47. Sher NA, Frantz JM, Talley AR, et al. Topical diclofenac in the treatment of ocular pain after excimer photorefractive keratectomy. *Refract Corneal Surg.* 1993;9:425–436.

48. David T, Serdarevic O, Savoldelli M, et al. Comparison of the effects of steroidal and non-steroidal antiinflammatory agents on corneal wound healing after photorefractive (PRK) for moderate myopia. *Invest Ophthalmol Vis Sci.* 1993;34(suppl): 705.

49. Morlet N, Gillies MC, Crouch R, Maloof A. Effect of topical interpheron alpha 2b on corneal haze after excimer laser photorefractive keratectomy in rabbits. *Refract Corneal Surg.* 1993;9:443–451.

50. Talamo JH, Gollamudi S, Green WR, et al. Modulation of corneal wound healing after excimer laser keratomileusis using topical mitomycin C and steroids. *Arch Ophthalmol.* 1991;109:1141–1146.

51. Liu JC, Steinemann TL, McDonald MB, et al. Effects of corticosteroids and mitomycin C on corneal remodeling after excimer laser photorefractive keratectomy. *Invest Ophthalmol Vis Sci.* 1991;32(suppl) Abstract.:1248.

52. Yamaguchi T, Sekiya Y, Noyori K. Effect of b-methasone, idoxuridine, and two collagen cross-linkage inhibitors on rabbit corneas after excimer laser photoablation. *Invest Ophthalmol Vis Sci.* 1991;32(suppl): 1248. Abstract.

6

Photorefractive Keratectomy for Moderate and High Myopia

Ronald Stasiuk

David Robinson

Hugh R. Taylor

Cathy McCarty

W. Bruce Jackson

Donald Johnson

Jae Ho Kim

DEFINITION

The definition of high myopia varies in the literature starting from -5.00 D[1-3] or -6.00 D[4-13] or -7.00 D[14,15] or -8.00 D[16-22] or -10.00 D[23-25] and is sometimes subdivided again at -15.00 D spherical equivalent at the spectacle plane. These arbitrary definitions are linked to a number of factors relating to the treatment of high myopia, such as poorer results achieved with high myopic corrections, including increased haze, more regression, increased risk of loss of best corrected visual acuity (BCVA), and slower recovery with surface ablation. Because of these poorer results with conventional ablation, new strategies (e.g., multizone/multipass ablations) are currently being employed. For consistency the definition in this book of moderate myopia is myopia from -6.00 to -10.00 D and of high myopia is myopia greater than -10.00 D.

PREOPERATIVE INDICATIONS AND CONTRAINDICATIONS

A careful preoperative history and a complete ocular examination are essential before treating patients for high myopia.

Indications for Treatment

- Age of 18 years or older.
- Stable spherical or cylindrical manifest refraction (change of 0.5 D or less per year from the date of the baseline exam)
- Signed informed consent document

Contraindications in Patients with Moderate/High Myopia

- Progressive myopia
- Stable myopia leaving less than 300 μm of corneal stroma after ablation
- Keratoconus (may be a cause of high myopia and/or astigmatism) with thin corneas
- Unstable keratometry readings
- Untreated retinal pathology (e.g., peripheral breaks)
- Less than 1 month since treatment of other eye for more than -10 D or less than 1 week for -6 D to -9.99 D.

Compared with low myopia, there has been a higher retreatment rate of patients with moderate and high myopia (13% for moderate myopia and 19% for high myopia versus 5% for low myopia on

VisX laser[26]), higher frequency of loss of one and two lines of BCVA, a lower percentage of patients gaining unaided 20/20 and 20/40 vision, and a higher percentage of patients with corneal haze.[26]

TECHNIQUES

Early techniques using small optic zones resulted in significant haze with regression, as reported by Seiler and Buratto, using the Summit laser systems. The zone sizes used were as small as 3.5 mm.[27,28] More recently, several techniques have evolved to reduce haze and regression, using multiple and larger optic zones with better edge tapering using multizones. Another purpose has been to achieve smoother surface ablation by limiting the amount of correction per pass and doing multiple passes.

Pop and Aras[29] published a comprehensive study using their original technique of multipass, multizone photorefractive keratectomy (PRK). Their idea was to reduce the depth of ablation further by using up to seven multiple zones, ranging from 3.50 to 6.00 mm, and single or multiple passes for each single zone, with a maximum correction of 4.00 D per zone. They also emphasized the use of more ablation in the smaller zones. These principles provided several clinical benefits:

- Fewer central islands by allowing more passes over the central zone
- Better centration, as the beam is recentered with each pass
- Less haze and regression with initial surgery
- Equilibration of surface temperature
- Smoother ablation bed due to superimposed zones
- Reduced depth of ablation
- More tapered edge
- Better clinical results.

A technique developed by Donald Johnson using the VisX 20/20 laser is a method of laser epithelial removal called *transepithelial ablation.*[30]

The scanning slit excimer lasers, such as the Meditec MEL-60, the Nidek EC-5000 and the Chiron Technolas 117, employ varying optic zones for correction of moderate and high myopia, with

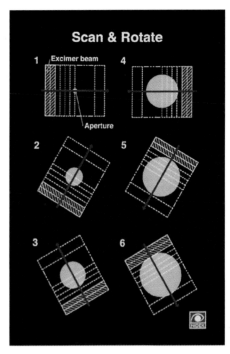

Fig. 6.1. Example of scanning laser system in which a linear-shaped laser beam sweeps the corneal surface in six directions each cycle, homogenizing the peaks and valleys which typify excimer-generated ultraviolet light energy. (Courtesy of Nidek Technologies Inc., Gamagori, Japan).

large transitional or blend zones. Potential benefits of scanning laser systems (Fig. 6.1) include reduction of intraoperative rise of corneal tissue temperature (Fig. 6.2) and reduction of acoustical shockwaves.

Using the Aesculap-Meditec Mel-60 laser, Menezo et al.[31] reported an ablation with an optical zone diameter of 5 mm and a tapered transition zone extending to 7 mm. Current optic zones used with Nidek lasers are shown in Table 6.1.

RESULTS OF TREATMENT WITH VARIOUS LASERS

Summit Excimer UV 200 Laser

Buratto and Ferrari[28] in Italy reported early experience with the Summit Excimer UV 200 laser. They

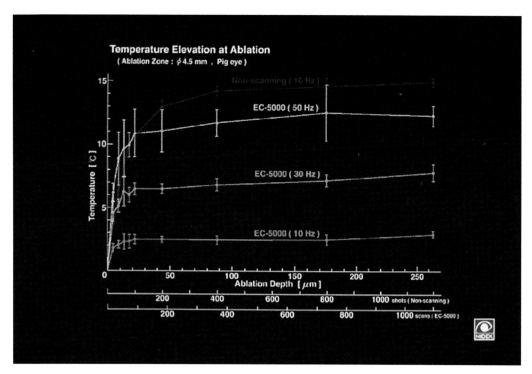

Fig. 6.2. The temperature elevation of the corneal surface with scanning is lower than that with non-scanning. (Courtesy of Nidek Technologies Inc., Gamagori, Japan).

Table 6.1. Optical and Transition Zones used with the Nidek EC-5000 Laser

Myopia Correction	Optical Zone (mm)	Transition Zone (mm)
−0.50 to −8.00 D	5.5	7.0
−8.00 to −11.00 D	5.0	6.5
−11.00 to −15.00 D	4.5	6.0

studied 40 eyes in 37 patients, correcting myopia from −6.00 D to −10.00 D over a 2-year period. PRK results showed that 35% of patients achieved a final refractive outcome within ± 1 D; 72% showed significant regression after 6 months, with 84% having corneal haze exceeding +1.

Buratto and Ferrari used single ablation zones between 3.9 and 4.5 mm in diameter, an older technique that results in significant postoperative haze and myopic regression with high-myopia PRK.[28] This was confirmed by similar reports by Gartry et al.,[32] Machat and Tayfour,[5] Shimizu et al.,[10] and Murta et al.,[13] using the Summit laser.

The erodable mask delivery system was incorporated into the laser optical hardware pathway by Summit Technology in the Apex Plus laser after initial trials with a mask contact lens showed poor results. Carones et al.[33] from Italy presented results with an initial series of 58 eyes using this system with 6-month results. Mean myopic correction was −5.96 ± 2.00 DS (range, −0.50 to −10.50 D) utilizing multizone software with three zones of ablation: 5.0, 6.0, and 6.5 mm. At 6 months, the mean refractive error achieved was +0.83 ± 0.88 D; 89% of the best cases had uncorrected vision of 20/25 or better. Any associated astigmatism was treated sequentially after correction of myopia using the appropriate mask. This technique appears to pro-

Table 6.2. Results of Excimer Laser Surgery for Moderate and High Myopia Employing the Summit Laser

Reference	Laser Model	No. of Eyes	Length of Follow-up Period (months)	Size of Ablation (Zones)(mm)
Gartry[32] (1992)	Excimed UV 200	a. 20 b. 20 c. 20	12	4.0
Kim[14] (1993)	Excimed UV 200	67	12	5.0
Machat[5] (1993)	Excimed UV 200	28	3–16	5.0
Buratto[6] (1993)	Excimed UV200	40	24	Single 4.3 to 4.9
Rogers[24] (1994)	Excimed UV 200 LA	27	3–16	3.6 to 4.5 and 5.0
Kim[42] (1994)	Excimed UV 200	19	6–14	2 zones: 4.5 5.0
Carones[33] (1995)	Apex Plus	58	6	3 zones: 5.0 6.0 6.5

vide good initial results, with no significant regression. However, longer-term follow-up and treatment of moderate and high myopia need to be carefully evaluated.[34] Published results of Summit excimer laser surgery for moderate and high myopia are shown in Table 6.2.

VisX Laser
Melbourne Excimer Laser Group Results–20/20B
With the VisX 20/20 excimer laser with V2.7 software, treatments for myopia of more than −5 D spherical equivalent (SE) and 10 D SE or less used two zones (5 and 6 mm), and treatments of myopia

Definition of Myopia (D)	Percent Within 1 D/2 D Target	Percent 20/40 Uncorrected	Percent Loss ≥2 Lines BCVA
a. >−5.00 b. >−6.00 c. >−7.00	a. 50%/NA b. 40%/NA c. 20%/NA	a. 63% b. 63% c. 25%	3% of all degrees of myopia
−7.25 to −13.50	52%/NA	63%	18%
−6.00 to −8.75	61%/93%	68%	0%
−6.00 to −10.00	35%/NA	N/A	40%
−10.25 to −20.50	75% at 12 mo/NA	N/A	3/7 eyes with 12 mo follow-up
−7.00 to −13.50	N/A	67%	11% decrease in BCVA
−0.50 to −10.50	N/A	89% 20/25 or better	N/A

exceeding −10.00 D used three zones (4.5, 5.0, and 6.00 mm). Myopic correction was equally divided among the zones.

Twenty-seven ophthalmologists in the Melbourne Excimer Laser Group reported results after 12 months of follow-up on 189 moderate myopes (−5.01 to −10.00 D) and 41 high myopes (exceeding −10.00 D). The percentage of moderate myopes within ± 1.00 D and ± 2.00 D of emmetropia at 12 months was 57% and 90%, respectively; corresponding results for high myopes were 39% and 56%. At 12 months, 25% of the moderate myopes had uncorrected vision of 20/20 or better, 71% had 20/40, and 87% had 20/60. Correspondingly, 2% of high myopes had uncorrected of 20/20, 27% had 20/40, and 54% had 20/60.

With BCVA at 12 months, 96% of moderate myopes and 68% of high myopes had 20/20 or better versus 97% for moderate myopes and 78% for high myopes preoperatively. Eight percent of moderate myopes and 22% of high myopes lost two or more lines of BCVA at 12 months. High myopes were significantly more likely to lose BCVA ($\chi = 0.08$, $p = .008$).

Mean corneal haze peaked at 1 month for moderate myopes and at 3 months for high myopes postoperatively. Severe haze in anterior corneal stroma ≥grade 2 was present in 4% of moderate myopes and 2% of high myopes. Results are summarized in Table 6.3A.

VisX Multipass, Multizone PRK–20/20B

Pop and Aras[29] used a VisX 20/20 laser at two sites, one with V2.7 software and the other with V4.01 software which incorporated pretreatment. Of 315 eyes treated, 105 had moderate myopia (−6.00 to −10.00 D) and 40 had high myopia (−10.00 to −27.00 D); the rest had lower myopia. At 6 months, 95.5% of low myopes, 84.8% of moderate myopes, and 59.5% of high myopes were within ±1.00 D of emmetropia. These percentages increased to 100% of low myopes, 91.3% of moderate myopes, and 74.8% of high myopes within ±2.00 DS of the intended spherical correction.

Unaided vision of 20/40 or better was 92.0% and 60% in the moderate- and high-myopia groups, respectively. Unaided vision of 20/25 was 75% and 25.7% in both groups, respectively. Mean corneal haze at 1 month was similar for all treatment subgroups. At 6 months, haze values were 0.14, 0.35, and 0.59 for the low-, moderate-, and high-myopia groups, respectively. A control group treated with the one-pass multizone technique had a significantly higher mean haze value.

Loss of two lines or more of BCVA was significantly lower than in other reported series, with only 2% of moderate myopes and 6% of high myopes being affected. At 6 months, 84.8% of moderate myopes and 59.5% of high myopes were within ±1 D of intended correction. Results are summarized in Table 6.3A.

VisX Transepithelial Multipass, Multizone PRK–20/20B

The development of the transepithelial, multipass, multizone technique by Johnson has been a gradual process that is still being refined and standardized. The method of removing the epithelium with the laser is performed by observing the epithelium disappear under low illumination. As the epithelial tissue is ablated, a vapor fluorescence can be observed. When all of the coloration is gone, Bowman's membrane has been reached. Using the initial technique of Johnson, the nature of the VisX 20/20 laser beam and V2.7 software caused the periphery of the ablation to absorb more energy, inducing a curvature change on the corneal surface. The induced convexity was estimated to be equal to 1 D which was incorporated into the multipass multizone nomogram of Johnson. In 1996 the technique was refined to remove the epithelium so that it ablated uniformly without the induced curvature change. This involved doing a PRK treatment on the surface of the epithelium to compensate for the greater peripheral absorption, and then proceeding in phototherapeutic kertectomy (PTK) mode to remove the remaining tissue. The results of Johnson and coworkers using personalized nomograms with the V2.7 software are listed in Table 6.3B.

VisX Transepithelial Single Pass, Multizone PRK–Star C

Jackson and collaborators developed the transepithelial PRK technique using the STAR laser that incorporated the Vision Key version 4 software with semi-automated system calibration and concentration of laser pulses in the central 2.5 mm to prevent central islands. Epithelial removal is accomplished by focusing the laser on the surface of the epithelium and performing a PTK ablation of 45 μm at 6 mm with the machine aligned to the center of the pupil. After 45 μm of epithelium are removed, a Paton spatula is used to remove any fluid and debris from the ablation area. The edge of the spatula serves as a windshield wiper blade to achieve uniform hydration of the surface. The surface is not wiped with a Weckcell sponge. The ablation is performed using a single pass of the standardized VisX multizone program. For correction of 6–10 diopters, two zones are used (5.5 mm and 6 mm). For correction of over 10 diopters, 3 zones are used

Table 6.3A. Results of Excimer Laser Surgery for Moderate and High Myopia Employing the VisX 20/20 B Laser

Reference	Laser Model	No. of Eyes	Length of Follow-up Period (months)	Size of Ablation (Zones) (mm)	Amount of Myopia (SE)	Percent within 1 D/ 2 D Target	Percent ≥(20/40)/(20/20) Uncorrected	Percent Loss ≥2 Lines BCVA
Carson[3] (1995)	20/20 B	a. 194	6	2 or 3 zones: 4.5, 5.0,	a. −5.00 to −10.00	a. 67%/89%	a. 71%/NA	a. 13%
		b. 53		6.0	b. −10.25 to −21.00	b. 38%/49%	b. 31%/NA	b. 13%
Melbourne Group (1996)	20/20 B	a. 189	12	2 zones: 5.0 and 6.0	a. −5.00 to −10.00	a. 57%/90%	a. 71%/NA	a. 8%
		b. 41	12	3 zones: 4.5, 5.0, 6.0	b. −10.25 to −21.00	b. 39%/56%	b. 27%/NA	b. 22%
Pop[29] (1995)	20/20 B	145	6	Mz/Mp* 3.5 to 6.0		20%/25%		
		a. 105			a. −6.00 to −10.00	a. 84%/91%	a. 92%/75%	a. 2%
		b. 40			b. −10.00 to −27.00	b. 59%/74%	b. 60%/25.7%	b. 6%
Aron-Rosa[15] (1995)	20/20 B	37	6	5.0 to 6.0	>−7.00	67%/74%	64%/62%	2.8%

*Multizone/multipass.

Table 6.3B. Results of Laser Surgery for Moderate and High Myopia using the Transepithelial Multipass-Multizone Technique

Reference	Laser Model	No. of Eyes	Preop Myopia Mean ± SD	Follow-up Period (mo)	Type of Ablation	Definition of Myopia(D)	Percent Within 0.5/1 D/2 D Target	Percent 20/25 20/40 UCVA	Loss ≥2 Lines BCVA	Gain ≥2 Lines BCVA
Johnson (1996)	VisX 20/20B	155	−7.12 ± 1.23 D	6	Transepithelial multipass/ multizone	−6 to −9.87	83.5% 76.1% 96.8%	58.1% 81.3%	1.9% (3 patients)	1.3%
Johnson (1996)	VisX 20/20B	36	−11.21 ± 1.22 D	6	Transepithelial multipass/ multizone	−10 to −14.74	47.2% 52.8% 83.3%	44.5% 66.8%	2.8% (1 patient)	5.6%
Johnson (1996)	VisX 20/20B	3	−16.96 ± 0.44 D	6	Transepithelial multipass/ multizone	>−15	66.7% 66.7% 100.0%	0 33.3%	—	33.3% (1 patient)

(5mm, 5.5 mm, and 6 mm). Modifications in the STAR include reduction of the blowers to decrease airflow around the eye, reduction of lighting to prevent dehydration and improved visualization of the pupil throughout the entire procedure for high myopia using oblique illumination and a ring illuminator for focus. Jackson also has incorporated pauses of 10–15 seconds between treatments at the different zones to allow the patient to relax and to cool the cornea.

Recent clinical results achieved by Jackson and coworkers[35] with the STAR excimer laser system from VisX appear to have provided superior results in 60 eyes, with mean preoperative myopia of −5.42 D (range, −1.50 to −19.25 DS) and follow-up periods ranging from 6 months to 18 months. At 6 months, 20/25 or better uncorrected vision was obtained in 83% and 33% in the −6.00 to 10.00 D subgroup and the over −10.00 D subgroup, respectively, using the Vision Key software with the STAR laser.[35]

Comparing different models and softwares of VisX, Agapitos and collaborators[36] reported that in subgroups with myopia of 6.00 to −10.00 D, 33% achieved 20/25 or better uncorrected vision with the V2.7/2.9 software compared to 65% with the Vision Key software on the VisX 20/20 B laser and 83% with the STAR laser. Results are listed in Tables 6.3C and 6.3D.

Aesculap-Meditec MEL-60 Excimer Laser

Menezo and coworkers[31] presented a study in 1995 using the Aesculap-Meditec MEL-60 excimer laser. A total of 133 eyes of 103 patients with myopia, ranging from −6.00 to −22.00 D, were treated using the scanning laser. Two groups were compared: group A, with a mean preoperative refraction of −9.59 ± 1.79 D (−6.00 D to −12.00 D, 88 eyes), and group B, with a mean preoperative refraction of −14.69 ±5.27 D (−12.50 to −22.00 D, 45 eyes).

Group A had a mean postoperative refraction of −0.29 ± 1.47 D at 1 month, −0.85 ± 1.68 D at 3 months, −1.17 ± 2.04 D at 6 months, and −0.56 ± 0.74 D at 1 year. Anterior stromal corneal haze peaked at 1 month. Haze did not significantly reduce the BCVA. In group A, 78% of the eyes were within ±1 D of emmetropia, with no cases of decreased visual acuity.

In contrast, group B showed a mean postoperative refraction of −1.34 ± 2.02 D at 1 month, −0.76 ± 2.08 D at 3 months, −3.88 ± 2.32 D at 6 months, and −5.50 ± 5.00 D at 1 year. In this group, 37% of the eyes were within ±1 D of emmetropia; three patients (6.06%) lost two lines of BCVA (preoperatively, all were below −15.00 D).

Because of the poorer predictability of results in group B, with a wider standard deviation, greater haze and regression, and significant loss of BCVA, the authors suggested that further improvement in the surface ablation technique was needed or that alternative treatment should be instituted.[31]

In a prospective multicenter study, Ditzen et al.[9] treated 325 eyes between 1990 and 1991 with the Aesculap-Meditec MEL-60 excimer laser. High-myopia patients were divided into two extra groups: group 3, between −10.25 and −15.00 D (87 eyes), and group 4, with more than −15.00 D (48 eyes), with a 6- to 12-month follow-up period. Maximum attempted spherical correction in both groups was −13.00 D. The maximum optical zone on the cornea was 5.00 mm. Average regression in group 3 was −2.00 D at 12 months, which appeared to be leveling off. In group 4 it was −5.00 D and progressing.

The authors concluded that ablation depth is the main factor in regression after PRK for myopia. Also, the shorter the reepithelialization time, the less likely it is that haze and regression will occur.

Although this was an early study, with a single zone of treatment and without a larger transitional zone or multizone, the results appeared to be encouraging for myopia between −10.25 and −15.00 D. At 12 months, mean refraction was −2 ± 2.8 D.

Published results of Meditec excimer laser surgery for high myopia are shown in Table 6.4.

Nidek Laser

The Nidek EC-5000 laser utilizes ablation zones up to 6.5 mm and continuously blends ablated and unablated areas in an area up to 9.0 mm. Rich and collaborators treated 100 myopes with the Nidek (EC-5000) laser; 73% had low myopia (below −6.00 D), 25% had moderate myopia (−6.01 to −9.99 D), and 2% had high myopia (−10.00 to 15.00 D). No patients had haze of more than +1.

Table 6.3C. Results of Excimer Laser Surgery for Moderate Myopia Employing the VisX 20/20B and STAR Excimer Lasers

Laser Model	No. of Eyes	Length of Follow-up Period (months)	Size of Ablation (mm)	Definition of Myopia (D)
VisX 20/20B 2.72 Jackson (1996)	1. 20	1.6	5.5–6.0	1. −6 to −10
	2. 22	2. 12		2. −6 to −10
	3. 26	3. 18		3. −6 to −10
VisX 20/20B Vision Key Jackson (1996)	1. 70	1. 6	5.5–6.0	1. −6 to −10
	2. 48	2. 12		2. −6 to −10
	3. 32	3. 18		3. −6 to −10
VisX Star Model C Jackson (1996)	1. 25	1. 6	5.5–6.0	1. −6 to −10
	2. 10	2. 12		2. −6 to −10
	3. 4	3. 18		3. −6 to −10

Preoperative Myopia (D) and Range	Postoperative Myopia (D) and Range	Attained Refractions (+0.5D, 1D, 2D)	UCVA ≥20/20 20/25, 20/40	Loss of 1, 2, >2 Lines BCVA
1. −7.51 ± 1.02 (−9.88 to −6.13)	1. −0.21 ± 0.95 (−1.75 TO +2.25)	1. a) 65.0% b) 80.0% c) 100.0%	1. a) 19.0% b) 33.3% c) 90.5%	1. a) 33.3% b) 14.3% c) 0.0%
2. −7.38 ± 1.00 (−9.88 to −6.13)	2. −0.30 ± 0.69 (−1.75 to +0.88)	2. a) 63.6% b) 86.3% c) 99.9%	2. a) 43.5% b) 69.6% c) 87.0%	2. a) 21.4% b) 4.3% c) 0.0%
3. −7.59 ± 1.00 (−9.88 to −6.13)	3. −0.43 ± 0.54 (−2.00 to +0.63)	3. a) 3.1% b) 96.2% c) 100.0%	3. a) 38.5% b) 69.2% c) 96.2%	3. a) 30.8% b) 7.7% c) 3.8%
1. −7.63 ± 1.13 (−10.00 to −6.13)	1. −0.45 ± 1.38 (−5.75 to +1.75)	1. a) 54.3% b) 77.2% c) 100.0%	1. a) 49.3% b) 62.0% c) 81.7%	1. a) 20.5% b) 5.5% c) 5.5%
2. −7.59 ± 0.93 (−9.50 to −6.13)	2. −0.23 ± 0.92 (−4.63 to +1.00)	2. a) 58.3% b) 91.6% c) 99.9%	2. a) 58.3% b) 70.8% c) 93.8%	2. a) 18.4% b) 0.0% c) 2.0%
3. −7.57 ± 1.03 (−9.88 to −6.13)	3. −0.32 ± 0.58 (−1.50 to +0.75)	3. a) 68.8% b) 84.4% c) 100.0%	3. a) 46.9% b) 81.3% c) 100.0%	3. a) 18.8% b) 6.3% c) 0.0%
1. −7.81 ± 1.10 (−10.00 to −6.25)	1. +0.27 ± 0.63 (−0.75 to +1.50)	1. a) 64.0% b) 84.0% c) 100.0%	1. a) 52.0% b) 68.0% c) 92.0%	1. a) 8.0% b) 12.0% c) 0.0%
2. −7.39 ± 0.99 (−8.88 to −6.25)	2. +0.48 ± 0.68 (−0.50 to +1.75)	2. a) 50.0% b) 90.0% c) 100.0%	2. a) 54.5% b) 63.6% c) 100.0%	2. a) 0.0% b) 0.0% c) 0.0%
3. −7.44 ± 1.2 (−9.00 to −6.25)	3. +0.09 ± 0.45 (−0.50 to +0.50)	3. a) 100.0% b) 100.0% c) 100.0%	3. a) 50.0% b) 75.0% c) 100.0%	3. a) 0.0% b) 0.0% c) 0.0%

Table 6.3D. Results of Excimer Laser Surgery for High Myopia Employing the VisX 20/20B and STAR Excimer Lasers

Laser Model	No. of Eyes	Length of Follow-up Period (months)	Size of Ablation (mm)	Definition of Myopia (D)
VisX 20/20B 2.72 Jackson (1996)	1. 11	1. 6	5.0, 5.5, 6.0	1. >−10
	2. 11	2. 12		2. >−10
	3. 10	3. 18		3. >−10
VisX 20/20B Vision Key Jackson (1996)	1. 24	1. 6	5.5, 5.5, 6.0	1. >−10
	2. 19	2. 12		2. >−10
	3. 9	3. 18		3. >−10
VisX Star Model C Jackson (1996)	1. 7	1. 6	5,0, 5.5, 6.0	1. >−10
	2. 6	2. 12		2. >−10
	3. 2	3. 18		3. >−10

Preoperative Myopia (D) and Range	Postoperative Myopia (D) and Range	Attained Refractions (+0.5D, 1D, 2D)	UCVA ≥20/20 20/25, 20/40	Loss of 1, 2, >2 Lines BCVA
1. −13.41 ± 3.74 (−22.50 to −10.13)	1. −1.64 ± 2.66 (−9.13 to +1.13)	1. a) 27.3% b) 36.4% c) 100.0%	1. a) 25.0% b) 33.3% c) 58.3%	1. a) 41.7% b) 16.7% c) 0.0%
2. −13.56 ± 3.76 (−22.50 to −10.13)	2. −2.42 ± 2.85 (−8.50 to +1.00)	2. a) 27.3% b) 45.5% c) 100.0%	2. a) 18.2% b) 18.2% c) 54.5%	2. a) 63.6% b) 0.0% c) 9.1%
3. −12.66 ± 2.43 (−16.00 to −10.13)	3. −2.23 ± 2.63 (−8.75 to +0.00)	3. a) 40.0% b) 40.0% c) 100.0%	3. a) 22.2% b) 44.4% c) 55.6%	3. a) 40.0% b) 20.0% c) 0.0%
1. −12.94 ± 3.45 (−21.50 to −10.25)	1. −0.52 ± 1.39 (−3.25 to −4.38)	1. a) 33.3% b) 66.6% c) 100.0%	1. a) 12.0% b) 36.0% c) 80.0%	1. a) 12.0% b) 12.0% c) 0.0%
2. −12.13 ± 2.10 (−17.13 to −10.25)	2. −0.28 ± 1.09 (−3.00 to +1.88)	2. a) 73.7% b) 73.7% c) 100.0%	2. a) 20.0% b) 30.0% c) 85.0%	2. a) 10.0% b) 30.0% c) 0.0%
3. −12.43 ± 2.62 (−17.13 to −10.25)	3. −0.79 ± 0.64 (−1.50 to +0.00)	3. a) 55.6% b) 66.7% c) 100.0%	3. a) 30.0% b) 50.0% c) 100.0%	3. a) 20.0% b) 20.0% c) 0.0%
1. −11.79 ± 1.12 (−13.79 to −10.63)	1. +0.50 ± 0.91 (−1.00 to +1.50)	1. a) 42.9% b) 42.9% c) 100.0%	1. a) 0.0% b) 14.3% c) 100.0%	1. a) 28.6% b) 0.0% c) 14.3%
2. −12.81 ± 3.65 (−20.13 to −10.63)	2. −0.88 ± 0.89 (−0.00 to +2.25)	2. a) 16.7% b) 66.7% c) 100.0%	2. a) 0.0% b) 16.7% c) 83.3%	2. a) 0.0% b) 33.3% c) 0.0%
3. −11.31 ±0.80 (−11.88 to −10.75)	3. +0.38 ± 0.53 (−0.00 to +0.75)	3. a) 0.0% b) 100.0% c) 100.0%	3. a) 50.0% b) 100.0% c) 100.0%	3. a) 0.0% b) 0.0% c) 0.0%

Table 6.4. Results of Excimer Laser Surgery for Moderate and High Myopia Employing the Meditec Laser

Reference	Laser Model	No. of Eyes	Length of Follow-up Period (months)	Size of Ablation (Zones) (mm)	Definition of High Myopia (D)	Percent within 1 D/ 2 D Target	Percent 20/40 Uncorrected	Percent Loss ≥2 Lines BCVA
Menezo[31] (1995)	MEL 60	a. 133 b. 88 c. 45	12	Tapered 5.0 to 7.0	−6.00 to −22.00 a. −6.00 to −12.00 b. −12.00 to −22.00	± 1D a. 78% b. 37%	26%(b)	3%

BCVA was within ± one line of the preoperative level in 100% of myopes at 6 months after treatment. Uncorrected vision of 20/20 or better occurred in 66.7% of patients, with vision of 20/25 or better occurred in 71.7% at 6 months postoperatively. All patients were within ±2.00 D of emmetropia. The mean refractive error was −0.10 D at 6 months.[37]

Results of Nidek excimer laser surgery for moderate and high myopia are shown in Table 6.5.

Schwind-Keratom Excimer Laser

Storch et al.[38] presented a pilot study of 25 patients with more than 6 months of follow-up using the Schwind-Keratom excimer laser in Israel. The mean preoperative SE was −5.70 ± 3.17 D (range, −1.75 to 13.00 D), which reduced to a mean postoperative result of −0.69 ± 0.88 D (range, 0 to 3.00 D); nine eyes were overcorrected from +0.35 to +2.75 D (mean, +0.92 ± 0.91 D).

The optical performance and quality of the cornea, as measured by the corneal indices on topography, stabilized by the second month. Ninety-two percent of patients had uncorrected vision of 20/40 or better. No patients had any clinically significant loss of BCVA.[38]

REGRESSION

Recent studies show that high and even low myopia may regress in a small percentage of patients after 2 years. Havid et al.[39] followed 681 eyes for more than 24 months after PRK treatment by the Aesculap-Meditec C excimer laser in Israel. They found that 40 eyes (5.8%) continued to regress after 2 years; 40% of this group had low preoperative myopia up to −6.00 D, with an average regression of −0.55 D in 18–24 months and −0.42 D in 24–30 months after treatment. As expected, 60% of the patients had high myopia between −6.00 and −12.00 D. This group regressed by −0.57 D in 18–24 months and by −0.18 D in 24–30 months, suggesting that remodeling and healing, as well as regression, cannot be fully predicted in some patients. Perhaps with the use of new algorithms, better scanning systems, multizones, or tapered transition zones, the results may improve.[40]

Medical treatment for haze and regression may eventually help improve the results of refractive surgery. Gillies et al.[34] in a prospective, double-blind, randomized pilot study of 30 patients, concluded that topical interferon alpha 2b (Schering Plough) gives a more predictable refractive result, with less regression and better contrast sensitivity after excimer laser PRK. A larger study may provide more significant results. The VisX 20/20 excimer laser was used at the Melbourne Excimer Laser Centre in Australia.

POSTOPERATIVE MANAGEMENT

First Week after PRK

Immediately after PRK, the following medications are applied as a statim dose: 2% homatropine, 0.1% diclofenac (Voltaren), and 1% chloramphenicol or tobramycin. Then, either a patch is applied or a dis-

Table 6.5. Results of Laser Surgery for Moderate and High Myopia Employing the Nider Laser

Reference	Laser Model	No. of Eyes	Preop Myopia Mean ± SD	Follow-up Period (mo)	Size of Ablation	Definition of High Myopia (D)	Percent Within 0.5/1 D/2 D Target	Percent 20/25 20/40 UCVA	Loss ≥2 Lines BCVA	Gain ≥2 Lines BCVA
World Nidek 9 Centers (1996)	Nidek	65	−7.21 ± 1.45	6	Up to 6.5 mm	−6 to −10	55.6% 71.4% 84.1%	64.6% 84.6%	6.1%	12.4%
World Nidek 9 Centers (1996)	Nidek	28	−9.59 ± 1.51	6	Up to 6.5 mm	>−10	7.1% 14.3% 42.9%	25.0% 46.4%	3.5%	17.9%
Gimbel (1996)	Nidek EC-5000	81	−9.28 ± 1.4	6		>−8	54.3% 92.6% 97.5%	79.0% 91.0%	2.5%	4.9%
Gimbel (1996)	Nidek EC-5000	12	−9.44 ± 1.14	12		>−8	25.0% 41.7% 91.7%	33.3% 75.0%	0	0

posable soft contact lens is used for 48 hr and removed. During this time, topical antibiotics are continued without nonsteroidal anti-inflammatory drugs or corticosteroids until the epithelium is healed, usually for 48–72 hr. Oral analgesics, hypnotics, and antiemetics are prescribed if required. The patient is evaluated regularly until reepithelialization occurs.

Subsequent Weeks

Topical lubricants are used, and steroids are used routinely in a reducing dose over 1 to 4 months. Stasiuk prefers to use steroids only if regression or haze develops. The patient is evaluated at 1, 3, 6, and 12 months.

At the Melbourne Excimer Center the second eye is treated within a week if myopia is less than −10.00 D or after 1 month if myopia is greater than −10.00 D, and only when both the patient and the ophthalmologist are happy with the result of the first PRK. However, there is considerable variation among centers in deciding when the second eye should be treated.

COMPLICATIONS

These are summarized in the Table 6.6. The most common problems are haze, regression which may be associated with haze, significant loss of BCVA, and secondary steroid glaucoma.

HIGH MYOPIA: MANAGEMENT OF COMPLICATIONS AFTER PRK

1. *Glaucoma* normally occurs secondary to prolonged use of topical steroids in a steroid responder. If steroids must be used, ocular hypotensives such as beta blockers may be necessary, with close supervision, since high myopes are at risk for optic nerve damage. Glaucoma usually reverses on cessation of topical steroids.

2. *Retreatment* is frequent for higher levels of preoperative myopia and is indicated for significant haze combined with regression. See Chapter 8 for further information.

   a. Myopic regression without much haze may respond to a prompt short course of topical steroids, which may be gradually tapered.

   b. In patients who do not react to steroids, retreatment PRK is considered. The patients need to be off steroids for at least 3 months, with stable refraction and sufficient corneal thickness, so that a minimum of 300 μm remains after retreatment in order to avoid ectasia. No retreatment is done before 6 months after PRK.

   c. Retreatment is performed with transepithelial laser ablation with full refractive correction PRK.

   d. Cases with regression and significant haze respond less favourably.

Table 6.6. Complications of PRK in Moderate and High Myopia

Myopia	Moderate (−5.1 to −10.00 D)	High (>−10.00 D)
Loss ≥2 lines BCVA	8%	22%
Glaucoma	7%	10%
Monocular diplopia	0.4%	1.7%
Haloes	0.8%	0
Microbial keratitis	0.4%	0
Iritis	0	1.7%
Retreatment	10%	27%
Hyperopia >1D	3%	5%

Source: Data from the Melbourne Excimer Laser Group (1996).

e. Pop and Aras[40] reported on 83 eyes treated for myopic regression with the VisX 20/20 excimer laser. The first group of 50 eyes had little haze (+1 D or less), with a mean sphere of −2.63 D before retreatment, which reduced to −0.23 D (± 0.5 D) at 1 year. At 6 months, 94% of the eyes were within ±1.00 D of the intended correction, the mean haze being +0.2. The second group of 33 eyes had marked haze, with a mean of +2.7. The mean sphere was −3.49 D, which corrected to +0.31 D (± 0.93 D) at 1 year after retreatment. Only 54% of the eyes were within ±1.00 D of the intended correction at 6 months and had a mean haze of +1.2. Pop and Aras recommended that retreatment in this group be postponed and that only half of the refraction be corrected.[40]

f. PRK during pregnancy is another cause of severe haze and regression with PRK.[41] Postmenopausal women taking hormone replacement therapy have significantly lower uncorrected visual acuity than control groups.[41]

3. *Hyperopia*

a. Overcorrection generally resolves but may take considerable time, especially in higher myopia PRK.

b. There is less transient hyperopia with the new multipass/multizone techniques and with scanning lasers.

c. In the early postoperative period, topical steroids should be withheld. The use of a temporary hyperopic disposable soft contact lens may avoid aniseikonia or presbyopic symptoms.

d. Permanent overcorrection may be treated either with the holmium: YAG laser or the hyperopic PRK.

4. *Loss of BCVA*

a. This is one of the main concerns with PRK treatment for high myopia. The most common cause is irregular epithelial healing and central islands.

b. Severe haze in the anterior stroma is often associated with regression, and may con-

tinue for 1–3 years after PRK and reduce the BCVA.

c. Very flat corneas (less than 33 D) after PRK can also result in aspheric aberrations.

d. Recent improvements in technique, better software, and the use of scanning lasers have reduced the incidence of significant loss of BCVA. Pop and Aras,[29] using the multipass/multizone approach for cases with more than −10 D, found that two or more Snellen's lines of BCVA were lost in 5.4% of patients compared to our Melbourne results of 22% when an earlier three-zone V2.7 software technique was used.

REFERENCES

1. Taylor HR, Guest CS, Kelly P, et al. Comparison of excimer laser treatment of astigmatism and myopia. *Arch Ophthalmol.* 1993;111:1621–1626.

2. Taylor HR, Kelly P, Alpins N. Excimer laser correction of myopic astigmatism. *J Cataract Refract Surg.* 1994;20:243–251.

3. Carson CA, Taylor HR. Excimer laser treatment of high and extreme myopia. *Arch Ophthalmol.* 1995; 113:431–436.

4. Sher NA, Chen V, Bowers RA, et al. The use of the 193-nm excimer laser for myopic photorefractive keratectomy in sighted eyes. A multicenter study. *Arch Ophthalmol.* 1991;109:1525–1530.

5. Machat JJ, Tayfour F. Photorefractive keratectomy for myopia: preliminary results in 147 eyes. *Refract Corneal Surg.* 1993;9:S16–S19.

6. Buratto L, Ferrari M. Photorefractive keratectomy for myopia from 6.00D to 10.00D. *Refract Corneal Surg.* 1993;9:S34–S36.

7. Salorio DP, Costa J, Larena C, et al. Photorefractive keratectomy for myopia: 18 month results in 178 eyes. *Refract Corneal Surg.* 1993;9:S108–S110.

8. Les Jardins SL, Auclin F, Roman S, et al. Results of photorefractive keratectomy on 63 myopic eyes with six months minimum follow-up. *J Cataract Refract Surg.* 1994;20:228–238.

9. Ditzen K, Anschütz T, Schröder E. Photorefractive keratectomy to treat low, medium and high myopia: a multicenter study. *J Cataract Refract Surg.* 1994; 20:234–238.

10. Shimizu K, Amano S, Tanaka S. Photorefractive keratectomy for myopia: one year follow-up in 97 eyes. *J Cataract Refract Surg.* 1994;10:S178–S187.

11. Orssaud C, Ganem S, Binaghi M, et al. Photorefractive keratectomy in 176 eyes: one year follow-up. *J Refract Corneal Surg.* 1994;10:S199–S205.

12. Sabetti L, Spadea L, Fuecese L, et al. Measurement of corneal thickness by ultrasound after photorefractive keratectomy in high myopia. *J Refract Corneal Surg.* 1994;10:S211–S216.

13. Murta JN, Proenca R, Velze RAV, et al. Photorefractive keratectomy for myopia in 98 eyes. *J Refract Surg.* 1994;10:S231–S235.

14. Kim JH, Hahn TW, Lee YC, et al. Photorefractive keratectomy in 202 myopic eyes: one year results. *Refract Corneal Surg.* 1993;9:S11–S16.

15. Aron-Rosa DS. Clinical results of excimer laser photorefractive keratectomy: a multicenter study of 265 eyes. *J Cataract Refract Surg.* 1995;21:644–652.

16. Sher NA, Barak M, Daya S, et al. Excimer laser photorefractive keratectomy in high myopia. A multicenter study. *Arch Ophthalmol.* 1992;110:935–943.

17. Cho YS, Kim CG, Kim WB, et al. Multistep photorefractive keratectomy for high myopia. *Refract Corneal Surg.* 1993;9:S37–S41.

18. Kim JH, Hahn TW, Lee YC, et al. Clinical experience of two-step photorefractive keratectomy in 19 eyes with high myopia. *Refract Corneal Surg.* 1993;9:S44–S47.

19. Heitzmann J, Binder PS, Kassar BS, et al. The correction of high myopia using the excimer laser. *Arch Ophthalmol.* 1993;111:1627–1634.

20. Maguen E. Salz JJ, Nesburn AB, et al. Results of excimer laser photorefractive keratectomy for the correction of myopia. *Ophthalmology.* 1994;101:1548–1557.

21. Sher NA, Hardten DR, Fundingland B, et al. 193-nm excimer photorefractive keratectomy in high myopia. *Ophthalmology.* 1994;101:1575–1582.

22. Tong PPC, Kam JTK, Lam RHS, et al. Excimer laser photorefractive keratectomy for myopia: six month follow-up. *J Cataract Refract Surg.* 1995;21:150–155.

23. Dausch D, Klein R, Schröder E, et al. Excimer laser photorefractive keratectomy with tapered transition zone for high myopia. A preliminary report of six cases. *J Cataract Refract Surg.* 1993;19:590–594.

24. Rogers CM, Lawless MA, Cohen PR. Photorefractive keratectomy for myopia of more than −10 dioptres. *J Refract Corneal Surg.* 1994;10:S171–S173.

25. Krueger RR, Talamo JH, McDonald MB, et al. Clinical analysis of excimer laser photorefractive keratectomy using a multiple zone technique for severe myopia. *Am J Ophthalmol.* 1995;119:263–274.

26. Taylor HR, McCarty CA, Aldred GF. Predictability of excimer laser treatment of myopia. *Arch Ophthalmol.* 1996;114:248–251.

27. Seiler T, Derse M, Pham T. Repeated excimer laser treatment after photorefractive keratectomy. *Arch Ophthalmol.* 1992;110:1230–1233.

28. Buratto L, Ferrari M. Photorefractive keratectomy or keratomileusis with excimer laser in surgical correction of severe myopia: which technique is better? *Eur J Implant Ref Surg.* 1993;5:183–186.

29. Pop M, Aras M. Multizone/multipass photorefractive keratectomy: six month results. *J Cataract Refract Surg.* 1995;21:633–643.

30. Alio JL, Artola A, Perez-Santonja JJ. Spanish clinical experience after 5,000 consecutive PRK and LASIK cases. *A Decade of Excimer Laser Meeting.* Monaco, March 15–16.

31. Menezo JL, Martinez-Costa R, Navea A, Roig V, Cisneros A. Excimer laser photorefractive keratotomy for high myopia. *J Cataract Refract Surg.* 1995;21:393–397.

32. Gartry DS, Muir MGK, Marshall J. Excimer laser photorefractive keratectomy. 18 month follow-up. *Ophthalmology.* 1992;99:1209–1219.

33. Carones F, Venturi E, Brancato R. Compound myopic astigmatism correction using an erodable mask in-the-rail excimer laser delivery system. *ISRS Abstract.* 1995;October, pp.30–31.

34. Gillies M, Garret S, Shina S, Morlet N, et al. Topical interferon alpha 2b for fibrosis after excimer laser PRK. *RACO Abstract.* 1994;September, p. 85.

35. Jackson WB, Mintsioulis G, Agapitos P, Norton S, et al. Excimer laser PRK using the VisX STAR. *ISRS Abstract.* 1995;October, p. 37.

36. Agapitos P, Mintsoulis G, Jackson WB, et al. Excimer laser PRK: a software comparison using the Alcon VisX excimer laser. *ISRS Abstract.* 1995; October, p. 34.

37. Rich LR, MacRae SM. American experience using the Nidek EC-5000. *ISRS Abstract.* 1995;October, p. 35.

38. Storch RL, Cohen S, Reiser R. Compound myopic astigmatism PRK using an elliptical ablation technique: one year experience. *ISRS Abstract.* 1995; October, p. 31.

39. Havid D, Nemet P, Brak B, et al. How long can regression continue after PRK for myopia. *Ophthalmology*. 1995;108:102–104.

40. Pop M, Aras M. PRK retreatments due to regression with an excimer laser: a one-year follow-up. *Ophthalmology*. 1995;108:102–109A.

41. McCarty CA. Relation of hormone and menopausal status to outcomes following excimer laser photorefractive keratectomy in women. *Aust New Zealand J Ophthalmol*. In press.

42. Kim JH, Sah WJ, Hahn TW. Excimer laser surgery of ophthalmology in Korea. *27th International Congress of Ophthalmology (IOS)*. Toronto, June 26–30, 1994.

7

Prevention and Management of Complications of Photorefractive Keratectomy

David S. Gartry
Ronald Stasiuk
David Robinson

A large amount of clinical data now exists in relation to excimer laser photorefractive keratectomy (PRK) and has been reviewed in the preceding chapters. This chapter addresses further the known complications of PRK and their prevention and management.

Considerable individual variation in response to PRK exists because of differences in wound healing from patient to patient. Although the excimer laser removes corneal tissue with unprecedented precision, wound-healing factors play a major role in the subsequent variable outcome. However, while there are side effects following PRK, very few sight-threatening complications have been encountered. Nonetheless, maximum follow-up at present is about 7 years. It has been concluded provisionally from available data that for lower degrees of myopia, serious longer-term side effects such as late-onset, sight-threatening infection, corneal decompensation, or permanent, clinically significant scarring, while not impossible, are unlikely.

REGRESSION

Regression is the tendency of the treated eye to lose some of the effect of the surgery within the first few months after surgery. This is due to wound healing and is more marked in patients with high myopia. In fact, the most useful predictor of regression identified to date is the amount of preexisting myopia, although there is a correlation with age in that older patients tend to regress less. In addition, the individual variability in corneal wound healing and the incidence of complications after PRK increase as greater amounts of myopia are treated.[1-7] Individual variation, standard deviation or variance in the data, increase with attempted correction. There are even instances in early studies of high myopia treatment in which patients have regressed completely to their original level of myopia.

There are several possible explanations for this regression. The ablation zone diameter in the early studies, using lasers manufactured generally by Summit Technology, was limited by technical constraints to 4 mm. Other centers that commenced studies later used upgraded lasers and were able to utilize larger ablation zones (on average, 5 mm). Subsequently, results of a controlled trial have revealed that regression is indeed reduced, and therefore predictability improved, when a larger zone is used.[8]

There are differences between lasers produced by different manufacturers or even between identical lasers. Every effort should be made to comply with the manufacturer's recommendations with regard to calibration tests, usually performed at the outset of each treatment session. The results of these tests of ablated calibration/test filters and perspex discs carried out by the manufacturer should provide feedback to the surgeons involved, and the necessary changes to laser algorithms can be made. Uniformity of laser performance between treatment sessions and between different centers can therefore be achieved.

It is possible that geographical and racial differences may have an influence on regression, and therefore on refractive outcome and on the incidence of complications. It has been suggested that ultraviolet (UV) light exposure following PRK can have a deleterious effect on the refractive outcome. This theory has been used to explain anecdotal reports of patients who regressed disproportionately following a holiday involving high UV exposure. A small but statistically significant difference between patients treated in the winter months compared with those treated in the summer months has been shown recently. Those treated during the former period had a better refractive outcome (Stevens et al., unpublished data, poster presentation at the annual congress of the Royal College of Ophthalmologists, Birmingham, UK, 1995). Again, this is difficult to reconcile with the results of Australian groups who report universally good results in spite of the hot climate.[9,10] Further study in which actual UV exposure is monitored in the post-PRK period is required before valid conclusions can be made.

The mechanism of regression is likely to be twofold: epithelial hyperplasia and anterior stromal remodeling (Fig. 7.1). Individual variation is likely to exist in relation to both of these wound-healing elements. In addition, from early work, it was hypothesized that epithelial hyperplasia might be more influential in promoting regression when relatively small ablation zone diameters were used. This hypothesis was based on the general observation that corneal epithelium "fills" small corneal facets relatively easily following injury, leaving a smooth surface contour. With larger-diameter PRK ablation zones, and particularly with transition zones, the effect of epithelial hyperplasia is reduced.

A questionnaire survey of 182 patients from two early cohorts revealed that regression was the major cause of dissatisfaction following PRK rather than complications such as haze and loss of best corrected visual acuity (BCVA). It is also interesting that a successful outcome in the first eye is not always followed by the same result in the second eye. Patients should be made aware, therefore, that there are no guarantees that both eyes will heal in the same way. Regression is key to the continued acceptance of PRK, and it is helpful to provide guidelines for patient selection in terms of preoperative myopia. Longer-term results from centers using larger ablation zone diameters and refined algorithms are likely to endorse the current view that greater efficacy (because of less regression) is achieved with current lasers. Nevertheless, in the absence of long-term data from these newer lasers, a conservative view should be taken. It is extremely important to counsel patients carefully prior to PRK and perhaps to eliminate those with unrealistic expectations. Even in patients with lower degrees of myopia, it is not possible to guarantee a successful outcome. Several surgeons who have pioneered the technique of surface PRK state that at present, one should be cautious with treatments for more than about 6 D of myopia.[5] Retreatment for regression is discussed in the following chapter.

NIGHT HALO EFFECTS

The aspheric shape of the refracting surfaces of the human eye, principally those of the cornea and lens, acts to minimize the potentially large optical aberration that would otherwise affect the retinal image produced by such a powerful optical system (spherical aberration, coma, oblique astigmatism, curvature of field, distortion). The overall refracting power of the eye is on the order of +60 D, with the front corneal surface contributing about +48 D, or approximately 75% of the total. As stated above, the cornea is therefore one of the main candidates for alteration in refractive surgical procedures, since relatively small curvature changes result in relatively large changes in refractive status. Alteration of corneal curvature, however, is likely to change the

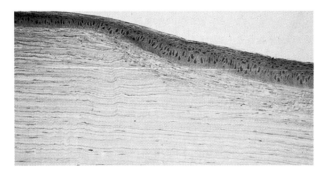

Fig. 7.1. Histopathology of cornea demonstrating regression. Note epithelial hyperplasia and anterior stromal remodeling. (Courtesy of S. J. Tuft, M.D., Moorfields Eye Hospital, London, England.)

aspheric shape of the cornea and increase optical aberration.

Following PRK, the central cornea is relatively flat, while the midperipheral cornea remains unaltered. Aberration effects are possible as a result of the demarcation between the central ablation zone and the untreated cornea. Early studies documented these effects.[2–5] It was found that when the surgery is particularly effective, a halo around lights at night may be noted, especially by patients with large pupils. This halo is an exaggerated form of positive spherical aberration and is a consequence of the relatively small diameter of the PRK ablation zone used in early studies, which typically was only 4 mm. The halo effect was experienced by about 80% of patients post-PRK and in 10% of cases was sufficiently problematic to prevent treatment of the other eye. It was found to be highly correlated with the overall change in refraction (Fig. 7.2), i.e., those patients with a large change in refractive status experienced the greatest halo effect. Halo was therefore noted more commonly in the first few weeks after PRK, since it was during this period that the maximal difference in refraction between the central and midperipheral cornea was present. As regression proceeded (loss of the effect of surgery) during the first few months, the halo effect decreased; in patients with total regression, the effect disappeared completely. Early studies using 4-mm-diameter ablation zones found, as expected,

a high correlation between pupil size and halo effect (Fig. 7.3); patients with larger pupils were much more likely to complain of halo. In addition, and as predicted, the halo effect is considerably reduced, although not eliminated completely, when the more powerful second-generation lasers, which utilize larger diameter ablation zones, are used.[8] Interestingly, in the questionnaire survey of patients from the early cohorts described above, the main cause of dissatisfaction was regression—cited by almost all of the 15% of patients who were unhappy with the outcome of PRK[5]—not halo.

The size of the treatment zone and centration of the zone are intimately related. With the early 4-mm ablation zone diameters, centration was critical. Decentered zones induced both astigmatism and asymmetrical halo effects which were most disabling, especially when driving at night. The most common diameter zone at present is 6 mm. Even with this increased diameter, optimal results are achieved when attention is paid to accurate centration. Effective retreatment (see the next chapter) for regression in patients who exhibit moderate regression without an aggressive haze response is possible, but the retreatment of a significantly decentered PRK ablation zone is difficult.[11] A simple repeat ablation using a second, accurately centered zone results in overlapping ablation areas leading to a multifocal cornea and does not restore normal corneal shape. Rigid gas-permeable contact

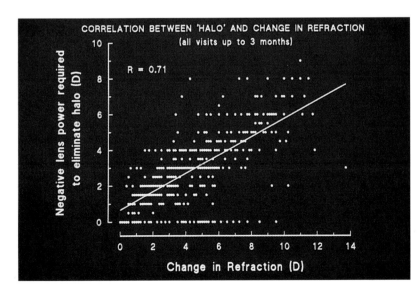

Fig. 7.2. Graph demonstrating the high correlation between halos and change in refraction in eyes that underwent PRK with a 4 mm ablation zone.

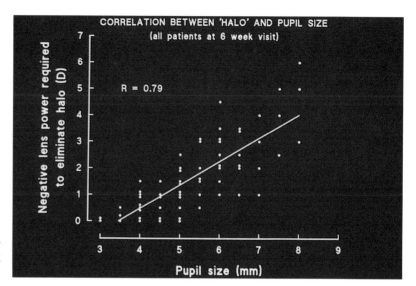

Fig. 7.3. Graph demonstrating a high correlation between pupil size and halo effect after PRK with a 4 mm ablation zone.

lens correction is of some benefit for these patients, but adequate retreatment for decentered zones will probably require topography-controlled ablations utilizing eye-tracking devices with scanning or "flying spot" lasers so that only the area of cornea that needs ablation receives exposure. Improved algorithms incorporating blended transition zones with large ablation diameters will minimize unwanted induced aberration effects. However, at present, it is important to fully inform the patient about the likelihood and the implications of the halo effect. Younger patients with large pupils who have more than 4 or 5 D of myopia (in whom PRK might produce a large difference between central and paracentral corneal power) should perhaps be excluded at this stage.

CORNEAL HAZE/SCARRING

A variable amount of anterior corneal haze, detected on slit lamp examination, develops in most patients (>95%) at about 1 month post-PRK. This diffuse haze increases to a maximum up to about 5 or 6 months, and then becomes more reticulate and fades over the first year (although it may not disappear completely). As with other complications, the incidence and severity of this haze increase as higher degrees of myopia are treated (Fig. 7.4). It is presently debatable whether this increased haze is due to deeper ablations (Fig. 7.5) or to the healing qualities of the more highly myopic eye. (See the following chapter for details on retreatment.)

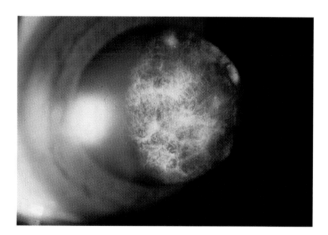

Fig. 7.4. Severe haze after PRK.

The deposition of iron within the basal epithelial cell layers has also been noted in long-term PRK corneas (Fig. 7.6a). This almost certainly represents subtle changes in corneal contour, since iron deposition occurs in most conditions in which tear flow is altered because of corneal irregularity (Stocker's, Ferry's, and Hudson-Stahli lines). It is also commonly encountered following radial keratotomy (Fig. 7.6b).

In considering the treatment of anterior stromal haze, some surgeons initially advocated repeat PRK to remove the layer of scarring responsible for reduced BCVA. It is known, however, that reablation of a severely affected cornea can result in further generation of anterior stromal haze and a tendency to further loss of BCVA. It would seem

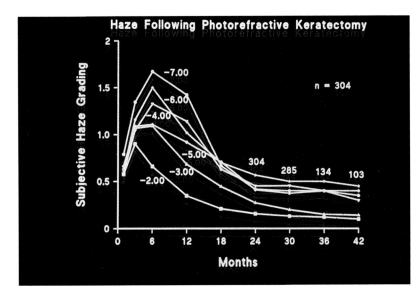

Haze Following Photorefractive Keratectomy

Fig. 7.5. Correlation between haze and amount of correction attempted after PRK with small ablation zones.

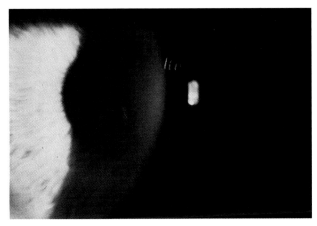

A

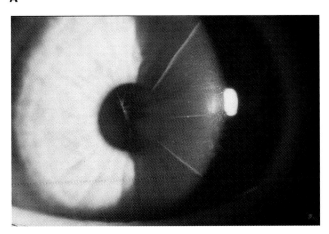

B

Fig. 7.6. (a) Iron deposition within the basal epithelial layer after PRK. (b) Iron deposition within the basal epithelial layer after radial keratotomy.

prudent, in the worst cases, to wait for several years, if necessary, for the haze to diminish. Irregular astigmatism can be corrected, at least in part, by the use of a rigid contact lens.

LOSS OF BCVA

In some patients, the period of maximal haze coincides with a significant loss of BCVA (up to three to four lines in rare cases in which higher degrees of myopia have been treated or retreated). It is possible that, due to this haze and/or irregular astigmatism, there may be some permanent deterioration in BCVA (see the tables in Chapters 5 and 6). Longer-term (2-year) studies have shown that BCVA improved with time in these patients, particularly between the 6th and 12th months (Fig 7.7a, b).

WOUND INFECTION AND DELAYED HEALING

Several cases of bacterial keratitis have been reported in the literature, one occurring the day after surgery,[12] one 2 days later,[13] one 3 days later,[14] one 6 days later,[13] and one 9 weeks later, which the authors felt might be associated with long-term topical corticosteroid use.[15] In the first three cases there was a rapid response to intensive topical antibiotics, but in the two cases that occurred later postoperatively a dense stromal scar resulted in a BCVA of 20/150 and counting fingers

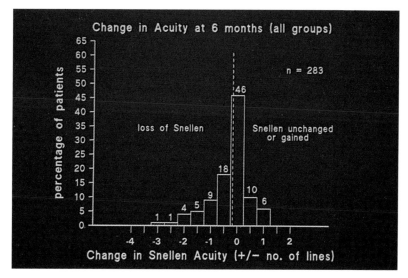

A

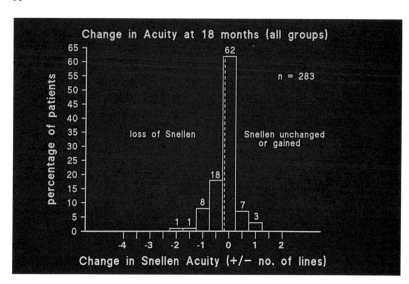

Fig. 7.7. Change in best-corrected visual acuity at (a) 6 months and (b) 18 months after PRK.

B

at 1 meter. These cases emphasize the need for adequate postoperative surveillance, particularly during recepithelialization. Bandage soft contact lenses may incrase the risk of contamination and bacterial keratitis.[13] In addition, it is well recognized that excimer laser radiation can reactivate latent herpes simplex virus (HSV) and that a careful history is therefore important.[16,17] Even when a careful history is elicited, it is important to note that at Moorfields Eye Hospital in London there have been two cases of HSV reactivation in patients with no known previous infective episode. While it is often

stated that excimer laser radiation at 193 nm (far UV) acts as a sterilizing source, it is evident that infection can occur in the early postoperative period when an epithelial defect exists, in spite of instillation of a broad-spectrum antibiotic. It is also of concern that a 62-year-old patient with systemic lupus erythematosus required a penetrating keratoplasty (PK) following delayed epithelial healing which resulted in a noninfectious, perforating corneal ulcer,[18] and a second patient needed a PK because of a decentered ablation zone and corneal scarring.[19]

EPITHELIAL PROBLEMS

An estimated 20–25% of patients experience some form of corneal surface discomfort following PRK, particularly in the first few postoperative months. This is hardly surprising considering the fact that, prior to laser exposure, the corneal epithelium is completely debrided across the central 7 mm or so of the cornea to allow for a 6-mm ablation zone. It is perhaps surprising, however, that more patients do not suffer frank recurrent erosion syndrome. Since Bowman's layer is removed during all but the least myopic PRK procedures, it would seem that the new epithelium strongly attaches at the basal cell level of the underlying newly ablated stromal surface. In addition, excimer laser PTK is said to be successful in 60–70% of patients treated for recurrent erosion syndrome due to trauma or basement epithelial dystrophies. Mild foreign body sensations on waking following PRK are undoubtedly due to epithelial irregularities in the first few postoperative months. These symptoms usually last for only seconds or minutes and normally are not sufficiently problematic to deter patients from undergoing a PRK procedure in the second eye. It would also seem that such symptoms disappear over time.

PTOSIS

This complication is relatively rare, but it can be most troublesome. In the first few months post-PRK, a slight ptosis has been reported in about 1–2% of patients and has been ascribed to the use of topical corticosteroids during this early period. More persistent ptosis is likely to be due to alterations in the levator complex of the upper lid, which presumably are caused by stretching at the time of speculum insertion. Needless to say, the PRK surgeon should be aware of the importance of gentle lid speculum insertion and should avoid undue pressure on the lids.

CORNEAL TOPOGRAPHICAL ABNORMALITIES/CENTRAL ISLANDS

The definition of a central islands varies but essentially involves an increase in central corneal power of at least 1.5 D comprising at least 2.5 mm of the central cornea.

Table 7.1. Classification of Central Islands

Grade	Height	Diameter
A	<3 D	<3 mm
B	≥3 D	<3 mm
C	>3 D	≥3 mm

Source: Ref. 19.

Classification

Levin et al.,[20] in a recent analysis of 400 PRK patients in Melbourne, classified central islands (Table 7.1) according to size in diameter and power. The smallest island is grade A, which is less than 3 mm in diameter and less than 3 D in power, compared to the largest, grade C, in which the power is more than 3 D and may involve at least 3 mm of central corneal diameter.

Figure 7.8 shows the larger grade C central island, with the difference topographical map on the right demonstrating a pre- and postoperative subtraction map and a very large central island. The corneal statistics are abnormal, particularly the Surface Regularity Index and the Surface Asymmetry Index, both of which are >0.5. Normally, these indices should be <0.5. The potential visual acuity was slightly impaired. These indices are related to corneal smoothness or lack of smoothness.

Initially, the central corneal epithelium is relatively thin and often is associated with hyperopia.

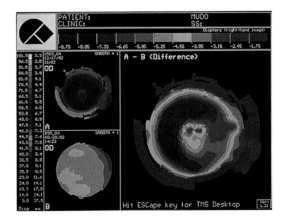

Fig. 7.8. Large central island, Grade C (topographic difference map).

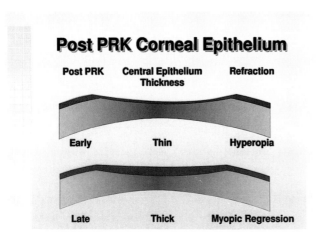

Fig. 7.9. Post PRK corneal epithelium.

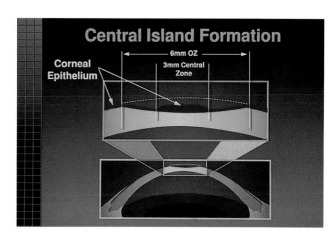

Fig. 7.11. Central island formation.

Later, with healing and remodeling, the epithelium thickens—up to three times or more in thickness—and may be associated with myopic regression (Fig. 7.9).

Etiology of Central Islands

There are a number of theories about the etiology of central islands. The most popular one postulates a hydration problem in which there is more fluid than normal in the central cornea, resulting in central stromal underablation with a subsequent bump (Fig. 7.10) or associated development of epithelial hyperplasia (Fig. 7.11).

Assouline and collaborators demonstrated that shock wave–induced deformation and subsequent

dynamic alteration of convection forces applied to emitted particles may be a principal mechanism underlying the formation of central islands, regardless of any biological response of the ablated tissue.[21]

Several laser manufacturers have found that central islands can be almost totally eliminated by applying extra central pulses. Other factors, such as degradation or mirrors and abnormal or excessive epithelial healing, may play a role—and perhaps the etiology is multifactorial.

Incidence of Central Islands

The incidence of central islands varies with different excimer lasers and with the technique involved. Central islands are more common in lasers with wide beam delivery systems. Lin's analysis showed that without software changes to allow for the delivery of extra central pulses, there was an incidence of central islands at 1 month after PRK of about 26% that diminished to 2% at 12 months.[22,23]

In Melbourne, Levin et al.[20] reported on over 400 patients and found an incidence of central islands of about 1% 6 months postoperatively. Most large islands improved, but smaller ones were less likely to change. Predominantly, these were grade A islands (the smallest variety); the least common were the more severe grade C islands. There was no statistical difference between PRK and photoastigmatic keratectomy (PARK) patients.

Central islands are rarely found in patients treated with scanning lasers. Central islands have

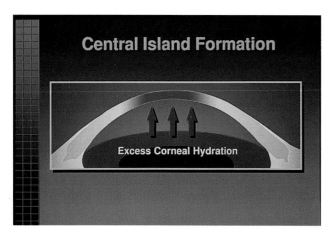

Fig. 7.10. Central island formation showing excess corneal hydration.

been reported after laser in situ keratomileusis (LASIK) and automated lamellar keratoplasty (ALK) procedures, presumably due to extra hydration of the stromal bed after the initial lamellar corneal flap.[24]

Clinical Symptoms of Central Islands

Symptoms generally are related to impaired quality of vision, such as monocular diplopia, blurred vision, haloes, glare, and ghosting. Refraction is not significantly affected in most cases.

VisX 20/20B laser pretreatment in the central 2.5-mm optical zone for a correction of about −1.00 D to −1.50 D reduced the incidence of central islands significantly. At the Hong Kong VisX users' meeting, Kinoshita found no central islands when he used the pretreatment software with his VisX laser (V4.0 vs. V3.2). Changing optics frequently may also be beneficial (S. Kinoshita, oral presentation, Fourth Alcon/VisX Users' Annual Meeting, Hong Kong, 1995).

Kinoshita showed an increase in the incidence of central islands with centripetal removal of epithelium compared to centrifugal debridement, in which the epithelium is removed centrally and toward the periphery. The latter technique probably allows more corneal hydration centrally.

Treatment of Central Islands

A conservative approach is preferred, since most patients improve with time, and the incidence of central islands at 1 year is very low—2% in Lin's series, and 1% at 6 months with Levin et al.[20,22,23]

In cases of severe persistent central islands, surgery can be considered. Contact lens use, pharmacological treatment with corticosteroids, and mechanical debridement are not effective. The best treatment is to use an excimer PRK to correct the island after measuring the size (in millimeters) and height (in diopters) of the central island on the topographical subtraction map. The best procedure is probably to wait at least 6 months, and preferably 12 months, as most patients do improve. Refer to the next chapter for a detailed discussion of excimer laser retreatment.

REFERENCES

1. Gartry DS, Kerr Muir MG, Marshall J. Photorefractive keratectomy with an argon fluoride excimer laser: a clinical study. *Refract Corneal Surg.* 1991;7: 420–435.

2. Gartry DS, Kerr Muir MG, Marshall J. Excimer laser photorefractive keratectomy—18 month follow-up. *Ophthalmology.* 1992;99:1209–1219.

3. Gartry DS, Kerr Muir MG, Lohmann CP, Marshall J. The effect of topical corticosteroids on refractive outcome and corneal haze after photorefractive keratectomy. *Arch Ophthalmol.* 1992;110:944–952.

4. Gartry DS, Kerr Muir MG, Marshall J. The effect of topical corticosteroids on refraction and corneal haze following excimer laser treatment of myopia: An update. A prospective, randomized, double-masked study. *Eye.* 1993;7:584–590.

5. Gartry DS. Excimer laser treatment of myopia—the present position. *Br Med J.* 1995;310:979–985.

6. Ficker LA, Bates AK, Steele ADMcG, et al. Excimer laser photorefractive keratectomy for myopia: 12 month follow-up. *Eye.* 1993;7:617–624.

7. Epstein D, Fagerholm P, Hamberg-Nystrom H, Tengroth B. Twenty four month follow-up of excimer laser photorefractive keratectomy for myopia. *Ophthalmology.* 1994;101:1558–1564.

8. O'Brart DPS, Gartry DS, Lohmann CP, et al. Excimer laser photorefractive keratectomy for myopia: comparison of 4.0- and 5.0-mm ablation zones. *J Refract Corneal Surg.* 1994;10:87–94.

9. Taylor HR, Guest CS, Kelly P, Alpins NA. Comparison of excimer laser treatment of astigmatism and myopia. *Arch Ophthalmol.* 1993;111:1621–1626.

10. Rogers CM, Lawless MA, Cohen PR. Photorefractive keratectomy for myopia of more than −10 diopeters. *J Refract Corneal Surg.* 1994;10(suppl): S171–S173.

11. Gartry DS, Larkin DFP, Flaxel CJ, et al. Retreatment for significant regression following excimer laser photorefractive keratectomy (PRK)—a randomised, double-masked trial. *Invest Ophthalmol Vis Sci.* 1995;36:S190.

12. Maguen E, Salz JJ, Nesburn AB, et al. Results of excimer laser photorefractive keratectomy for the correction of myopia. *Ophthalmology.* 1994;101: 1548–1557.

13. Amayem A, Tawfik Ali A, Waring GO III, Ibrahim O. Bacterial keratitis after PRK. *J Refract Surg.* 1996;12:642–644.

14. McDonald MB, Frantz M, Klyce SD, et al. Central photorefractive keratectomy for myopia: the blind eye study. *Arch Ophthalmol.* 1990;108:799–808.

15. Sampath R, Ridgway AEA, Leatherbarrow B. Bacterial keratitis following excimer laser photorefractive keratectomy: a case report. *Eye.* 1994;8:481–482.

16. McDonnell PJ, Moreira H, Clapham TN, et al. Photorefractive keratectomy for astigmatism. Initial clinical results. *Arch Ophthalmol.* 1991;109:1370–1373.

17. Pepose JS, Laycock KA, Miller JK, et al. Reactivation of latent herpes simplex virus by excimer laser photokeratectomy. *Am J Ophthalmol.* 1992;114:45–50.

18. Seiler T, Wollensak J. Myopic photorefractive keratectomy with the excimer laser. 1 year follow-up. *Ophthalmology.* 1991;98:1156–1163.

19. Colin J. Greffes de cornee apres keratectomie photorefractive au laser excimer. *J Fr Ophthalmol.* 1992; 15:437.

20. Levin S, Carson CA, Garrett SK, Taylor HR. Prevalence of central islands after excimer laser refractive surgery. *J Cataract Refract Surg.* 1995;21: 21–26.

21. Assouline M, Moossavi J, Muller-Steinwachs M, et al. Central steep island following photorefractive keratectomy. *Invest Ophthalmol Vis Sci.* 1996;37: S573.

22. Lin DJC. Corneal topographic analysis after excimer photorefractive keratectomy. *Ophthalmology.* 1994; 101:1432–1439.

23. Lin DJC, Sutton HF, Berman M. Corneal topography following excimer laser photorefractive keratectomy for myopia. *J Cataract Refract Surg.* 1993;19: S149–S154.

24. Price FW. Central islands of corneal steepening after automated lamellar keratoplasty for myopia. *J Refract Surg.* 1996;12:36–41.

8

Photorefractive Keratectomy Retreatment

John A. van Westenbrugge
Howard V. Gimbel
Geoffrey B. Kaye

INTRODUCTION

Ever since the first photorefractive keratectomy (PRK) procedures were done, there has been a need to consider retreatment. Certain cases of radial keratotomy (RK) with residual refractive error and overcorrected epikeratophakia have also been managed using PRK. The more recently developed laser in situ keratomileusis (LASIK) procedures also involve retreatment, especially during the algorithm development and learning curve of this technique. There are a number of reasons for retreatment and a variety of methods to achieve it.[1–4]

As a result of the rapid advances in technology and the authors' exposure to a number of different lasers (Fig. 8.1), retreatment has involved many different combinations of lasers (Table 8.1). Initial retreatments in 1991 were with the Summit ExciMed upgraded software, primarily to enlarge the optical zone to 5.0 mm, after prior treatment with the Summit using the original 4.5-mm optical zone. The VisX laser enabled the development of techniques for the retreatment of residual myopia, astigmatism, and optical zone enlargement. As higher corrections were attempted with the VisX, the incidence of central island, regression, and haze increased. From this, experience was gained in treating these phenomena with the VisX laser. At present, the authors do most of their PRK, phototherapeutic keratectomy (PTK), and retreatment with the Nidek and Novatec lasers.

Retreatment techniques have undergone significant and sometimes rapid evolution. The authors have been generous in their use of retreatment, per-

forming it whenever necessary to achieve complete patient satisfaction (Table 8.2). Retreatment was deferred only if the amount of correction involved was too small, if the approach required was too difficult or untested, or if future advances in technology which would be of benefit in a given case were anticipated. The retreatment rates were lower when the newer laser systems were used for the primary PRK procedures.

All the methods that were used for each problem area will be described. Methods which have not been successful are included also so that new investigators in this area may either avoid them or modify them to improve their success rates.

INDICATIONS FOR PRK RETREATMENT

Retreatment techniques may be grouped into the following categories:

1. *Simple undercorrection.* These are cases in which the corneal response is unexpectedly less than desired on initial treatment.
2. *Simple overcorrection.* These are cases in which the corneal response is unexpectedly greater than desired on initial treatment.
3. *Simple regression.* These are cases resulting in myopia which develops slowly during the healing phase but without significant haze.
4. *Haze with regression.* This is by far the most common category. Haze takes on different patterns in different cases. The type of laser used can also influence the haze pattern.

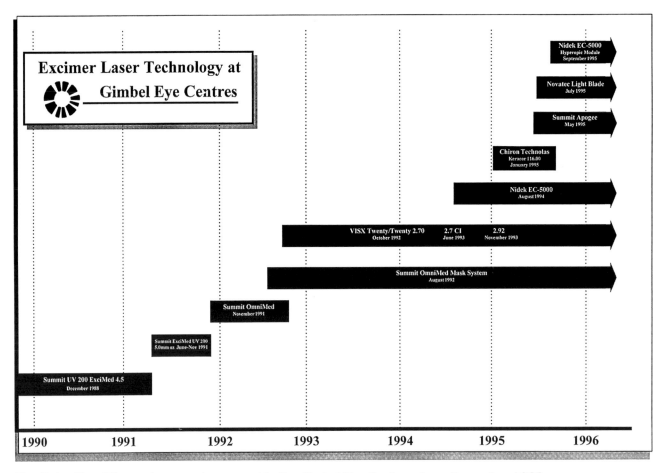

Fig. 8.1. The different laser systems used in the Gimbel Eye Centres, from December 1988.

Table 8.1. Gimbel Eye Centre Excimer Laser Experience, June 1990 to January 1996 (Minimum 3-Month Follow-up After the Primary Procedure)

	Primary Surgery	Repeat Surgery*	
	n	*n*	%
Myopia and astigmatism	7901	1467	18.6
LASIK myopia and astigmatism	189	42	22.2
Total	8090	1509	18.7

*Mean time to retreatment is 6.0 ± 2.2 months.

Table 8.2. Incidence of Retreatment in Primary Myopic PRK, June 1990 to January 1996 (All Laser Systems)

Preoperative	Repeat PRK (%)*
−0.00 to −2.00	6.45
−2.01 to − 4.00	6.50
−4.01 to −6.00	16.02
−6.01 to −8.00	18.50
−8.01 to −10.00	28.57
−10.01 to −12.00	29.13
−12.01 to −14.00	33.70
−14.01 to −16.00	49.50
−16.01 ≤	27.70

*Percent retreatment with a minimum of 3 months after primary PRK.

5. *Haze without regression.* Haze by itself is very rare. It is almost invariably accompanied by regression. There are a handful of cases in which either haze occurs without regression, due to an unusually even distribution of the regrowth of tissue, or the patient is initially overcorrected and haze and regression settle to a state of emmetropia with haze.

6. *Small optical zone.* Night vision effects have been a problem for certain patients, particularly those whose eyes were treated with optical zones as small as 4.5 mm. Although this effect has markedly decreased as we have expanded the optical and transition zones, it may still be present in some patients with larger pupils and high corrections.

7. *Decentration.* Decentration is divided into two categories:

   a. *Primary (iatrogenic) decentration.* This is usually a reflection of inexperience by the surgeon and is fortunately rare after an initial set of cases.

   b. *Secondary decentration.* This is related to an asymmetrical healing response, often with arcuate or segmental peripheral haze. This is a rare complication with scanning delivery systems.

   Primary and secondary decentration can be differentiated easily with serial corneal mapping. Both types of decentration seen on corneal mapping are usually accompanied by astigmatism.

   Different authors have used different parameters to define decentration. Also, some refractive surgeons center their ablations on the visual axis and others on the center of the pupil. This adds another variable in determining what constitutes decentration. Various methods have been devised for measuring decentration. Some use an arbitrary measure of 1 mm of decentration from the center of the pupil for purposes of statistical analysis. The authors have generally relied on corneal mapping as a guide and have used the pupil center as the intended center of treatment. The degree of decentration required to make a clinical impact varies widely, depending on the pupil size, the amount of correction, the attempted astigmatism correction, and the am-

bient light under which clinical parameters are measured.

Clinically significant primary decentrations are rare and tend to occur in the surgeon's early cases. The number of decentrations should decrease further in the future once reliable eye tracking technology becomes available.

8. *Central island.* The central island was encountered largely after using the VisX and Chiron Technolas lasers to treat wider optical zones.[5] The authors also encountered some central islands with the use of a 6.5-mm zone with the Summit OmniMed and Summit Apex Plus lasers.

The usual symptoms noted by a patient with a central island include ill-defined visual disturbances and blurring, ghosting, and/or monocular diplopia despite excellent Snellen visual acuity. Retreatment is undertaken at least 4 months, but more often 6 months, after initial laser treatment.

EPITHELIUM

At this point, it is appropriate to provide a more extensive discussion of the epithelium because our understanding of its nature and its variations plays a significant part in our strategy for a number of PRK retreatment techniques.

Doing PRK has provided some new knowledge of the nature of the epithelium. Manual removal of the epithelium is rarely done in normal practice except to clear loose or irregular epithelium from an injury site or recurrent corneal erosion. While doing PRK, epithelium is removed from relatively normal corneas. Most practitioners generally clear a slightly larger area than the treatment zone in order to accommodate small movements of the eye when treatment is applied. The nature of the epithelium appears to vary widely. In some cases, it is very firmly adherent. This is generally true in younger patients. Occasional patients, more often in the older PRK population, have an epithelium so loose that it comes off in one sheet with a few sweeps of the instrument. It is often so loose that one is prompted to question the patient about symptoms of recurrent corneal erosion.

One phenomenon of interest which can be encountered when removing epithelium on initial treatment for 6-mm or larger zones is a loose area of epithelium located superiorly from about 10 o'clock to 2 o'clock, extending from approximately the 6-mm zone margin to the superior limbus (or superior pannus, if present) (Fig. 8.2). This loose zone is often present even when the remainder of the corneal epithelium was relatively adherent.

When doing epithelial removal for retreatment after PRK, the pattern is significantly different. A loose superior zone is still found if it was present previously. Of interest is the fact that there is an annular region of loose epithelium between the original peripheral untouched epithelium and a firmly adherent area located centrally in the deeper part of the PRK treatment zone. The annular area was 1 to 2 mm in width and appears to bridge across the margin of the original treatment zone, suggesting that epithelium is, at least for some time postoperatively, less adherent in the zone where excimer laser ablation had been shallow at the periphery or where epithelium had been previously removed without excimer ablation. This tends to confirm the usefulness of excimer laser treatment for recurrent corneal erosion, suggesting that if ablation is deep enough, there will be firm adherence of epithelium.[6] It also gives some clue to a postoperative phenomenon described by many patients which resembles recurrent corneal erosion: a feeling of "sticking" of the eyelid in the morning, with pain if the eyelid is opened rapidly, as well as sensitivity or tenderness on touching or rubbing the eye. These findings suggest that the annular loose area of epithelium may be responsible for these symptoms.

The observation of loose epihelium must be considered when doing astigmatic keratotomy after PRK. We have noted that the optical zone marker at 6 to 7 mm for astigmatic keratotomy can loosen the epithelium for the entire circumference of the zone marker if pressed firmly and not quickly removed. Due to the relative movement of the eye and the marker, the epithelium may be loosened and even torn, and significant symptoms may develop. Also, when the diamond knife is passed across the cornea, the epithelium often drags, tearing in a wake rather than being cut. This tearing may be minimized by lifting the blade and repuncturing the epithelium in a number of segments for the astigmatic keratotomy. This procedure leaves little bridges across the epithelium and does not cause the big wake-like tear of epithelium.

Another characteristic of the epithelium which has been demonstrated in the course of retreatment is the *epithelial smoothing principle*. By this, we mean that the epithelium tends to be thicker over any relative depression in the corneal stroma and thinner over any relative elevation of the corneal stroma. This basic characteristic of the epithelium is evident to anyone who has ever followed a small defect in the corneal stroma and found the smoothing effect of epithelial fill-in to be present. This phenomenon is frequently encountered when doing transepithelial ablation, especially in PRK retreat-

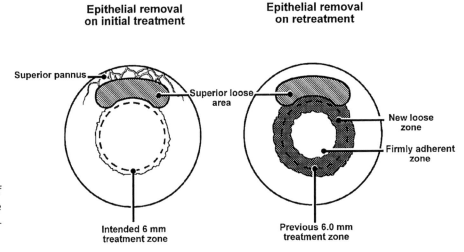

Fig. 8.2. Superior loose area of epithelium often found at the time of epithelial removal and new annular loose zone found after PRK.

ments and also for PTK procedures. Being aware of this principle works to one's advantage both in accomplishing things that could otherwise not be as easily accomplished and in avoiding undesired side effects. Some of the applications of the epithelial smoothing principle are demonstrated in the discussion of various retreatments in this chapter.

STEROIDS

The role of steroids after PRK is controversial. Several studies have concluded that there is no significant difference between steroid-treated and non-treated groups.[7] From clinical experience of the authors, they believe that steroids still play a significant role in improving the outcome for a significant number of patients.

The conclusions of previous studies were reached legitimately but are possibly in error for the following reasons:[8,9]

1. The total number of patients involved was too small to determine the small but significant proportion of patients for whom steroids do make a large difference.
2. The steroids were not used for a long enough period of time to fully suppress the haze and regression responses initiated by the PRK procedure.[9–11]

With regard to the first point, the clinical impression of the authors is as follows:

1. Some 70% of patients could do without steroids entirely, with little or no noticeable effect.
2. Thirty percent of patients would have some significant effect.
3. Of the 30%, 25% would have a modest effect (such as a 1.00 D regression for a −6 D correction, with some mild haze that is only marginally optically significant).
4. Of the 30%, 5% would show significant haze and regression (such as 3.00 to 5.00 D of regression for a −6 D correction, with optically significant haze).
5. Of the above-mentioned 5% of patients, 1% or 2% (1–2% of the whole treatment group)

would show the largest amount of regression, with a tendency to recurrent regression in the face of retreatment.

The above figures are only approximations based on clinical impressions. If they are accurate, it would be difficult to determine statistically the effect of steroids in the small, significantly subgroup of responders.

With regard to the second point, 3 or 4 months of treatment with steroids may not be sufficient to entirely suppress the haze and regression responses of the small, strongly responding subgroup.[12] Many patients who have required retreatment for haze or regression did well and varied little from the norm while they were on steroids during their first 3 months. Their responses started at about the fourth month and continued to the sixth month or beyond. In treating some patients in whom haze or regression tended to recur but who eventually achieved a successful and satisfactory outcome, the following sequence was used. In this example, the patient was a 34-year-old male.

1. Initial refractive error — −6.50 D

   Epithelial removal — Manual

   Treatment — Summit ExciMed laser for full correction of −6.50 D with optical zone diameter of 5.0 mm.

   Medication — 0.1% dexamethasone (Maxidex Alcon, Ft. Worth, TX)
   qid × 1 month
   bid × 1 month
   qd × 1 month

   Result — Regression starting at the fourth month and continuing to the seventh month, with a refractive error of −3.25 D and marked haze.

2. Refractive error — −3.25 D

   Epithelial removal — Laser

Retreatment	VisX Twenty/Twenty laser for full correction of −3.25 D with optical zone diameter of 5.0 mm.
Medication	None. This was shortly after publication of the initial study indicating that steroids did not appear to make a significant difference.[8]
Result	Regression starting at the second month and progressing to −3.50 D by the third month.

3. Refractive error   −3.50 D

Epithelial removal	Laser
Retreatment	VisX Twenty/Twenty laser for full correction of −3.50 D with optical zone diameter of 6.0 mm
Medication	0.1% fluorometholone (FML, Allergan, Irvine, CA) and ketorolac tromethamine (Acular, Allergan, Irvine, CA) initially qid and then tapering slowly at monthly intervals for 12 months.
Result	Very slow regression to −2.00 D, with only some mild, patchy areas of haze and best corrected visual acuity (BCVA) retained at 20/20.

4. Refractive error   −2.00 D

Epithelial removal	Laser
Retreatment	VisX Twenty/Twenty laser for full correction of −2.00 D with optical zone diameter of 6.00 mm.
Medication	FML and Acular, initially qid and then tapering slowly at monthly intervals for 12 months.
Result	Emmetropia with BCVA of 20/15 2 years later.

Table 8.3. Example of a Typical FML and Acular Extended Tapering Dosage Schedule

Month	Drop Schedule
1	qid
2	tid
3	bid
4	bid, qd, alternating
5	qd
6, 7	q2d
8, 9	q3d (or 2×/week
10–12	q week

The slow tapering of steroids and nonsteroidal anti-inflammatories requires further explanation. The strength of the initial medication was not decreased, nor was the initial tapering delayed, until the drops were being used twice daily. At that stage the schedule was slowed, sometimes treating twice daily or daily on alternating days to avoid an abrupt decrease in dosage (Table 8.3). This program may be shortened or extended, depending on the haze and regression response of the eye.

PRK RETREATMENT TECHNIQUES

The gain or loss of BCVA at 3 months after PRK retreatment with the Nidek EC-5000 for all categories is shown in Table 8.4.

Simple Undercorrection

This is the easiest retreatment to perform and is still undertaken regularly. Never trust a new laser, whether a new model or an individual machine. On average, the authors have found greater achieved than attempted corrections with the early Summit machines and the Nidek. Fortunately, these were consistent and the algorithm was adjusted. Never trust a new eye. Even when algorithms have been worked out for individual machines fairly consistently, individual eyes can still show overresponses. During the early part of any trial, we tended to approach every new machine as having the potential for overcorrection. They still use conservative parameters even for familiar machines, especially for first eyes, for higher corrections, and for patients over 30 years of age. Undercorrections are frequent.

Table 8.4. Three-Month BCVA Following Repeat PRK Excimer Laser Surgery, 1995–1996 (*N* = 267*)

| | | Gain | | | | | | Loss | | | |
| | | 2 Lines | | 1 Line | | Same | | 1 Line | | 2 Lines | |
Reason	*n*	*n*	(%)	*n*	(%)	*n*	(%)	*n*	(%)	*n*	(%)
Simple undercorrection	78	—	—	15	(19.2)	58	(74.4)	3	(3.8)	2	(2.6)
Simple overcorrection	24	4	(16.7)	2	(8.3)	17	(70.8)	1	(4.2)	—	—
Simple regression	60	5	(8.3)	3	(5.0)	47	(78.3)	4	(6.7)	1	(1.7)
Haze with regression	33	6	(18.2)	10	(30.3)	15	(45.5)	2	(6.1)	—	—
Haze without regression	11	3	(27.3)	4	(36.4)	4	(36.4)	—	—	—	—
Small optical zone	3	—	—	—	—	3	(100.0)	—	—	—	—
Decentration (1°/2°)	12	—	—	1	(8.3)	10	(83.3)	1	(8.3)	—	—
Central island	46	14	(30.4)	15	(32.6)	16	(34.8)	1	(2.2)	—	—

*All repeat surgery performed using the NIDEK EC-5000.

The authors retreat refractions as small as −0.75 D, depending on the patient's subjective visual complaints and objectives (e.g., specific career requirements).

In a simple undercorrection, the epithelium is removed manually with an No. 57 blade (Alcon, Ft. Worth, TX), as for initial treatments, and the residual refractive error is retreated. The authors perform these retreatments early, usually shortly after the 1-month visit. They defer them only if there is some concern about the reliability of the refraction at 1 month. This early treatment is based on the assumption that most eyes tend to heal without significant haze or regression response. There is little advantage in waiting for a long time to see how the eye will respond before considering treatment. After 1 month, it is highly unusual for the refraction to become hyperopic. Most cases will continue to shift toward myopia if they shift at all. For this reason, there has been little need for evolution in this form of retreatment.

Complications are usually similar to those encountered after primary treatment. There is occasional overcorrection, although this is less likely when smaller amounts are being treated. The authors tend to be more conservative in retreating older (presbyopic) patients for this reason.

Simple Overcorrection

Simple overcorrection is simple in name only. Hyperopic correction with the excimer laser using a

7.0-mm treatment zone has been under development for some time. Only in 1995 did treatment zones of 9.0 to 9.5 mm become available on a number of machines. The authors have had some early experience in treating hyperopia using these laser zones, and have used the Nidek EC-5000, Novatec LightBlade, and Summit Apex Plus for retreatment of overcorrected myopes as well as primary hyperopes.

The basic technique is straightforward. The Alcon No. 57 blade is used to clear the epithelium out to 9.5 mm and a pattern of 5.5 to 6.5 mm optical zone with a blend to 9 or 9.5 mm is used as the treatment algorithm. Of approximately 50 operations performed, 30 have been retreatments of PRK overcorrection. One result, which appears to be consistent, is that a 50% greater effect was obtained when treating after initial PRK than when treating primary hyperopia. At this time, it is not known whether this result is peculiar to the algorithm of certain lasers or whether is is consistent with all hyperopia treatments with any laser. This should be kept in mind when treating myopic overcorrections. If astigmatism is concurrently treated, there is a significant further hyperopic shift.

Simple Regression

This is a regression to myopia without significant haze. It tends to occur somewhat more slowly and later than the typical regression with haze response. New stromal tissue probably is laid down subepithelially, but slowly enough that there is insufficient disorganization to cause the appearance of haze.

Initially, the authors attempted to treat simple regression in the same fashion as a simple undercorrection but consistently obtained overcorrections. This occurred probably because, with manual removal of the epithelium, some of the new stromal tissue was removed as well as the potentially thickened epithelium. When retreatment was performed according to the refraction, undesirable additional flattening of the cornea occurred because both the manual removal of tissue and the excimer ablation were contributing to overall stromal tissue removal.

In many cases of retreatment, a larger-diameter optical treatment zone was used. This may also have contributed to the overcorrection effect by reducing the *divot* effect, a subset of the epithelial smoothing principle (see the section on epithelium). This refers to the commonly observed phenomenon in which a small (often steep-sided) defect is completely filled in by epithelium. Sometimes after an injury causing such a defect, there is still a small dip in the epithelium which may be revealed by fluorescein pooling. This dip tends to fill in slowly, often to the point where no evidence of the original injury remains. From time to time, one uncovers such stromal defects, or divots, when removing epithelium immediately prior to laser treatment when no corneal injury had been evident prior to the procedure. When these divots are wider and/or shallower, a long-term dip or flat spot may be retained on the epithelial surface despite significant epithelial thickening, creating a facet.

When smaller zone excimer laser treatments (e.g., 3.0 mm) were done in early studies—or even 4.5 mm, (especially for fairly high refractive errors such as −4.00 to −6.00 D)—there often was significant undercorrection due to central epithelial thickening in the treatment zone. This response was similar to that occurring with a small divot-like defect (Fig. 8.3).

Evidence for this comes from cases with small zone correction that showed relatively rapid early regression (4 to 8 weeks postoperatively) and immediate short-term reversal by simple epithelial removal. As the optical zone is enlarged and there is a more gradual transition from center to periphery, the amount of central epithelial thickening is reduced. Some overcorrections resulting from treatment of simple regression without haze may be

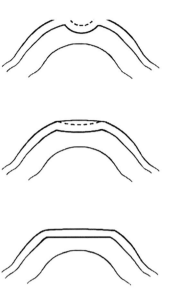

Fig. 8.3. The three diagrams present stromal defects of equal depth but increasingly greater width, showing that epithelium tends to be thicker in small-diameter stromal defects than in larger-diameter defects. The dotted line indicates what the epithelial thickness would have been in the region of the defect if the epithelial thickness had been uniform over the entire cornea.

attributed to optical zone enlargement, and the associated diminished central epithelial thickness compared to the epithelial thickness after the first (smaller optical zone) treatment.

Treatment of simple regression should be categorized with treatment for regression with haze. It is therefore important that one not be deceived by the relative lack of haze and consider this the same as a simple undercorrection. If myopia is seen sometime after PRK, it is important to have interim follow-up information on whether this myopia was present from early in the postoperative period or whether there has been gradual myopic regression. If there was a slow regression, it should be treated in the same manner as regression with haze.

If there has been a relatively rapid progression to myopia during the second month, one should consider the rapid portion of the regression to be related to epithelial thickening rather than stromal regrowth. This should be taken into account when considering retreatment, especially if the retreatment involves an expansion of the optical zone.

Haze with Regression

This is the most common problem encountered and often the most difficult one to deal with. Regression with haze tends to occur increasingly with higher amounts of correction and has been one of the primary motivations for the development of LASIK.[13] Depending on the success of LASIK in the future and the use of laser delivery techniques such as scanning (which the authors believe results in a lower incidence of haze), regression with haze could become a relatively uncommon reason for retreatment.

Haze originates from regrowth of stromal collagen in an irregular, noncrystalline pattern, and is usually associated with a change in the refractive status of the eye. The pattern of haze determines its refractive effect (Fig. 8.4). If it is centrally situated, there is a myopic effect. A hyperopic effect is caused by an annular, more peripheral haze pattern. An arcuate pattern leads to an astigmatic effect. Sometimes the haze starts out in an annular pattern, giving rise to a hyperopic shift. Later, it may progress centrally, causing regression of the refractive status to emmetropia or even myopia (Fig. 8.5).

The authors have not encountered a significant case of haze or regression when treating myopia under −4.00 D. Even with high amounts of correction, most patients have relatively clear corneas with small amounts of regression, if any. There do appear to be specific patients who show a regression with haze response. These patients may share some predisposing systemic or genetic factor, possibly analogous to that of the patient who is steroid responsive and has a high pressure in response to steroids. Some patients have persistent recurrence of haze and regression. They have required a number of retreatments, often at different stages in the evolution of the authors' retreatment regimen (see the patient example in the section on steroids). Their eyes do not appear to have suffered any cumulative ill effects from these retreatments. In future, such multiple retreatments should become less common in our practice for three reasons:

1. Many higher corrections are done (above −9.00 D) with LASIK.
2. Current retreatment techniques are significantly more effective than earlier techniques.
3. There is a lower incidence of regression with haze with the scanning slit delivery system (Nidek).

The authors' retreatment of regression with haze has evolved through six steps. These will now be described.

1. *Manual removal of epithelium with retreatment of residual refractive error.* As indicated above in the discussion of regression without haze, this technique has resulted in overcorrections, sometimes rather large ones (e.g., 5.00 D). The presence of a large regression with haze generally indicated a significant amount of stromal regrowth. With manual removal of the epithelium, a rather rough, irregular surface was often encountered, especially if the haze pattern was reticular. Presumably the major reason for the large subsequent overcorrection was that a significant amount of stromal regrowth tissue was removed with manual removal. When the additional excimer laser treatment was added, the total effect was excessive.

2. *Manual removal and scraping of haze.* Manual removal of epithelium and scraping of haze has left a smooth stromal bed when performed early (usually 6 to 8 weeks postoperatively).[14,15] Most often, surgical treatment has been delayed until attempts with topical steroids have failed and significant regression of the refractive correction has occurred. Possibly early debridement of haze before it becomes fibrous and attached to the stroma may be useful in cases where the early refractive result was optimum.

In a few cases of well-established haze, the authors attempted to do manual removal alone. They did not find a plaque-like entity that could be cleanly peeled off. Most often a rather rough, irregular surface remained and a large regression effect recurred. In other cases, the authors encountered only a partial peeling of an area of haze, raising the concern of irregular astigmatism, decentration, and asymmetry. A rough stromal surface may tend to induce a stronger healing response, with haze and regression, compared to a smooth surface. This means that a rough surface left after manual removal would tend to produce a stronger repeat regression with haze response. Initial treatments that involved distinct steps (such as the diaphragm controlled steps of the early Summit and VisX lasers) also appeared to induce a haze response. This might be related to the concentration of step cuts across the parallel collagen fibers. With the normal spherical pattern imposed on the cornea, wider steps occur centrally with relatively narrower

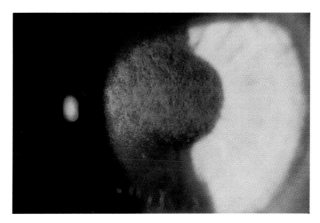

Fig. 8.4a. Haze with regression 8 months after PRK for myopia prior to retreatment (color photograph).

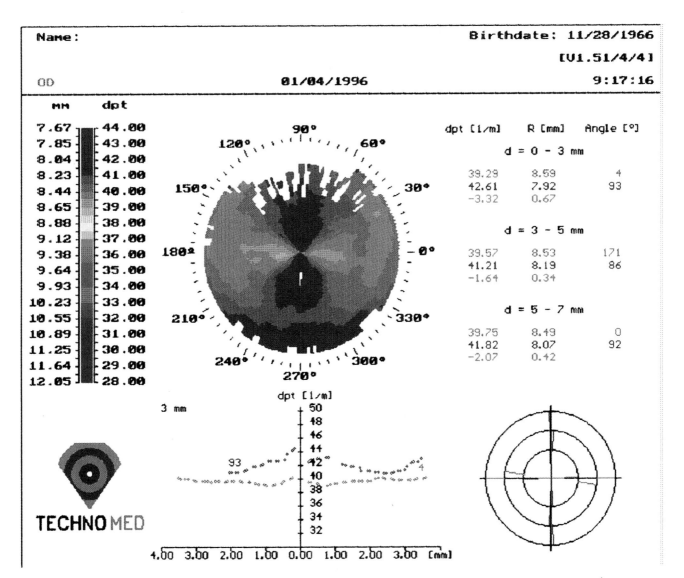

Fig. 8.4b. Preoperative corneal map showing astigmatism and central steepening. BCVA was $20/30^{-1}$ with refraction of $-5.75/-2.50 \times 3°$.

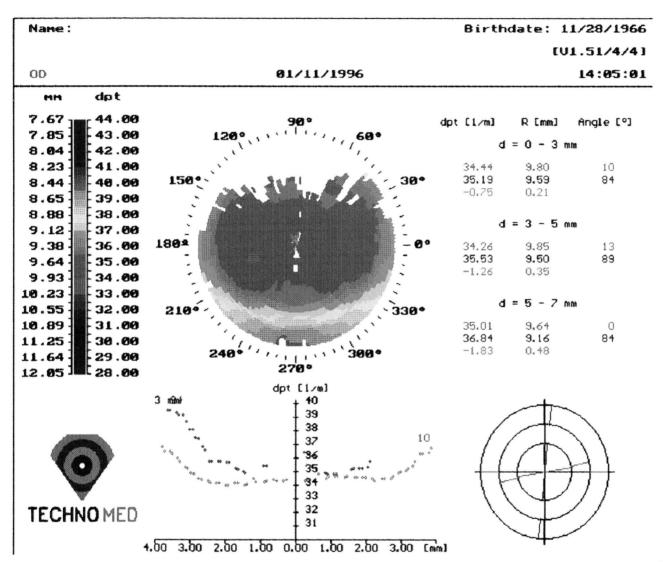

Fig. 8.4c. One month after PTK and myopic PRK retreatment with the Nidek laser, the BCVA improved to 20/20^{+2} with refraction of +0.25/−1.00 × 40°. The corneal map shows central flattening with decreased astigmatism already at 2 weeks p/o.

steps peripherally, giving more cuts across the parallel collagen fibers in the periphery (Fig. 8.6). The overlapping of these steps because of saccades during treatment may be the explanation for the development of peripheral haze (annular and arcuate) in many patients. This theory is also consistent with the observation that the multizone, multipass technique and scanning lasers give rise to less haze, presumably because of a smoother surface.

3. *Manual removal of epithelium with limited excimer laser retreatment based on pachymetry.* Because of the large number of overcorrections obtained by earlier methods of retreatment, the authors decided to do pachymetry immediately before retreatment and then immediately after manual removal of the epithelium. The theory was that if there was some degree of epithelial thickening as well as removal of stromal tissue along with the epithelium, the amount of tissue removed could be documented and retreatment parameters could be adjusted. For example, in a patient with 5.00 D of regression with haze, one might envision the following scenario:

a. Preoperative pachymetry which measured 500 μm.

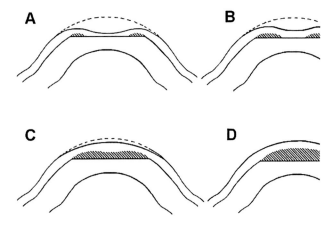

Fig. 8.5. This is an example of how one might obtain a hyperopic shift from early haze development when this occurs in an annular fashion. If the development of central haze catches up to the peripheral haze (as it often does), the initial hyperopia may disappear, giving way to an ultimate myopic regression with haze.

b. Manual epithelial removal performed.

c. Repeat pachymetry measurement of 430 μm, implying removal of 70 μm of tissue.

d. One would allow 50 μm to account for epithelial thickness and another 20 μm to indicate additional tissue removed. Approximately 10 μm of tissue removal, either manually or by PTK, gives 1 D of refractive effect. In this example, one would reduce the expected 5.00 D of retreatment by 2.00 D to only 3.00 D of retreatment.

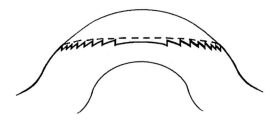

Fig. 8.6. This diagram shows the increased concentration of steps at the periphery of a myopic cut, with the benefit of some vertical exaggeration. Each ablation step is the same depth, and each segment has a curvature parallel to the original corneal curvature above, producing a pattern in which there is more roughness per unit area peripherally than centrally.

This technique presented two difficulties:

a. Following manual removal, there was still a rough surface which could contribute to a repeat regression with haze response.

b. Although the authors used two different ultrasonic pachymeters, Pach-Pen XL (Bio-Rad, Santa Ana, CA) and DGH 2000 (DGH Technology Inc., Frazer, PA), the roughness of the surface after epithelial removal often prevented readings of how much tissue actually had been removed. The authors continued to have unpredictable results, especially overcorrections.

4. *Retreatment after laser removal of epithelium, with pachymetry.* Having observed with previous excimer laser removals of epithelium that there was a distinctly blue fluorescent pattern, the authors decided to remove epithelium with the excimer laser using the blue fluorescence to determine the endpoint of treatment. When nonfluorescence was reached over most or all of the zone, the treatment was stopped and pachymetry was repeated. This provided a smoothing effect because higher points of stroma were ablated first (epithelial smoothing principle). There was a smoother surface allowing a more consistent second pachymetry reading, and we had a more controlled and measured removal of tissue (obtaining information on epithelial removal from both the amount noted from the reading given by the excimer laser and by pachymetry).

Using the 10 μm per diopter rule, the amount of treatment applied with the laser was tailored. The problems encountered with this technique were still those of frequent overcorrection and the presence of central island with the use of the VisX laser for retreatment.

5. *Retreatment after laser removal of epithelium using a standard 50-μm ablation.* Because of the variability of retreatment results using fluorescence as an endpoint when using the VisX laser, a standard 50-μm removal of epithelium was adopted and retreatment for the measured refractive error was then performed.

The authors were still plagued largely by overcorrections and the persistence of central islands with this technique. One illustrative case that brought the source of central islands to our attention was one in which the residual refractive error was only 1 D. Normally, even with lasers that are prone to creating central island abnormalities, one would not expect an optically significant or topographically evident central island with just 1 D of correction. The central island was created in the process of laser epithelial removal. It also underlines the importance of being fully aware of the characteristics of the excimer laser one is using.

For standard VisX PRK procedures based on Machat's work,[16] the authors decided on a 2.5-mm central island treatment consisting of 50% of the primary treatment (e.g., for a 5.00 D treatment we would add an additional 2.5 D of treatment in a 2.5-mm central zone). The authors found that this markedly reduced our incidence of central islands, but some patients appeared to get a significant refractive effect, causing overcorrections.

With newer software versions (2.92), the incidence of central islands was markedly reduced because of the incorporation of additional central pulses to compensate for the central island tendency. Despite the new software for refractive purposes, the central island tendency was still fully in effect when the laser was in the PTK mode. Additional elements to our retreatment algorithm were developed using the following reasoning:

a. The amount of central island effect was considered to be at least equivalent in PTK mode to the same depth in PRK mode. A PRK treatment for a 6-mm zone with the VisX taken to a depth of 50 μm was equal to 3.33 D. This would normally have called for a 1.66 D central island ablation in the PRK mode.

b. The central island effect was expected to be greatest when the larger area pulses (close to 6 mm in diameter) were used in PRK mode. Because all the pulses were 6 mm in diameter for the PTK mode, a larger area central island was expected. The authors therefore expanded the area over which the central island treatment was applied from 2.5 mm to 3 mm.

After settling on a 50-μm standard ablation for epithelial removal and treating 1.66 D over a 3-mm optical zone, the authors were no longer getting central islands with retreatment.

Despite standardization of the epithelial removal and elimination of central islands, overcorrections still occurred. The authors thought that they were getting faster ablation of the stromal regrowth than of the original stromal structure. An arbitrary 50% reduction of the measured refractive error was introduced and found that for a significant propor-

tion of patients this brought the refraction to emmetropia. In some patients this resulted in undercorrection, but by using the same standardized transepithelial ablation pattern, retreatment could be done in the early postoperative period (about 1 to 2 months).

A modification of this technique, which has proved useful and reasonably predictable in cases where there is a wider area of haze, is as follows: If after the initial 50 μm of transepithelial ablation significant haze with a large peripheral component remained, additional PTK is applied over the full (6.00-mm) zone. When this was done, the authors subtracted 1 D from the total treatment for every 10 μm of further PTK. For example, for −5.00 D haze and regression, after the initial 50-μm epithelial ablation and central island pattern, if two additional 10 μm of treatment were added to eliminate haze over the entire treatment area, the total amount of treatment anticipated was reduced by 2.00 D. Fifty percent of the −3.00 D was treated, so that only −1.50 D of PRK was performed.

6. *Transepithelial ablation technique with the Nidek laser.* After settling on a transepithelial ablation technique with the VisX laser for treatment of regression with haze, the authors needed to develop a technique for the Nidek laser. The Nidek laser has a scanning pattern which gives a smoother ablated surface, but it also has a distinct Gaussian-like distribution of energy.

Because of the high energy level centrally and low energy level peripherally, ablation of 70 μm was necessary to achieve epithelial removal over the full zone. Because this exceeded the standard assumption of 50 μm for epithelial thickness by 20 μm, it was presumed that this would give 2.00 D of additional effect. In fact, it gave up to 3.00 D of refractive effect. For regression with haze situations in which the residual myopia was 3.00 D or more, this did not pose a significant problem. Enhancements for smaller amounts of myopia carried a large risk of overcorrection with this approach.

With the availability of hyperopic correction for the Nidek laser, changes in the transepithelial ablation approach were made. In order to obtain the most uniform removal of epithelium, a 50-μm PTK ablation (rather than 70 μm) is performed over the desired optical zone (usually 6 or 7 mm). This is followed by a hyperopic ablation that has an optical zone of 5.5 mm blending to 9 mm. In keeping with the previous reasoning, 2.00 D of hyperopic correction is used. Good results by enhancement with this method have been obtained and have markedly reduced the overcorrections for retreatments of myopia below 3.00 D.

Note the following precaution: when using transepithelial ablation, remember that epithelium tends to be thinner over the edge of a treatment zone of an eye previously treated with PRK (i.e., thinner over the shoulder of a treatment zone). Breakthrough to stroma may be seen over these peripheral areas in any of the following three circumstances:

a. When the transepithelial PTK ablation zone is larger than the original treatment zone, breakthrough will occur. If the ablation is perfectly centered, this will result in peripheral breakthrough almost simultaneously in a ring pattern before complete epithelial removal centrally. This can be useful for expanding the optical zone to some degree, but it is likely to give a myopic shift.

b. If the transepithelial ablation is decentered or if it is applied centrally over a previously decentered PRK ablation pattern, the peripheral breakthrough will occur in a crescent-like pattern. If the PTK pattern is decentered from the original PRK pattern, the crescent will occur in the direction in which the PTK is decentered relative to the center of the original PRK pattern. This can be useful in centering a decentered pattern. It can add to the original flattening effect, causing a hyperopic shift (or overcorrection) if the ablation breaks through centrally or has the potential to create minus cylinder in the axis 90° to the new, long axis of treatment (see the section on decentration).

c. If the previous PRK pattern involved treatment of astigmatism, a breakthrough crescent occurs on either side of the long axis of the original treatment ellipse. If continued, this ablation may reduce or eliminate the previously achieved astigmatic correction. This is also true for treatment after previous RK where the crescent of breakthrough is seen in the same axis as the transverse incisions.

Haze without Regression

Treatment of haze alone can be challenging, especially if the refraction is close to emmetropia. The

nature of haze tends to vary with its depth. Initial small amounts of haze, which consists of collagen laid down relatively close to the original unablated stroma, tends to be more uniform and finer in quality, with little significant optical effect. As further collagen is laid down it becomes more irregular, and a reticular structure develops with areas of epithelium between.

When treating haze, one should be careful not to be too aggressive in pursuing treatment to a completely clear cornea, as this increases the risk of inducing hyperopia. The current method of treating haze consists of doing a transepithelial ablation to remove epithelium by whatever method is appropriate for the laser used. The authors often find that merely ablating the initial 50 μm of tissue, intended primarily for epithelial removal, greatly reduces the rough reticular pattern (Fig. 8.7). If there is resid-

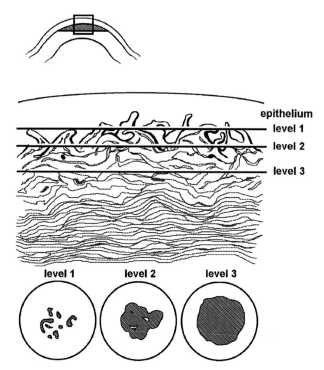

Fig. 8.7. This diagram demonstrates how the collagen regrowth becomes more disorganized the farther away it is from the original collagen structure, and how the reticular pattern of marked haze extends in an irregular fashion into the epithelium. The accompanying shaded patterns show the areas of nonfluorescence occurring within an ablation pattern, becoming more confluent as treatment progresses deeper into the stroma.

ual myopia and if the haze is concentrated more centrally, the haze is treated with a PRK pattern. Conservative parameters should be used. The authors have generally used 50% of the measured refractive error.

In the absence of any refractive error, 5- to 10-μm increments of PTK should be used to treat haze. One should keep in mind that in a 6- or 7-mm zone (depending on the beam profile of the laser used), every 10 μm will give approximately 1.00 D of hyperopic shift. In these cases, a hyperopic PRK treatment pattern is used following the removal of haze with PTK. After the treatment of haze, the authors recommend using a long, slow taper of steroids and nonsteroidal anti-inflammatories, as discussed in the section on steroids.

Small Optical Zones

Many different optical zone sizes have been used over the course of PRK experience. Currently, the authors use the Nidek laser with an optical zone varying from 5.5 to 6.5 mm, most commonly with a transition zone that extends to 7 mm. At times, they expand the transition zone to 8 or even 9 mm in eyes with large pupils and low corrections.

There are certain considerations related to optical zone size:

- *Quality of vision, especially at night.* Patients with smaller optical zones may often complain of visual aberrations at night, but not usually during the day (Fig. 8.8a). Aberrations are described as starbursts, halos, and/or blur. It is not uncommon for some patients to experience the full range of these effects. These night vision phenomena increase in incidence with any treatment zone decentration.

There is only a rough correlation between pupil size and night vision effects. In other words, some patients who have rather large pupils do not have significant complaints of night vision effects, and others who appear to have relatively small pupils may have significant complaints. Three major factors that may affect the accuracy of observations:

1. There may be considerable variation in the accuracy of judging pupil size. The only reliable instrument for judging pupil size in darkness may be an infrared camera or a similar device that does not stimulate a pupil response. Such an instrument can accurately measure pupil size in darkness or near-total darkness, such as one might encounter on a country road at night.

2. Patient responses may be subjective. There is often great difficulty in communicating exactly the difference between starburst, halos, and blur, especially when there is some residual refractive error complicating the assessment. Rarely does one encounter a patient with sufficient artistic skills to draw the exact patterns experienced.

3. It is difficult to quantify the severity of the effect. As with other parameters such as astigmatism, there may be great variance in a patient's ability to tolerate certain visual effects. In other words, two patients who are experiencing the same amount of visual aberration will vary significantly in their description of its severity because of their different tolerance levels.

Despite the above limitations, the authors have an impression of the incidence of significant night vision effects for the various optical zones used in their patients:

1. 4.5 mm: 20%.
2. 5 mm: 12%.
3. 6 mm: 5%.
4. 6.5-mm optical zone with a transition zone to 7 mm: 1–2%.
5. 6.5-mm optical zone with a transition zone to 8 or 9 mm: 0%.

In only a very few instances were these effects significant enough to prevent the patient from engaging in night driving.

The starburst and halo effect could potentially come from three sources:

1. Residual refractive error. This would give rise to a blurry circle, which some patients might interpret as a starburst.
2. Edge effect. This would consist of light scatter from the edge of the optical zone (Fig. 8.8b).
3. Peripheral myopia, with pupils that dilated beyond the optical zone. This may produce a separate myopic focus from the untreated peripheral cornea which would create a larger, blurry circle image or halo around the primary image (Fig. 8.8c).

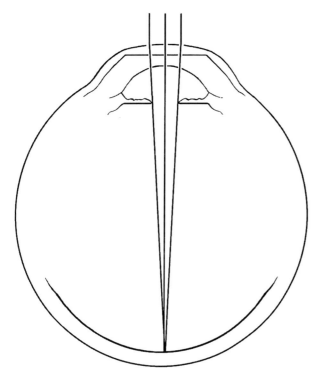

Fig. 8.8a. Daytime conditions with a small pupil and no light scatter or optical aberration following myopic PRK.

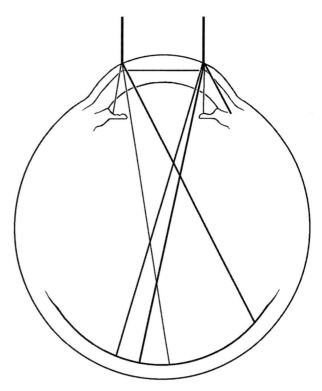

Fig. 8.8b. Demonstration of the edge effect causing variable scatter of light rays which strike the cornea at the edge of the optical zone.

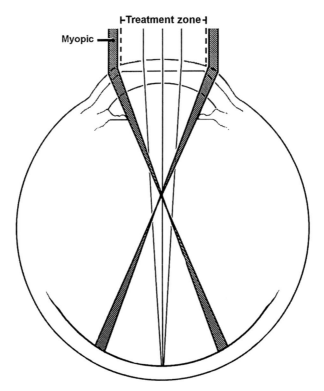

Fig. 8.8c. Peripheral myopia creating a halo or blurred circle image around the primary image.

Night myopia also has a significantly higher incidence in post-PRK patients than in the general population. This observation is based on cases in which the refraction is emmetropic, excellent daytime visual acuities are present, and maximally measured pupil sizes in dim light are small to moderate. Some of these patients nevertheless complain of blur occurring in dark conditions. This may be explained by the reduced positive asphericity and resulting spherical aberration.

- Size of the zone and degree of correction. One is limited by the degree of correction required when considering the optical zone size. Large corrections treated with large optical zones require the removal of a significant amount of corneal tissue and are likely to increase the risk of a regression with haze response.

Transepithelial Ablation to Enlarge the Optical Zone

This is a method described by Seiler and collaborators.[17] It takes advantage of the fact that epithelium tends to be thinner over the margins or shoulders of a previously treated area. By ablating through the epithelium with a larger optical zone size, one tends to break through the epithelium at the edges of the optical zone first. Peripheral stroma is removed,

and the size of the effective optical zone is expanded (Fig. 8.9). Seiler and coworkers stated that this could result in some return of myopia (usually about 1.00 D) because the corneal curvature increases with this technique. This effect can be used to advantage in some patients with a small degree of overcorrection. The authors have noted a refractive shift in the myopic direction of approximately 1.00 D.

While this procedure does tend to increase the optical zone, its effectiveness is limited. It does not create a dramatic improvement for people with severe night vision effects.

Late Completion of a Large Optical Zone

This is a method developed by Stephen Trokel (personal communication, 1996). The epithelium over the entire new treatment zone is removed. The original treatment is programmed into the laser. The patient is aligned under the laser and the treatment pattern commenced. The early pulses are blocked until the expanding pattern reaches the size of the original optical zone. The blocking of the beam is then discontinued, and the remaining pulses that normally would have been applied for the larger optical zone are applied over the entire original

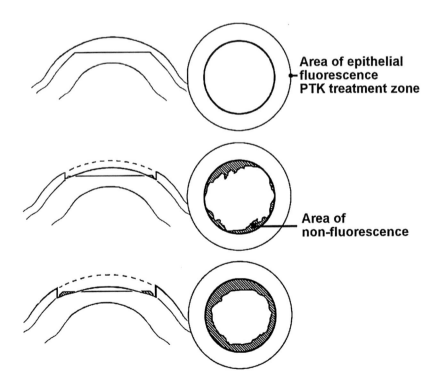

Fig. 8.9. Transepithelial ablation resulting in enlargement of the optical zone.

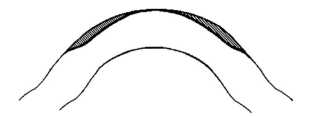

Fig. 8.10. Tissue removal in hyperopic ablation.

treatment area, expanding to the size of the new treatment zone. An example is as follows:

Original treatment	−5.00 D
Original optical zone	5 mm
New treatment zone available	6 mm

- Epithelium is removed to allow for the new 6-mm application; −5.00 D with a 6-mm zone diameter is programmed into the laser.
- The patient is positioned under the laser. Pulses are expended against another surface until the iris diaphragm expands to the 5-mm optical zone.
- The laser beam is no longer blocked, and pulses from the 5-mm zone expanding out to 6 mm are applied to the cornea.

Depending on the type of laser used, it is helpful to do a dry run on photo paper and actually measure when the sequence reaches the 5-mm diameter. Other lasers will give enough information to tell when the pulses have reached the 5-mm diameter. The new VisX Star excimer laser has this option (late completion of a large optical zone) as one of its programs.

Use of a Hyperopic Program to Treat Small Optical Zones

With the recent availability of farsighted corrections using the Nidek laser, the authors have elected to use the hyperopic capability to assist in expanding the optical zone (Fig. 8.10). The authors use a conservative approach, using an optical zone of 5.5 mm with a blend to 9 mm.

For example, in retreating a −6.00 D original correction in a 6-mm zone after removal of the epithelium, the authors use the hyperopic program and ablate for 3.00 D of correction with a 5.5-mm optical zone expanding to 9 mm. To counteract the effect of this added hyperopic correction, the authors arbitrarily calculated half of the hyperopic value of 3.00 D and do a further myopic correction of 1.5 D. Figure 8.11, which is somewhat exaggerated for purposes of illustration, shows that with expansion of the optical zone, the ablation does extend deeper into the cornea. This increases the chance of inducing haze and regression responses or thinning of the cornea. Pachymetry should be done prior to this treatment, and careful calculation performed to see how much additional corneal thinning would occur with this method. Never exceed 150 μm of stromal tissue removal.

Decentration

Decentration is among the most difficult problems to treat. One method has been suggested by Theo Seiler.[18,19] He uses a transepithelial ablation zone decentered in the direction opposite to the original decentration and continue ablation of epithelium until stroma appears (Fig. 8.12). This is generally in a crescent pattern, away from the center of the ini-

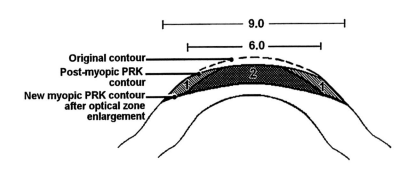

Fig. 8.11. Use of the hyperopic program to expand the optical zone. The shaded area labeled 1 indicates the area of tissue removed by the hyperopic treatment. The shaded area labeled 2 indicates additional myopic correction following the hyperopic treatment.

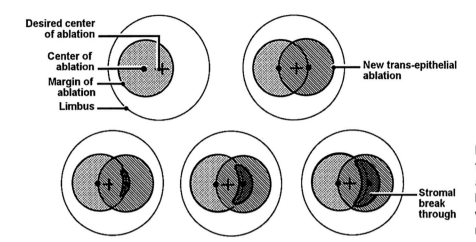

Fig. 8.12. This shows the new transepithelial ablation pattern and the subsequent stromal breakthrough pattern observed when treatment is applied for primary decentration.

tial decentered treatment. The technique tends to induce a hyperopic shift which may sometimes be large. Astigmatism may still be retained. These two conditions may themselves require further retreatments. A patient with significant symptomatic decentration should be advised of the possibility of multiple retreatment sessions.

Secondary decentration (i.e., in which the initial treatment was centered but an asymmetrical healing response has caused decentration to be apparent on corneal mapping) is treated with transepithelial ablation (Fig. 8.13). Usually the area of increased healing response shows breakthrough first, and this area is selectively ablated. The endpoint is determined as the point where breakthrough to stroma starts to occur in areas other than the areas of stromal regrowth with haze. This is generally effective in improving the status of the cornea both subjectively and topographically. One should be cautious in determining the amount to be treated at any one time and advise the patient that it may be best to do this treatment in more than one session. Only a small amount of the regrowth tissue should be removed at each epithelial ablation session, and approximately a month or more should be allowed for the epithelium to establish itself in a normal fashion (i.e., thinner over any elevated stromal areas and thicker over any depressions in stromal contour).

Central Island

Several theories have been proposed to account for central islands, and various definitions have been

proposed specifying the size, the number of diopters, and sometimes the decrease in BCVA. Sometimes the authors found central islands on topography, described frequently as a peninsula or isthmus pattern. They treated them simply on the basis of subjective complaints suggesting a central island and a history of treatment with a laser that is known to produce central islands. When this approach was used, these patients had complete resolution of their symptoms following treatment.

The initial treatment strategy was relatively simple and straightforward. Based on the corneal map, the size, location, and dioptric power of the central island were determined. The dioptric power was determined by reading the average power in the midperiphery of the treatment zone and was subtracted from the highest power of the central island.

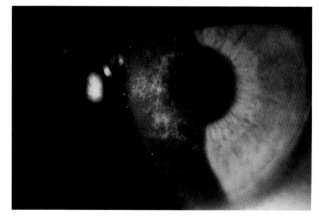

Fig. 8.13a. Haze with regression 14 months after PRK for myopia.

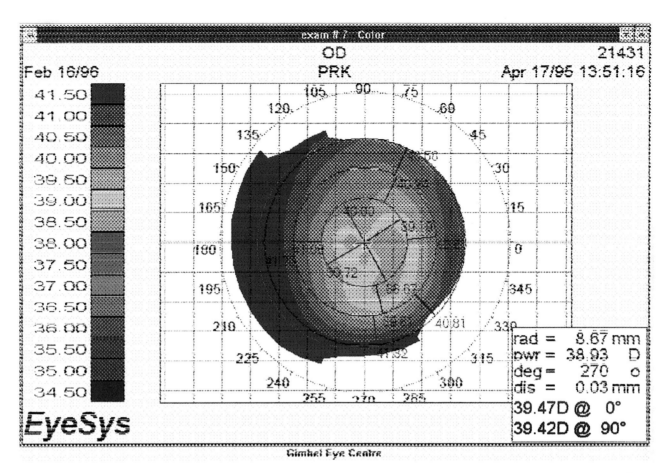

Fig. 8.13b. Preoperative corneal map showing secondary decentration of the optical zone. BCVA was $20/30^{-3}$ with refraction of -2.75 D.

Epithelium was then removed, and the illumination level under the microscope was adjusted so that the pupil size was equal to that shown on the corneal map. The margins of the pupil were used as a guide to positioning the central island treatment. A PRK pattern of treatment was applied using the dioptric power and optical zone determined from the corneal map. In the majority of these cases the central island was undertreated, sometimes leaving an optically significant residual central island.

The authors' current method of treatment for central islands uses the Nidek laser. They use transepithelial ablation, selecting an optical zone that will adequately cover the central island area, commonly 4.5 or 5.0 mm. In this situation, the higher central energy of the Nidek beam is advantageous. The limit of ablation is usually set at 70 μm. Treatment

is usually stopped well before this limit is reached and is based on the pattern of nonfluorescence as treatment progresses (Fig. 8.14). Breakthrough of the stroma is almost invariably central. Depending on the height and configuration of the central island, the dark nonfluorescent spot of ablation either maintains itself for a large number of pulses at about the same spot size (if the island is steep) or spreads out steadily and occasionally quickly (if the central island is shallow). Once the central area of nonfluorescence begins to approximate the size of the central island (as measured by corneal topography or as suspected on the basis of previous experience when the topography has not shown a central island), ablation is stopped. Also, ablation should be suspended if areas other than the center show breakthrough. If these additional sites of break-

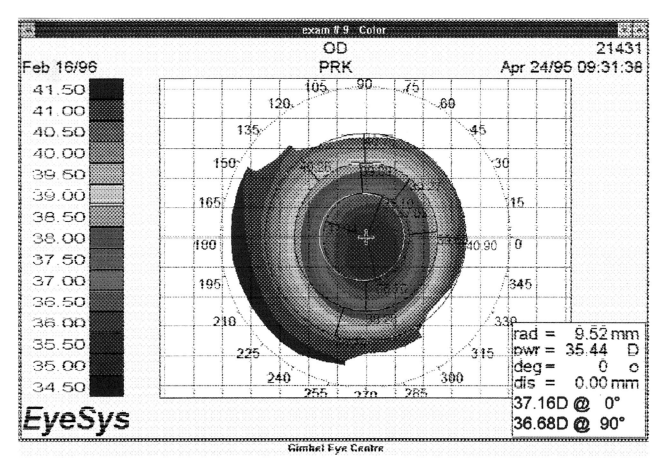

Fig. 8.13c. One week after PTK and PRK retreatment with the Nidek laser, the BCVA improved to 20/25 with refraction of +0.50/−0.75 × 85°. The postoperative corneal map shows improved centration of the optical zone.

through are at the far periphery and if one suspects that the entire central island has not been treated, one may stop the treatment and resume it with a smaller optical zone (e.g., going from a 5-mm treatment zone down to a 4-mm zone).

With the earlier method of central island treatment, the authors observed that 80% of patients showed a small to marked residual central island. With the new method of treatment using the Nidek laser, all patients are symptomatically improved, and over 80% show no central island at all after retreatment (Figs. 8.15, 8.16). In retrospect, with a better understanding of the epithelial smoothing principle (see the subsection on epithelium), one realizes that the undercorrection of the central island using the first method was likely due to the fact that the epithelium was thinner over the under-

lying stromal elevation of the central island, and perhaps somewhat thicker in the midperiphery. The corneal contour, as indicated by corneal mapping of the epithelial surface, would not have shown the true extent and elevation of the central island, and therefore the true dioptric elevation of the underlying stromal central island would have been hidden. In addition, the current method of treatment allows real-time observation and judgment of the completion of treatment.

PRK AFTER RK

Use of PRK after RK is a simple concept, but there are significant potential problems. Foremost among these, is a much higher incidence of haze and

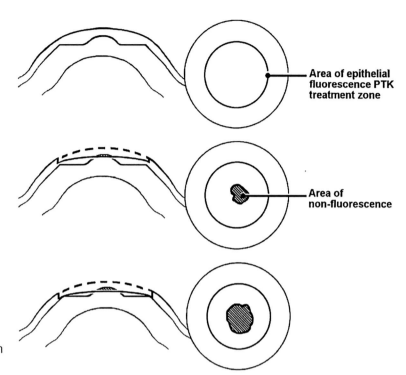

Area of epithelial fluorescence PTK treatment zone

Area of non-fluorescence

Fig. 8.14. Central island treatment with demonstration of central breakthrough.

regression than after PRK of the same amount in a previously unoperated eye[20] (Fig. 8.17). Although reports of this in the literature are few, it has been the authors' impression—and that of several of our Canadian and international colleagues—that this is the situation.[21,22] One theory is that with previous activation of keratocytes by the RK incisions, PRK causes much greater activation of new collagen formation than does PRK alone.

When manual removal of epithelium is done, there is some concern that the incisions may be reopened, contributing to regression and haze responses and/or to an increased effect of the original RK. When transepithelial ablation is used rather than manual removal of epithelium, there is often breakthrough in an unpredictable pattern due to irregular underlying stromal topography, potentially altering the end result. The authors found less regression and haze after transepithelial ablations.

In view of these factors, the authors recommend dividing the RK group into categories and varying the approach according to the situation. They also recommend using the steroid and nonsteroidal anti-inflammatory combination that are for strong recurrent haze and regression situations, tapering them for 9 months or longer, depending on the haze or

regression response shown (refer to the discussion on steroids).

One should warn patients with problems that are known to complicate RK, such as diurnal fluctuation or night vision effects, that these will not be remedied by PRK.

Prior to doing PRK after RK, one should perform a careful and complete refraction. These refractions are notoriously difficult to do because of the unstable nature of the cornea, diurnal fluctuation, accommodation, and the poor correlation between refraction and visual acuity in RK patients (we find that the visual acuity of most RK patients is better than one would routinely expect from the refraction). A manifest and cycloplegic refraction should be done at least once prior to PRK treatment. This refraction should be done as close to the same time of day as possible so that the relationship between the two may be established, minimizing the effect of diurnal variation. Several refractions should be performed throughout the day over as long a period from awakening to bedtime as possible. Afterward, a careful history should be taken, determining when the patient encountered the greatest decrease in vision. The patient should then be advised of the options for treatment, taking into account that correction of

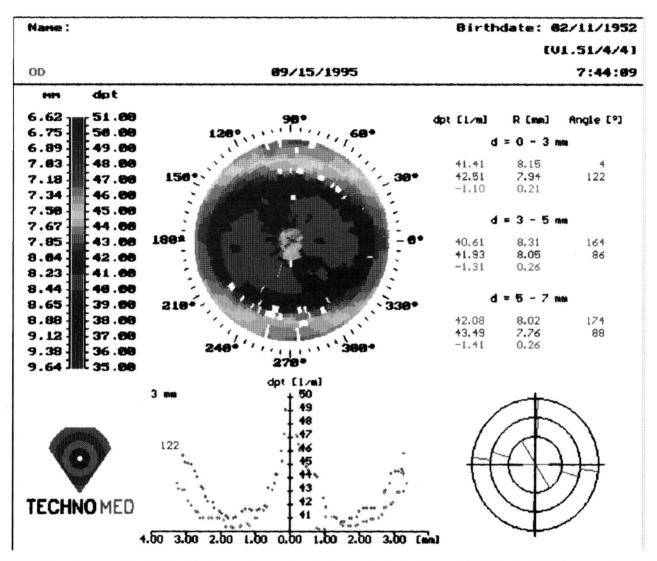

Fig. 8.15a. Preoperative TechnoMed corneal map showing a central island 4 months following PRK for myopia using the VISX 20/20 laser. BCVA was 20/25 +3 with refraction of +0.25 −0.50 × 37. The patient complained of decreased contrast sensitivity and ghosting.

the maximum amount of myopia at one point in the day may result in potentially significant hyperopia earlier in the day.

PRK Retreatment Categories After RK

Residual Spherical Myopia After RK Treatment of Spherical Myopia

This is the simplest problem to retreat and is fairly frequently encountered. In this situation, one can use transepithelial ablation to avoid disturbing the RK incisions. One should be familiar with the char-

acteristics of one's own laser when doing the transepithelial ablation. In doing manual removal of the epithelium, the strokes of the debriding instrument should be parallel to the incisions rather than across them.

After surgical epithelial removal, treat for the refracted amount of residual myopia. If a transepithelial ablation was done, the refractive effects of the ablation are taken into account. When a transepithelial ablation was done, breakthrough occurred in a radial pattern first, corresponding to the area around the incisions (Figs. 8.18A, 8.19).

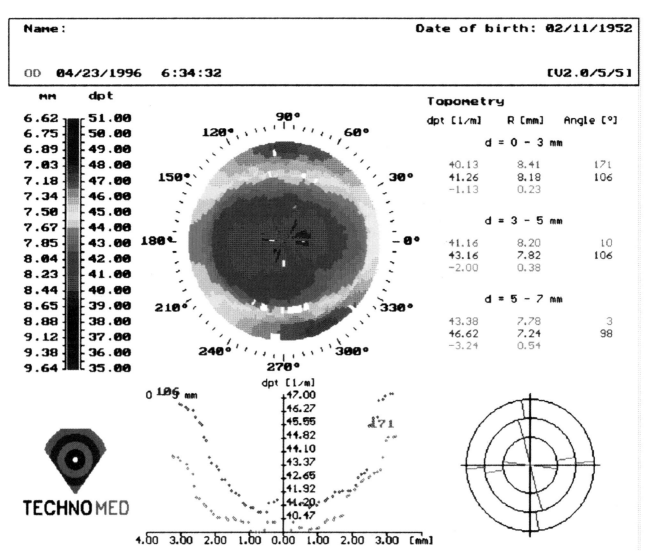

Fig. 8.15b. 6.0 months after PTK retreatment using the Nidek EC-5000, BCVA was 20/20, with refraction of +150 −1.25 × 37. Postoperative corneal map shows central flattening, with no evidence of the central island.

Myopia with Induced Astigmatism After RK Treatment of Spherical Myopia or Overcorrection of Astigmatism After RK Treatment of Myopia with Astigmatism

In both of these cases, transepithelial ablation is likely to show breakthrough over the shoulders of the newly flattened axis, rounding the cornea back to a more spherical shape. Decreasing the astigmatism with PTK is likely to induce a degree of hyperopic shift, depending on the beam profile of the laser used. It is important to be conservative with this approach because if an undereffect is achieved,

transepithelial ablation is easily repeated after 4 to 6 weeks to gain further effect. Careful note should be made of the number of microns ablated at the time of stromal breakthrough.

Myopia with Residual (Undercorrected) Astigmatism After RK and Astigmatic Keratotomy (AK) for Myopia with Astigmatism

In this situation, avoid transepithelial ablation because breakthrough of the shoulders on the steep axis of astigmatism tends to reverse some of the

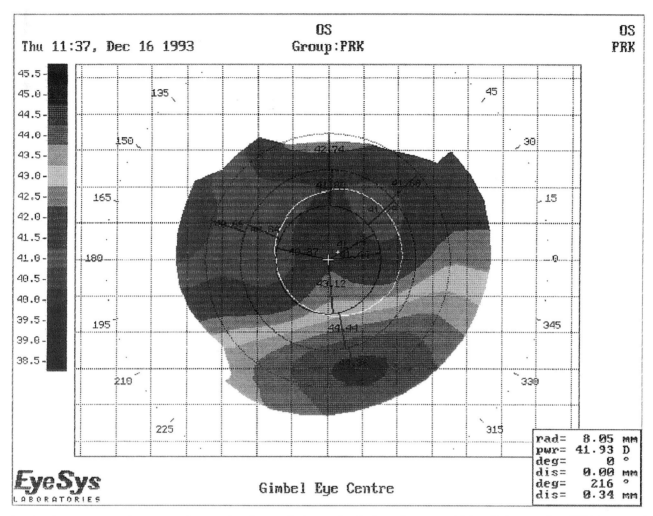

Fig. 8.16a. Preoperative corneal map showing an isthmus (variation of a central island) 1 year after PRK for myopia with the VisX Twenty/Twenty system. BCVA was $20/20^{-3}$ with refraction of $-1.25/-0.75 \times 7°$ and subjective complaints of ghosting and poor night vision.

astigmatism effect already obtained (Fig. 8.18B). The authors recommend surgical removal of the epithelium, with subsequent myopic and astigmatic ablation of the residual refractive error. A higher risk of haze and regression may be anticipated with surgical removal of the epithelium.

Residual Astigmatism After RK and/or AK for Myopia with Astigmatism (e.g., Plano/−2.00 D × 90)

Use the same technique as for the previous category. However, some degree of hyperopia should be anticipated and allowed for.

Hyperopia

Due to the possibility of progressive hyperopia in potentially large numbers of RK patients in the future, there is great interest in the potential ability of PRK to remedy this situation. There are two concerns:

1. Extensive removal of epithelium (because of the large area required for hyperopic ablation) over almost the whole length of RK incisions could potentially reopen incisions, causing increased effect, and possibly being the starting point for haze and regression responses.

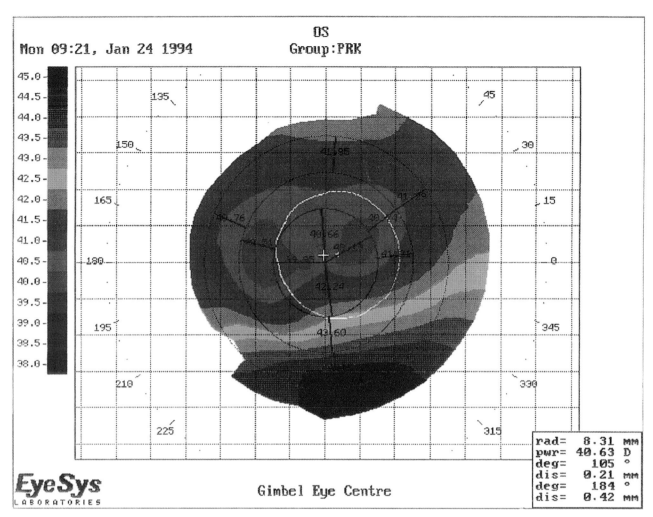

Fig. 8.16b. One month after PTK and PRK enhancement with the VisX Twenty/Twenty system, the BCVA was 20/20 with refraction of −0.25/−1.00 × 15°. The postoperative corneal map shows central flattening, with no evidence of the isthmus.

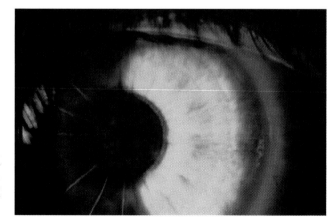

Fig. 8.17a. Haze with regression in an eye which had RK twice and PRK once for residual myopia. This photograph was taken 1 year after PRK enhancement with the VisX Twenty/Twenty system and demonstrates moderate haze.

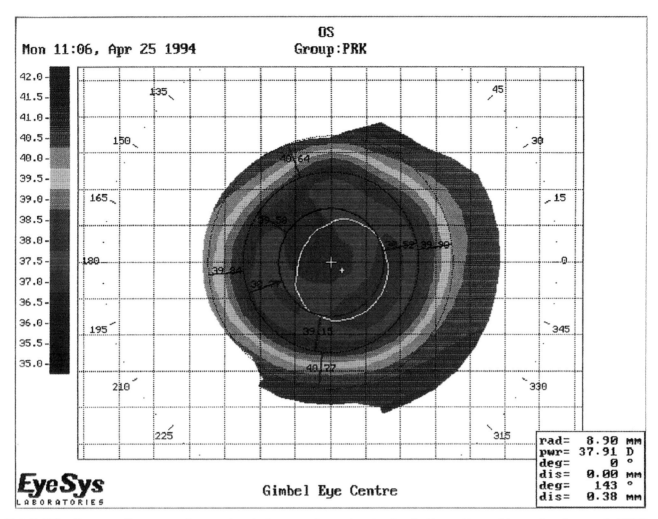

Fig. 8.17b. Preoperative corneal map showing a pseudo-peninsula due to the pattern of haze development. BCVA was $20/20^{-1}$ with refraction of $-1.25/-0.50 \times 75°$.

2. Hyperopia would thin a peripheral cornea already weakened by RK incisions. One potential concern is that despite correcting the hyperopia present at the time, such thinning would speed up further progression of the hyperopia, resulting in a quicker return of this situation several years later. Of course, if the hyperopia is disabling and the patient is not suited for or amenable to spectacle or contact lens correction, this may be the only available option.

PRK AFTER EPIKERATOPHAKIA

Some cases of epikeratophakia with Barraquer-Krumeich-Swinger (BKS) microkeratome with non-freeze keratomileusis and lenticule reshaping have resulted in a large overcorrection. The donor lenticules on these patients have been perfectly clear, with excellent correctable vision. The hyperopic results are undoubtedly due to contracture and thickening of the peripheral portion of the lenticule

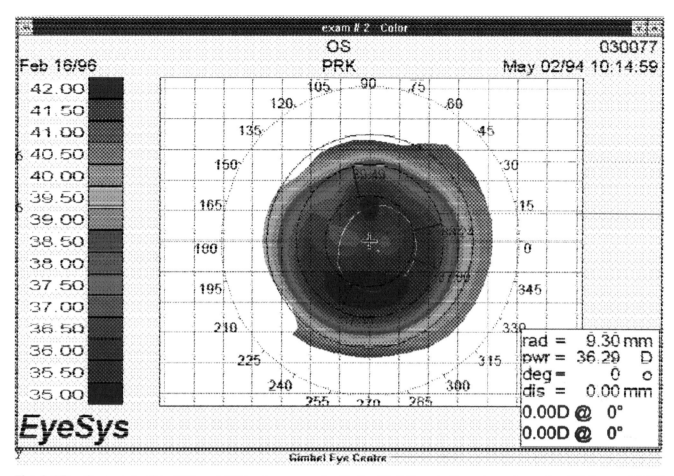

Fig. 8.17c. One week after PTK and PRK enhancement with the VisX Twenty/Twenty system, the BCVA was 20/25 with refraction of $+0.25/-1.00 \times 75°$. The postoperative corneal map shows central flattening and a more regular optical zone.

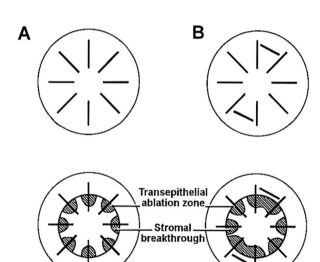

Fig. 8.18. (A) The pattern of stromal breakthrough in PRK enhancement after RK which tends to occur around the incisions, although rarely as symmetrically as illustrated. (B) A somewhat less symmetrical pattern in PRK enhancement after previous RK and astigmatism treatment with AK.

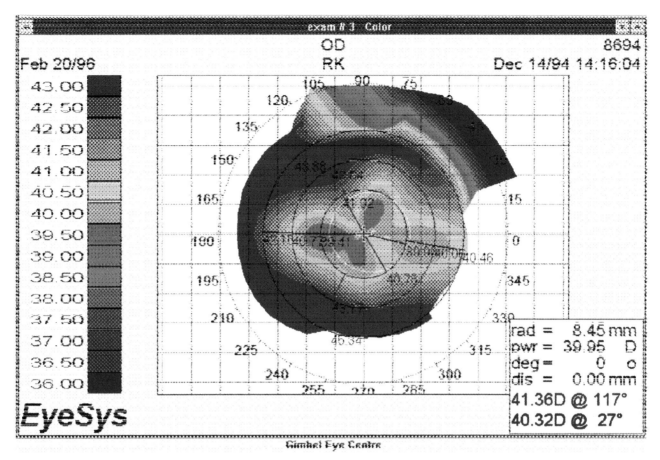

Fig. 8.19a. Pre-PRK corneal map of an eye which had previous eight-incision RK. The map shows a petaloid pattern centrally. BCVA was 20/20 with a refraction of −4.00/−0.75 × 90°. PRK was performed using the Nidek EC-5000.

that results in a plateau-shaped corneal surface (Fig. 8.20). Because of the clear graft and good quality of vision, the authors hesitated to remove these lenticules when laser technology was developing to reshape this grafted tissue.

When the authors first obtained the Summit ExciMed laser before any technology was available for hyperopic corrections, they shielded the central cornea with disks of increasing diameter to remove more peripheral tissue and obtain a hyperopic correction in one patient. This resulted in steep margins and a somewhat uneven surface, resulting in the development of moderate haze. Nevertheless, the refraction was improved. With the development of the ablatable mask by Summit on the OmniMed system in 1993, the authors tried this system for further correction in this patient and other overcorrected epikeratophakia patients. The size of the

ablatable mask and the optical zone corrected were not large enough to remove the full extent of the peripheral shoulder of tissue.

The next attempt to correct these patients involved the Nd:YLF picosecond Intelligent Surgical Laser (ISL). This obtained intrastromal ablation of tissue in overlapping arcs. The procedure was very tedious and somewhat imprecise because of the difficulty of staying in the same tissue plane with microsaccades, pulse pressure, and breathing movements of the head, even though the head was held firmly on the headrest of the slit lamp delivery system. Some change in curvature was obtained and no complications ensued, but the technique was abandoned while we awaited hyperopic PRK.

The authors have since successfully treated six patients with hyperopia from overcorrected myopic epikeratophakia using the Summit Apex Plus mask

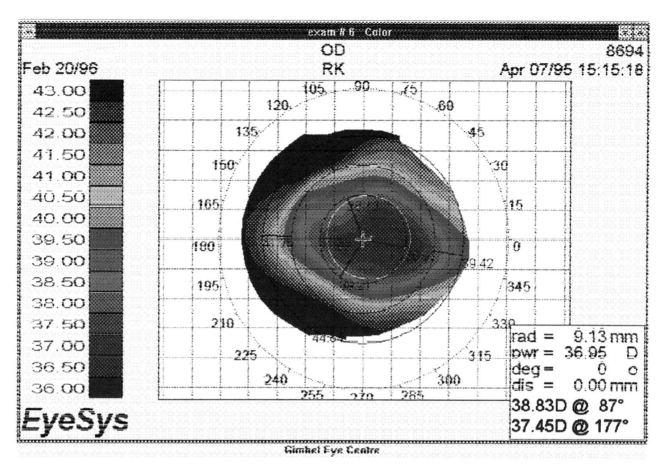

Fig. 8.19b. Four months after PRK enhancement, the BCVA was $20/20^{-3}$ with a refraction of $+1.25/-0.50 \times 30°$. The corneal map shows an enlarged, flattened, more uniform optical zone.

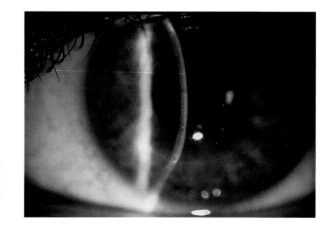

Fig. 8.20. Color photograph showing a plateau-shaped corneal surface with an epikeratophakia lenticule in place. The refractive error was $+8.75/-1.00 \times 150°$ 4 years after epikeratophakia surgery.

in rail system, the Nidek EC-5000 with hyperopic module, and the Novatec LightBlade. Following is an illustrative example of a sequence of treatments a 28-year-old male patient:

1. Initial refractive
   error   −11.50/−0.75 × 04
   BCVA   20/15
   Treatment   Epikeratophakia, June 1989
   Result   June 1992, +8.75/−1.00 × 150 with BCVA 20/20
2. Retreatment   ISL picosecond laser, nine treatments from June 1992 to June 1993
   Result   June 1993, +7.25/−2.25 × 145 with BCVA 20/15^{-3}
3. Retreatment   PTK with VisX (using the central epithelium as a mask), June 1993 (Fig. 8.21).
   Result   August 1993, +8.75
4. Retreatment   Summit OmniMed with 6.5-mm ablation zone and 5.00 D hyperopic mask, September 1993
   Result   December 1993, +6.25/−1.50 × 155 with BCVA 20/20
5. Retreatment   Summit OmniMed, with 6.5-mm ablation zone and 4.00 D hyperopic mask after PTK (with corneal masking by epithelium), December 1993
   Result   August 1995, +0.50/−1.75 × 161 with BCVA 20/20
6. Retreatment   Nidek PTK smoothing of cornea to improve the corneal contour, August 1995
   Result   January 1996, +0.75/−0.75 × 137 with BCVA 20/40, due to mild to moderate haze, which should improve over time

This case demonstrates the use of intrastromal ablation and PTK smoothing techniques using methyl cellulose, PTK smoothing using the epithe-

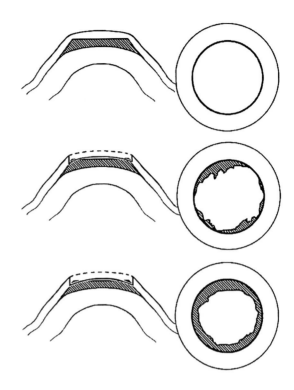

Fig. 8.21. PTK ablation pattern after epikeratophakia using the central epithelium as a mask.

lium as a mask, and the use of the ablatable mask for hyperopic corrections.

Such a case can be managed more easily by going directly to one of the current laser systems with hyperopic correction capability, using optical zones of 5.5 to 6.5 mm and blend zones out to 9.0 to 9.5 mm. Laser ablative technologies now allow us to recontour not only normal corneas, but also previously treated corneas, for improved focus and improved quality of vision.

LASIK RETREATMENT

LASIK is an emerging surgical technique which we are using for the refractive correction of high myopia. Initial reports on the results of this procedure indicate that it has advantages over PRK.[13,23–29] Postoperative pain and discomfort following LASIK are less, and stability of refraction is achieved earlier, providing faster visual rehabilitation. Since Bowman's layer is left intact, the risk of postoperative corneal haze is significantly decreased. Also, as the corneal epithelium is largely undisturbed, the risks of postoperative infection and infiltration of the cornea are diminished.

The authors use the automated corneal shaper (Chiron IntraOptics, Irvine, CA) to cut an 8.5-mm-diameter, 160-μm-thick flap on the anterior corneal surface. After the flap is lifted, excimer laser is applied to the corneal stroma beneath the flat, using the Nidek system in most cases. Since this is a new procedure, initially we were conservative in the amount of treatment applied to the cornea. For this reason, a significant number of our patients were undercorrected and required enhancements.

Enhancements are performed from as early as 2 weeks up to 6 months postoperatively. Gentian violet lines are placed at the temporal aspect of the flap, as with the original LASIK procedure, to allow perfect apposition of the flap after laser treatment. The procedure begins by carefully undermining the edges of the previously cut flap, using an intraocular lens positioning hook. It is advisable to examine the eye at the slit lamp and mark the edges of the flap with a gentian violet marker prior to attempting to lift the flap with the patient positioned supine at the laser. The cornea is kept well moistened while the hook is used to cut through the epithelium and to identify the entire edge circumference of the flap. After a few months, the stromal healing at the edges is quite secure and requires careful dissection. Once the epithelial seal and stromal healing at the edges of the flap are broken, the flap is easily lifted off its bed by blunt dissection with a spatula or, if necessary, by injecting balanced salt solution (BSS) beneath its edge, and gently lifting with the tip and shaft of the cannula. The spatula or a curved tying forceps is used to turn the flap. The fluid which was needed to dissect the flap is wiped to the edge of the stromal bed with a Paton spatula (Technolas C-5903, Germany) and absorbed with a Merocel sponge (Merocel Corp., Mystic, CT). Based on the residual refractive error, the laser is programmed to ablate the stromal bed. Myopic retreatment is straightforward. Retreatment for hyperopia requires shielding of the flap at the hinge when 9-mm blend zones are used. Patients often have difficulty seeing the fixation light because the stromal bed is roughened by the healing process, the dissection, and the fluid. Preoperatively, they are warned about this and are advised that the pinpoint light will become diffuse. They are instructed to remember to look at the center of the diffuse light during laser ablation.

Repositioning of the flap is performed as for a primary procedure.

In one case, which the authors attempted to enhance 10 months postoperatively, the flap was too adherent centrally to safely dissect completely. In this case, the flap was simply repositioned, with stabilization, when a new cut may be considered. It is advisable to use the microkeratome for a fresh cut in LASIK enhancements that are undertaken more than 6 months after the primary surgery.

Because the epithelium at the edges of the flap is irregular in an enhancement procedure (compared to the primary procedure, in which the cut in the epithelium is clean, having been made with a microkeratome blade), great care is needed to ensure that no epithelium encroaches beneath the flap. This epithelium is easily lifted from beneath the flap, using the cannula tip, a lens positioning hook, or a disposable needle tip. If the epithelial edges are trapped beneath the flap, this could predispose to epithelial ingrowth. Slit lamp examination is done for final inspection of the edges and interface before discharge. Patients are advised preoperatively that the rougher epithelial edges will probably result in somewhat more discomfort in the early postoperative period than they may have experienced after the primary LASIK procedure. Hydration of the flap and stromal bed may also delay the return of clear vision by a few hours.

Retreatment for interface debris follows the same technique, with the use of a Paton spatula to wipe the undersurface of the flap and the stromal bed. Irrigation is kept to a minimum to prevent flooding of the fornices and washing of mucus and debris into the stromal bed. Good drainage is maintained for the same reason.

Retreatment of wrinkles in the flap is not effective because of their permanence, even after 24 hr. For this reason, it is important for the eyes to be carefully inspected in the first hour postoperatively to determine that the flap is stable prior to the patients' departure. Patients should always be advised that if their vision becomes worse instead of better, or if there is any added irritation, they should return immediately.

Retreatment after a complicated LASIK procedure takes various forms. If the microkeratome failed to make a complete pass, the eye is allowed to heal for 3 months. The procedure is then repeated, usually without any evidence of the previous cut in the flap or bed. If the flap is excessively thin or irregular, or if the bed is irregular, the same approach is used, unless there is significant haze in the visual axis from the irregular surface healing. Haze occurs if the cut is so thin that Bowman's membrane is invaded. In these cases, surface PRK can be used to ablate through the haze, removing it, and to achieve the desired refractive effect. Manual debridement of the epithelium is not advised. Laser ablation of the epithelium is recommended, adjusting the PRK algorithm according to the breakthrough pattern. This depends not only on the corneal topography of the particular eye but also on the beam profile of the laser being used.

The authors have had to use this technique in only one case. In this eye, with a corneal diameter of 11 mm and an average keratometric value of 46.00 D, a thin flap with washboard-like ridges on the bed resulted during the primary LASIK procedure. The flap may have been buttonholed, but this was not appreciated at the time. The laser treatment for a correction of −8.75 D was performed and the flap repositioned. In the healing phase, mild haze developed in a patchy geographic pattern in the interface. The surface healing was irregular, suggesting that there may have been buttonholing of the flap. The edges of these microholes in Bowman's membrane curled inward, allowing slivers of epithelium under the edges. Three months postoperatively, the refraction was $-2.00/-0.25 \times 30°$ and the BCVA was $20/20^{-3}$.

PTK of the epithelium was performed as of this writing, with irregular stromal breakthrough encountered after 30 μm of ablation. PTK smoothing was continued to 50 μm, at which point the stromal breakthrough became confluent centrally in a 2.5-mm area. Slit lamp examination showed no trace of the epithelial ingrowth slivers. A myopic correction is expected from the central breakthrough. The technique may be repeated if necessary.

In one patient with an 11.5-mm-diameter cornea and an average keratometric value of 46.25 D, a particularly thin flap was inadvertently cut. A buttonhole occurred, and no laser treatment was done. The flap was simply repositioned. Epithelial downgrowth through the buttonhole occurred, leading to haze in the interface. In this case the flap was lifted approximately 1 month after the initial surgery, and the epithelial tissue was scraped from the stromal bed and flap with a No. 57 blade (Fig. 8.22). The flap was then carefully repositioned as in a primary

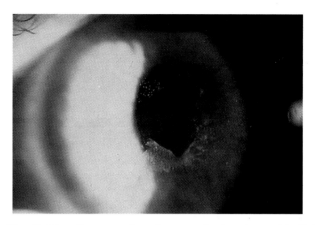

Fig. 8.22a. Preoperative photograph showing epithelial downgrowth which occurred through a buttonhole in the LASIK flap. The epithelial tissue was manually scraped from the flap and stromal bed with a No. 57 blade.

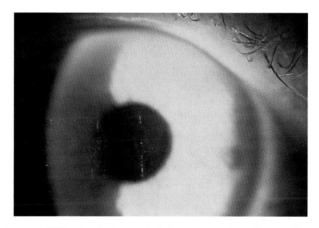

Fig. 8.22b. A photograph taken 6 weeks after epithelial tissue removal.

LASIK procedure. The edge healed without ingrowth. A repeated attempt at LASIK is planned after a few months of stabilization.

CONCLUSION

It remains to be seen whether the current advances in technology will become established enough to enable specific retreatment techniques to be subjected to controlled studies or whether we will need to continue to meet new challenges with responses based on intuition, observation, and our knowledge of the developing technology. Although PRK is still more of an art than a science, there is significant potential for treating almost any complication of PRK with the excimer laser itself.

In conclusion, the following recommendations can help increase the chance of ultimate success with retreatment:

1. Know your laser as well as you possibly can through a number of sources; other users may be an even better resource than the manufacturer.

2. Prepare patients for the possibility that retreatment may require more than one step, perhaps doing steps as many as 1 to 6 months apart. This allows for the last three recommendations.

3. Be conservative. Remove only small amounts of tissue at a time. In certain cases, it may be even appropriate to simply aim for a 50% effect with an initial treatment if there is significant uncertainty or numerous variables in a given situation.

4. If in doubt, do pachymetry to ensure that you still have a significant amount of corneal tissue to work with.

5. Avoid doing more than one step at a time whenever possible. Due to the variability and unpredictability in this situation, do not count on the response for a given step and base the next step on these assumptions. Frequently, these assumptions will either be incorrect or vary significantly from what was predicted.

REFERENCES

1. Lawless MA, Cohen PR, Rogers CM. Retreatment of undercorrected photorefractive keratectomy for myopia. *J Refract Corneal Surg.* 1994;10(suppl 2): S174–S177.

2. Seiler T, Derse M, Pham T. Retreated excimer laser treatment after photorefractive keratectomy. *Arch Ophthalmol.* 1992;110:1230–1233.

3. Epstein D, Tengroth B, Fagerholm P. Excimer retreatment of regression after photorefractive keratectomy. *Am J Ophthalmol.* 1994;117(4):446–456.

4. Hersh PS, Carr JD. Excimer laser photorefractive keratectomy. *Ophthalmic Pract.* 1995;13(4):126–133.

5. Peters DJ, Lim DTC. Central islands: which machines cause the least of these complications and why? *Ophthalmic Pract.* 1995;13(4):139–141.

6. O'Brart DPS, Kerr-Muir MG, Marshall J. Phototherapeutic keratectomy for recurrent corneal erosions. *Eye.* 1994;8(4):378–383.

7. O'Brart DPS, Lohmann CP, Klonos GJ. The effects of topical corticosteroids and plasma inhibitors on refractive outcome, haze and visual performance after photorefractive keratectomy. *Ophthalmology.* 1994;101(9):1565–1574.

8. Gartry DS, Kerr-Muir MG, Marshall J. The effect of topical corticosteroids on refraction and corneal haze following excimer laser treatment of myopia: an update. A prospective, randomized, double-masked study. *Eye.* 1993;7(4):584–590.

9. Fitzsimmons TD, Fagerholm P, Tengroth B. Steroid treatment of myopic regression: acute refractive and topographic changes in excimer photorefractive keratectomy patients. *Cornea.* 1993;12(4):358–361.

10. Tengroth B, Epstein D, Fagerholm P. Excimer laser photorefractive keratectomy for myopia. Clinical results in sighted eyes. *Ophthalmology.* 1993; 100(5): 739–745.

11. Gartry DS, Kerr-Muir MG, Lohman CP. The effect of topical corticosteroids on refractive outcome and corneal haze after photorefractive keratectomy: a prospective, randomized, double-blind trial. *Arch Ophthalmol.* 1992;110(7):944–952.

12. Caubet E. Course of subepithelial corneal haze over 18 months after photorefractive keratectomy for myopia. *Refract Corneal Surg.* 1993;(suppl):S65–S70.

13. Pallikaris IG, Saganos DS. Excimer laser in situ keratomileusis with photorefractive keratectomy for correction of high myopia. *J Refract Corneal Surg.* 1994;10(5):498–510.

14. Loewenstein A, Lipshitz I, Lazar M. Scraping of epithelium for treatment of undercorrection and haze after photofractive keratectomy. *J Refract Corneal Surg.* 1994;10(suppl):S274–276.

15. Machat JJ. PRK retreatment, indications and techniques. *Ocular Surgery News.* 1994;12(23):56.

16. Machat JJ. PRK retreatment, indications and techniques. *Ocular Surgery News.* 1994;12(24):44.

17. Seiler T, Kriegerowski M, Schnoy N. Ablation rate of human corneal epithelium and Bowman's layer with the excimer laser (193 nm). *Refract Corneal Surg.* 1990;6(2)99–102.

18. Seiler T, McDonnell PJ. Excimer laser photorefractive keratectomy. *Surv Ophthalmol.* 1995;40(2): 89–118.

19. Seiler T, Schmidt-Petersen H, Wollensak J: Complications after myopic phototherapeutic keratectomy primarily with the Summit excimer laser. In Salz J, McDonnell PJ, McDonald MB, eds. *Corneal*

Laser Surgery. St Louis, MO: CV Mosby; 1995: 131–142.

20. Gimbel HV, Sun R, Chin PK. Excimer laser photorefractive keratectomy after previous radial keratotomy. *Can J Ophthalmol*. In press.

21. Maloney RK, Chan WK, Steinert R. A multicenter trial of photorefractive keratectomy for residual myopia after previous ocular surgery. *Ophthalmology*. 1995;102(7):1042–1053.

22. Burnstein Y, Hersh PS. Photorefractive keratectomy following radial keratotomy. *J Refract Surg*. 1996; 12:163–170.

23. Pallikaris IG, Papatzanaki ME, Siganos DS. A corneal flap technique for laser in situ keratomileusis. *Arch Ophthalmol*. 1991;145:1699–1702.

24. Brint SF, Ostrick DM, Fisher C, et al. Six-months results of the multicenter Phase I study of excimer laser myopic keratomileusis. *J Cataract Refract Surg*. 1994;20:610–615.

25. Salah T, Waring GO, El-Maghraby A. Excimer laser keratomileusis in the corneal bed under a hinged flap: results in Saudi Arabia at the El-Maghraby Eye Hospital. In: Salz J, ed. *Corneal Laser Surgery*. St Louis, MO: CV Mosby; 1995;187–195.

26. Maldonado Bas A, Onnis R. Excimer laser in situ keratomileusis for myopia. *J Refract Surg*. 1995;11 (suppl):S229–S233.

27. Fiander DC, Tayfour F. Excimer laser in situ keratomileusis in 124 myopic eyes. *J Refract Surg*. 1995;11(suppl):S234–S238.

28. Gomez M. Laser in situ keratomileusis for myopia using manual dissection. *J Refract Surg*. 1995;11 (suppl):S239–S243.

29. Kremer FB, Dufek M. Excimer laser in situ keratomileusis. *J Refract Surg*. 1995;11(suppl): S244–S247.

9

Automated Lamellar Keratoplasty (ALK) and Laser in Situ Keratomileusis (LASIK)

Maria Clara Arbelaez

Juan J. Pérez-Santonja

Mahmoud M. Ismail

Jorge L. Alió

Ekktet Chansue

José Güell

Ray Jui-Fang Tsai

Howard V. Gimbel

INTRODUCTION

The concept of lamellar refractive surgery was introduced by José Barraquer[1] almost half a century ago. Myopic keratomileusis, as devised by Barraquer, involved flattening the anterior curvature of the cornea by removal of a stromal lamella. Laser in situ keratomileusis (LASIK)—the use of the microkeratome to make a corneal flap that gives access to the corneal stroma combined with ablation of the exposed stromal bed with an excimer laser—has become for many corneal surgeons the technique of choice to correct moderate and high levels of myopia. It was first described in 1990 by Pallikaris and coworkers, who created a corneal flap in rabbits with a microkeratome and then ablated the bed to achieve a refractive change.[2] In 1992, Buratto and associates used an excimer laser to remove tissue from a corneal button that had been placed under the laser.[3]

Some surgeons favor the LASIK technique to the extent that they perform it even on patients with low levels of myopia. The features of the LASIK procedure that may account for its increasing use include the very limited disruption of the epithelium and Bowman's membrane (Bowman's membrane is cut only at the periphery, and the epithelium dries somewhat but is not removed) that can lead to pain-free healing, central corneal haze-free healing, and rapid visual recovery. In addition, the predictability of the surgical outcome usually ranges from satisfactory to excellent due to the precise removal of stromal tissue inherent in laser technology. Furthermore, complications related to corticosteroid use are virtually eliminated because these drugs are usually used for only a very short time after LASIK. Thus the procedure has the potential to deliver the results that have long been the goal of refractive surgery—a high degree of predictability combined with a rapid and comfortable postoperative course.

Before photorefractive keratectomy (PRK) evolved and before LASIK came into use for the correction of high levels of myopia, automated lamellar keratoplasty (ALK) was virtually the only corneal procedure (after epikeratoplasty became increasingly unpopular because of its lack of predictability and poor optical results[4]) that could provide any degree of correction of these refractive errors. The predictability of ALK, however, was often less than desired,[5,6] and PRK performed with early models was also associated with a number of problems.[7,8] It was, in fact, the deficiencies of these techniques that provided an incentive to search for a better method, such as LASIK.

131

The level of success with ALK often depended on the surgeon who performed the procedure. Few studies have been reported in the literature, and no large, definitive, long-term clinical trial has been performed. The results of three studies published recently in peer-reviewed journals are summarized below.[9-11]

ALK FOR MYOPIA

Ibrahim et al.

An ALK study with the Automatic Corneal Shaper (Ruiz nomogram and complete cap resection) was conducted at the El Maghraby Eye Hospital in Jeddah, Saudi Arabia, on a consecutive series of 88 eyes with a mean preoperative spherical equivalent of 12.00 D of myopia.[9] Two of the four surgeons performing the surgery had experience with the ALK technique. Manifest refraction was the principal postoperative variable. The corneal cap was sutured into place for most eyes.

The surgery reduced the level of myopia in all eyes, but there was a tendency toward undercorrection, with 57% having a refraction of more than −1.00 D at 1 year. At 5 weeks, the mean refraction was −0.21 D, and by 1 year it was −1.86 D. At 1 month, 21% of the eyes were within ± 0.5 D of the planned correction, 38% were within ± 1.0 D, and 67% were within ± 2.0 D. At 1 year, the outcome ranged from −13.25 D to +4.6 D, and only 35% of the eyes were within ± 1.00 D of the planned correction, making the predictability of the refractive outcome only fair. Prior to surgery, almost half of the eyes had less than 20/40 visual acuity with spectacle correction. Following surgery, 21% had 20/40 or better uncorrected visual acuity. Refractive astigmatism was increased moderately by the procedure (mean, 0.5 D), primarily due to suturing. Many patients reportedly experienced postoperative glare and halos, but an incidence was not given. The disc–bed interface was persistently clear in most patients, and postoperative corticosteroid use was limited.

Because of undercorrection at 1 year of approximately 1.5 D, the authors suggested that a change in the algorithm may be needed. They concluded that predictability of outcome with this surgical procedure was poor and suggested that their study could be used as a benchmark for comparison with newer techniques of keratomileusis.

Price et al.

A single-center, two-surgeon, consecutive series of keratomileusis in situ for myopia using the Automatic Corneal Shaper was performed on 152 eyes by Price and associates.[10] The mean preoperative myopia value was −9.30 ± 3.10 D (range, −5.1 to −22.75 D). In the first 64 eyes the cornea cap was completely resected, but later in the study a flap was used (85 eyes), Radial and astigmatic keratotomies (retreatments) were performed in 50% of the eyes after the original keratomileusis procedure to enhance the results.

The mean follow-up period was 5.6 months, with a range of 1 to 20 months. One month postoperatively, 21% of the eyes were within ±0.5 D of the intended correction, 38% were within ± 1.0 D, and 67% were within ± 2.00 D. Before any retreatments, 6% of the eyes had 20/20 or better uncorrected visual acuity, 44% had 20/40 or better, and the rest had 20/60 to 20/200. Loss of two lines of best corrected visual acuity occurred in 6% of the eyes. An overall 5% shift of refraction in the myopic direction occurred between months 1 and 6. Few complications were observed.

The variability of the initial refractive results, requiring retreatment in more than half of the eyes, was noted to be a limitation of the technique.

Lyle et al.

This study was a prospective series of ALK for myopia in 128 eyes with a follow-up period of approximately 1 year.[11] One surgeon performed all of the surgeries, and the learning period was not omitted. The hinged flap technique was used in 17 cases in the latter part of the study. The Ruiz nomogram and the Automatic Corneal Shaper were used for the microkeratome resections. An undercorrection of up to 1.00 D was targeted for some patients. Departing from the methods recommended by Casebeer,[12] the surgeons performed a third lamellar cut if the second cut was insufficient to correct the myopia according to a pachymetry measurement. Since retreatments were performed for undercorrected patients, the data were presented for all patients (N = 128) and for the subset with no retreatments (N = 29).

The mean postoperative uncorrected visual acuity, expressed in decimal fractions for all patients, was 0.68 ± 0.22 (20/30) (range, 0.1 to 1.0). At the last follow-up exam, 86% of the eyes had uncorrected visual acuity of 20/40 or better. A total of 76.4% of eyes were within 1.0 D of emmetropia, and 93% were within 2.0 D.

For the subset of patients who had no post-ALK retreatments, the mean uncorrected visual acuity at approximately 1 year was 0.69 ± 0.21 (20/30), which was very similar to the value for all patients. The mean best corrected visual acuity postoperatively for the subset was 0.95 ± 0.10 (20/21). Two of the eyes (6.9%) lost two or more lines of best corrected visual acuity.

The mean preoperative cycloplegic spherical equivalent refraction for all patients of −7.48 ± 2.0 D (range, −1.75 to −13.25 D) was reduced to a mean of −0.39 ± 1.14 D at the last follow-up. The value for the subset of patients was −6.78 ± 2.45 D (range, −11.25 to −2.5 D) preoperatively, and postoperatively at approximately 1 year it was −0.46 ± 1.7 D (range, −4.75 to +4.0 D). Seventy-two percent were within ± 1.0 D of emmetropia, and 90% were within 2.0 D. Complications included 4% of eyes with an overcorrection greater than +1.0 D and epithelial ingrowth in the interface requiring surgical removal in 2%. Best corrected visual acuity of two lines or more was lost in 6.3% of eyes.

Good results were achieved in this study with at least 1 year of follow-up for all patients. With ALK surgery alone, uncorrected visual acuity was 20/40 or better in 86% of eyes, and 90% were within ± 2.0 D of emmetropia. The correction achieved at 3 months postoperatively (prior to any reoperations) was stable and close to the value recorded at the last visit. The authors concluded that ALK was a reasonably safe and effective technique for correcting moderate to high myopia.

LASIK FOR MYOPIA

Microkeratomes

The microkeratome was developed by José Barraquer in 1962. All microkeratomes consist of a fixation device that holds the eye and applanates the cornea against the undersurface of the device and a blade that carves a lamellar disc like a carpenter's

plane. In situ myopic keratomileusis with an automated microkeratome was first introduced by Luis A. Ruiz, M.D., of Bogota, Colombia, in the late 1980s. This instrument (Fig. 9.1) made it possible to control the speed of the pass across the eye so that more consistent cuts could be made, and ALK was developed based on this technology. From the time of the very first lamellar refractive procedures done by Barraquer,[13] accuracy and predictability have been a concern. Although the results of ALK have not been completely accurate or predictable, the Ruiz automated microkeratome, known today as the Automatic Corneal Shaper (Chiron Vision, Claremont, CA), greatly improved the keratomileusis technique and is the most popular system in use today. Other systems for performing the lamellar keratoplasty preceding the laser ablation include the Draeger lamellar rotary microkeratome, the MicroPrecision lamellar keratoplasty system, the Universal Keratome, the Clear Corneal Keratome of Guimaraes, and the Schwind Keratome.

The Automatic Corneal Shaper system consists of an electrical motor-driven automated microkeratome, which makes the speed of the pass across the eye constant, an adjustable suction ring for selecting the diameter of corneal tissue that will be resected (maximum diameter cut of 9.0-mm), a plate system with plates of different thicknesses to vary the depth of the resection, and a control unit with a vacuum pump for the suction ring and the power supply for the microkeratome. The electrical

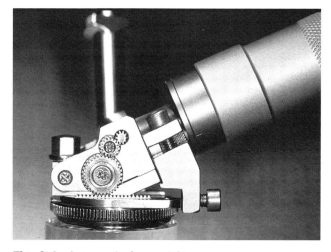

Fig. 9.1. Automatic Corneal Shaper.

motor powers the blade oscillation and the automated gear-driven system for passing the keratome head through the suction ring, and both are related. One interesting feature is the reverse position. With this position, the surgeon can perform a flap or hinged keratectomy by advancing the keratome head until it is mechanically stopped by a stop screw and then reversing direction.

The Draeger lamellar rotor microkeratome (Storz Instruments GMBH, Heidelberg, Germany) is a semiautomatic rotor keratome with a self-incorporated suction ring which operates with a rotational mode of its blade. The incision is carried out continuously, with accurate adaptation of the motorized feed to the circumferential speed of the rotor blade. The cutting thickness may be changed to 150, 250, or 350 μm by exchanging the spacer. This microkeratome has a transparent corneal applanation plate for selecting the diameter of the disc that will be resected.

The MicroPrecision microkeratome (Eye Technology, Inc., St. Paul, Minnesota) is a manual keratome with a high-speed turbine motor that powers the oscillation of the blade. The thickness of the disc is determined by fine-tuning the distance between a fixed plate and the blade using a differential micrometer. This system has multiple rings for selecting the appropriate disc diameter that will be resected.

The Universal Keratome (Phoenix Keratek, Inc., Scottsdale, AZ) is an automatic keratome with a self-incorporated suction ring. A high-speed electrical motor powers the blade oscillation, and a piston system promotes the blade advancement. The thickness and diameter of the disc are determined by a polymethylmethacrylate (PMMA) insert placed into the microkeratome head.

The Clear Corneal Keratome of Guimaraes (Belo Horizonte, Brazil) is a manual keratome that offers a large optical zone of 9.0-mm and uses a very thin 2-mm wide blade. The suction ring is on the same glass platform in which the blade is running. The microkeratome requires the use of only one hand and the force of the blade can be controlled with one finger.

Excimer Lasers for LASIK

The extreme precision of the excimer laser in shaping corneal stroma has been seen as a way to improve the results of lamellar refractive surgery.[14,15] The LASIK technique would ideally combine the accuracy of the excimer laser to remove corneal tissue with the ability of the microkeratome to access the inner stroma and preserve Bowman's membrane, reducing the effect of wound healing and some of the problems associated with PRK.

The original concept of using the excimer laser in myopic keratomileusis was driven by the early variable and poor results with the excimer for surface ablation (PRK) in patients with high myopia. Because of the depth of the ablation required, wound healing is very important in these patients. Scarring is more prominent, and regression caused by hyperplasia of the epithelium and new collagen production is also more or a problem. It is assumed that with laser lamellar keratoplasty, the healing process will be less intense, and therefore that less scarring and regression will occur.[16]

Chiron Technolas Keracor 117

Arbelaez et al.

Overview

In a study performed by Arbelaez and collaborators in Cali, Colombia, a third-generation excimer laser system, the Chiron Technolas Keracor 117, with new scanning software known as PlanoScan that allows the beam to scan or "skip" around the ablation area, was used. The features of this laser system are shown in Table 9.1. The beam of the Keracor 117 scans the cornea, moving a 2-mm spot rapidly across the ablation zone. It can ablate an 8-mm zone instead of the 7-mm zone ablated by the wide-field Keracor 116 model. The larger optical zone helps to reduce postoperative glare. The increase in pulse frequency from 10 Hz in the Keracor 116 model to 20 Hz in the Keracor 117 model allows a very rapid treatment time, which decreases the effects of temperature and humidity and permits

Table 9.1. Features of the PlanoScan Keracor 117 Excimer Laser

Beam size	2 mm
Beam energy density	120 mJ/cm^2
Pulse frequency	20 Hz
Beam tracking	Active
Maximum treatment size for myopia	8 mm
Maximum treatment size for hyperopia	9 mm

Table 9.2. Corneal Effects Seen with the Keracor 117 PlanoScan

- Less acoustical shock
- Less trauma
- Less edema
- Extremely smooth corneal ablation
- Prepared for topographic link

Table 9.4. Study Exclusion Criteria

- Anterior segment pathology
- Residual, recurrent, or inflammatory ocular disease or corneal abnormality
- Ophthalmoscopic signs of progressive or unstable myopia
- Unstable central keratometry readings
- Previous intraocular or corneal surgery in the eye to be operated on
- Blindness in the contralateral eye
- History of herpes keratitis
- Diagnosed autoimmune disease, connective tissue disease, or clinically significant atopic syndrome or diabetes
- Chronic systemic corticosteroid or other immuno-suppressive therapy and any immunocompromised situation
- Pregnancy

more consistent corneal hydration during the ablation. The beam produces less of an acoustical shock wave, as evidenced by the reduced plume. A very evenly ablated surface is the usual result, and central islands have not been seen. The corneal effects are summarized in Table 9.2.

Design and Methods

Preoperative Evaluation: Patients who provide informed consent for the procedure and who were likely to comply with the visit schedule were entered into the study, provided that they met the inclusion criteria shown in Table 9.3 and none of the exclusion criteria shown in Table 9.4.

The patient examinations include measurements of visual acuity with and without correction for distant and near vision. The use of soft contact lenses is discontinued for 3 weeks and rigid lenses for 4 weeks before the presurgical evaluation. Refractions are performed with and without cycloplegia, and ultrasonic pachymetry measurements of the central cornea were obtained. The eyelids and adnexa are examined for infection, signs of dryness, or exposure keratopathy. Deeply set globes, which can cause difficulty with the application of the suction ring, are noted. A detailed slit lamp examination is performed and intraocular pressure measured. The fundus is evaluated through a dilated pupil.

Table 9.3. Inclusion Criteria

- Spherical myopia of 0 to 14.00 D and refractive astigmatism of 0 to 6.00 D
- A stable refraction during the last year
- Age of at least 18 years
- Ability and willingness to return for scheduled follow-up examinations for 2 years after surgery

Surgical Procedure: Topical proparacaine or tetracaine is administered every 5 min four times for 20 min before surgery. Anxious patients receive 10 mg of Valium before the procedure and/or systemic sedation.

The Automatic Corneal Shaper is used to create the corneal flap, with a new blade inserted into the keratome head for each procedure. The blade holder and blade assembly are checked by rotating the probing shank between the thumb and forefinger to evaluate whether the gears turned freely. A 160-μm plate is inserted into the microkeratome, except for patients with more than 15.0 D of myopia, in whom a 130-μm plate is used. The motor is attached to the corneal shaper and the shaper is attached to the pneumatic fixation ring, and the forward and reverse motions are assessed.

Patient demographic and refractive data are entered into the computer terminal of the Chiron Technolas Keracor 117 excimer laser system. The system is activated, and a fluence test is performed before each procedure.

Surgical Technique: The anesthetized eye is irrigated with saline, and the eye and face are prepared and draped as for intraocular surgery. One drop of 0.5% Betadine is instilled, and a blepharostat that gives maximum exposure of the globe is put in place. To aid centration and help to reorient the disc in the event of complete cap resection, a specially designed corneal marker that has a pararadial line joining an internal 3-mm circle with an external 10.5-mm circle is dipped in gentian violet and placed on the cornea, with the inner circle concentric with the pupil.

The pneumatic fixation ring is applied to the globe, with the handle of the ring directed inferiorly for the right eye and superiorly for the left eye to aid exposure and avoid resting the instrument against the patient's nose. The surgeon can perform centering movements by using the fixation ring to move the cornea. Pressing the footpedal once activates the suction, and an intraocular pressure of 65 mm Hg or more should be obtained, as measured with a Barraquer tonometer on a dry cornea. This conical plastic instrument has a convex dome which magnifies the flat lower surface and the inscribed applanation ring. When the intraocular pressure is 65 mm Hg, the applanation circle created by the tonometer will exactly equal the diameter of the inscribed circle. If the pressure is lower, the applanation circle will be larger than the inscribed circle.

Prior to lamellar resection, the corneal shaper is inspected to be sure that a 160- or 130-μm plate has been inserted. A single drop of balanced salt solution (BSS) is placed on the underside of the shaper for lubrication. Placing the shaper head on the pneumatic fixation ring involves inserting the dovetail into the dovetail groove and lowering it into the horizontal position. Then the shaper head is inserted into a notch on the fixation ring until a tooth of the largest pinion is engaged in the dented rack.

When the forward pedal is depressed, the microkeratome moves forward to perform the lamellar incision and stops when the stopper is reached. The reverse pedal is then depressed to reverse the microkeratome, and the corneal shaper is then removed from the rack. Suction to the pneumatic suction ring is stopped by depressing the suction footpedal, but the ring is kept in position to stabilize inadvertent eye movements. The hinged corneal flap is folded over to the nasal side of the eye with an irrigation cannula.

The excimer laser is focused on the center of the corneal bed, and 30 sec later the laser is activated to perform the ablation. The stromal bed and the underside of the corneal flap are cleaned of cells by irrigation with a stream of filtered BSS while brushing the surfaces and suctioning the excess fluid. The flap is then gently replaced over the bed and irrigated continually to complete the cleaning of the interface and reposition the flap. The gentian violet pararadial mark on the cornea is aligned across the incision. The fixation ring is removed without disturbing the flap. To confirm adequate adhesion across the interface, the peripheral cornea is indented with forceps to check for the presence of striae passing from the periphery into the flap.

The lid speculum is removed. One drop of 0.3% tobramycin is instilled, and an eye shield is placed over the eye to prevent the patient from rubbing the globe and dislodging the flap. At the first postoperative visit, the eye is examined at the slit lamp to ensure that the flap is in place and that there are no significant interface opacities. For 1 week postoperatively, Flarex and Naphcon A, 1 gtt tid, are instilled. If at later visits it appears that the expected refractive outcome has not been achieved (≤20/40 uncorrected visual acuity with ≥1.0 D of residual refractive error), a repeat procedure (enhancement) can be performed 3 months after the initial surgery. If more than 1 year has passed since the initial procedure, the enhancement is approached as if the eye had no previous surgery. The same plate employed in the initial surgery is used, and the current subjective refraction is entered into the computer.

Results

A total of 237 eyes with mean spherical myopia of −3.6 D (SD, 2.4 D; range, 0 to −14.0 D) and 236 eyes with a mean level of cylinder of 1.3 D (SD, 1.2 D; range, 0 to 6.0 D) underwent LASIK surgery for the correction of myopia with or without astigmatism. Patients were grouped into categories of low myopia (−2.0 to −6.0 D, 198 eyes), moderate myopia (−6.5 to −10.0 D, 31 eyes), and high myopia (−10.5 to −14.0 D, 8 eyes). Postoperatively, patients were to be examined the next day, at week 1, and at months 1, 3, 6, 12, and 24.

Three months postoperatively, follow-up data were available for 97 eyes (79, 15, and 3 eyes in each of the refractive groups, respectively), representing 41% of the original study population of 237 eyes. The mean postoperative sphere was 0.34 D, with a standard deviation of 0.52 D and a range of −1.75 to 1.0 D. Both uncorrected and best corrected visual acuity results were very good: 96% of the low-myopia eyes and 82% of the moderate-myopia eyes had 20/40 or better vision without correction, and 100% of eyes in all of the preoperative myopia categories had 20/40 or better corrected acuity.

The accuracy was excellent: 88% of the low-myopia eyes and 67% of the moderate-myopia eyes were within ± 0.5 D, and 100% of the low group and 87% of the moderate group were within ± 1.0 D of the intended correction. In the high-myopia category, the number of patients available at follow-up was too small to report. Overall, 95% of the eyes were within ± 1.0 D of the intended correction. For cylinder, 93% were within ± 0.5 D of the intended correction. The procedure appeared to be safe, with 2% of the eyes losing one line of best corrected visual acuity in the low-myopia category and 9% of the eyes losing two lines in the moderate-myopia category.

A summary of the results is shown in Table 9.5.

Conclusions

Scanning beam technology with the PlanoScan Keracor 117 provides a wide, oscillating beam that has many clinical advantages. It uses a wide optical zone of 8 mm that reduces postoperative glare and produces a very smooth ablated surface. Topography shows the ablated surface to have very smooth contours, less postoperative fibrosis, and less regression. The short treatment time permits more consistent corneal hydration during the ablation, which also helps to produce a very evenly ablated surface without central islands.

In this study, 98% of the myopic eyes were corrected to within ± 1.0 D, and 93% of the astigmatism was corrected to within ± 0.5 D of the intended correction at 3 months. All of the eyes were corrected to within 1.5 D. Visual acuity of 20/40 or better was achieved in 100% of the eyes. Accuracy was better in the eyes with less than 10.00 D of myopia. Loss of lines of best corrected visual acuity was low in all groups.

Chiron Technolas Keracor 116

Guell et al.

Design and Methods

Forty-three eyes with myopia ranging from −7.0 to −18.5 D were operated on in this study of LASIK in which the Automatic Corneal Shaper and the Keracor 116 excimer laser were used in the multizone mode with a personally modified nomogram.[17] All of the procedures were performed by Guell in Barcelona, Spain using the same surgical technique. Procedures performed during the learning and nomogram-adjusting period of the first 3 months were excluded. The eyes were divided into a moderate myopia group of −7.0 to −12.0 D and a higher myopia group of −12.25 to −18.0 D. The cycloplegic refraction was used for surgery parameters.

Surgical Procedure: Patients are given diazepam and topical anesthesia. The personally modified laser multizone mode has the following characteristics: similar height for the different ablation zones, a blending zone of 6.8 mm, diameter of the inner zones varied to correspond with the desired maximum ablation depth, and ablation depth not exceeding 100 μm for corrections of up to −12.0 D and 120 μm for corrections of up to −18.0 D. The preoperative calibration test film verifies that 62 to 68 pulses are required for 95% removal of the area. A hinged 130-μm corneal flap is made with the corneal shaper for each case, and each microkeratome blade (sterilized for each case) is used for three procedures.

Results and Conclusion

Table 9.5 summarizes the results. The moderate myopia group (21 eyes) had a mean preoperative spherical equivalent refraction of −9.3 ± 1.3 D, with a range of −7.0 to −12.0 D and a postoperative mean refraction of −0.80 ± 0.79 D (range, −0.25 to −3.5 D). The mean preoperative spectacle-corrected visual acuity of 0.74 ± 0.20 (approximately 20/25 to 20/32) was 0.74 ± 0.18 postoperatively.

The higher-myopia group (22 eyes) had a mean preoperative spherical equivalent refraction of −14.86 ± 1.87 D, with a range of −12.25 to −18.0 D and a postoperative mean spherical refraction of −1.80 ± 1.29 D (range, plano to −5.25 D). The mean preoperative spectacle-corrected visual acuity of 0.50 ± 0.19 D (20/40) was 0.51 ± 0.18 D postoperatively. No overcorrections occurred in either group. A total of 85.7% of the eyes in the moderate-myopia group and 40.9% in the higher-myopia group were within ± 1.0 D of the intended correction. One eye in the higher group lost one line of spectacle-corrected visual acuity. No eye had visu-

Table 9.5. Summary of the Results of Recent LASIK Myopia Investigations

| | Arbelaez et al. (Chiron Technolas Keracor 117) Myopia | | | Guell and Muller[17] (Chiron Technolas Keracor 116) Myopia | | Chansue et al. (Aesculap Meditec) Myopia | | |
	Low	Moderate	High	Moderate	High	Low	Moderate	High
Number of eyes	198	31	8	43		33	40	27
Follow-up time		3 months		6 months			6–9 months	
Preop sphere		All levels						
Mean (SD)		−3.6 D (2.4 D)		−9.3 D (1.31 D)			−9.9 D (5.1 D)	
Range		Up to −14.0 D		−7.0 D to −12. D			−3.1 D to −19.3 D	
Postop sphere							Mean NA	
Mean (SD)		−0.34 D (0.52 D)		−0.80 D (0.79 D)			95% ± 1.0 D intended	
Range		−1.75 D to +1.0 D		Plano to −3.5 D				
Preop cylinder								
Mean (SD)		1.3 D (1.2 D)		1.25 D (0.75 D)			NA	
Range		0 to 6.0 D		0.50 D to 3.0 D				
Postop cylinder		Mean NA					NA	
Mean (SD)		93% ± 0.5 D		0.96 D (0.33 D)				
Range				0.50 D to 1.50 D				
BCVA				All levels				
20/40 or >	100%	100%	100%	71.4%	50%			
20/32 or >		NA		NA				
20/25 or >	96%	73%	100%	NA				
20/20 or >	94%	55%	67%	14.3%	4.5%			
VAsc								
20/60 or >		NA		NA			NA	
20/40 or >	96%	82%	—	71.4%	4.5%	100%	92.5%	88.9%
20/32 or >		NA		NA		90.9%	75.0%	59.3%
20/25 or >	83%	36%	—	NA		87.9%	60.0%	18.5%
20/20 or >	62%	9%	—	0%	0%	87.9%	55.0%	14.8%
Accuracy								
± 0.5 D	88%	66.7%	NA	52.3%	13.6%	78.8%	65.0%	51.9%
± 1.0 D	100%	87%	NA	85.7%	40.9%	100%	95.0%	88.9%
± 1.5 D	100%	100%	100%	NA			NA	
± 2.0 D	100%	100%	100%	90.4%	63.6%	100%	100%	92.6%
Gain of BCVA	2%	9%	0%	14.3%	22.7%	0	22.5%	11.1%
Loss of BCVA	4%	9%	0%	0%	4.5%	0	0	0

Notes:

NA = not available.

Low myopia = −2.0 to −6.0 D (all investigators); moderate myopia = −6.5 to −10.0 D (all investigators except Salah et al., for whom moderate myopia = −6.12 D to −12.0 D, and Guell and Muller, for whom moderate myopia −7.0 D to −12.0 D; high myopia = −10.5 to −14.0 (Arbelaez et al.); −12.25 to −18.5 D (Guell and Muller); −10.5 to −18.5 D (Chansue et al.); −10 to −15 D (Tsai et al.); −12.1 to −20.0 D (Salah et al.); very high myopia = >−15 D (Tsai et al.).

| Tsai et al. (Nidek EC-5000) Myopia | | | | Salah et al.[19] Summit Omnimed) Myopia | | | Pérez-Santonja et al. (VISX 20/20) Myopia −8.0 to −20.0 D | Gimbel et al. (Nidek EC-5000) Myopia All Levels |
Low	Moderate	High	Very High	Low	Moderate	High		
18	39	32	19	40	29	19	120	47
	6 months				5.2 months All levels		6 months	6 months
−4.8 D	−8.6 D	−13.3 D	−19.1 D		−8.24 D (4.4 D)		−13.6 D (3.3 D)	−11.9 D (4.6 D)
	−2.1 D to −16.0 D				−2.0 D to −20.0 D		−8.0 D to −20.0 D	−8.0 D to −27.25 D
	Mean at 6 months				Mean at 5.2 months		Mean at 6 months	
−0.05 D	−0.31 D	−0.23 D	−0.25 D		+0.22 D ± 1.42 D		+0.18 D ± 1.66 D	−1.02 D (1.68 D)
	0.0 to +5.0 D							−5.0 D to +2.00 D
	3 D or less				75% 1.5 D or less 0.0 to 4.0 D		0.83 D (0.40 D) 0.0 to 1.5 D	1.5 D (1.0 D) 0 to 4.25 D
	NA				Mean decrease 0.25 D ± 64 D inc. 1.25 D to dec. 2.0 D		0.85 D (0.50 D)	0.71 D (0.65 D) 0 to 2.00 D
					43.4% NA NA 44.6%		NA	
94.4%	89.7%	90.6%	52.6%		NA		50% 20/40 or better	74.5%
83.3%	82.%	68.7%	31.6%	26.4%	44.8%	36.8%		NA
	NA				NA			NA
72.2%	51.3%	43.7%	10.5%		NA			59.6%
38.9%	38.5%	15.6%	5.3%	68.4%	17.5%	0%		21.3%
								31.9%
83.3%	66.7%	46.9%	42.1%	63%	NA	NA	60% within ± 1.0 D	61.7%
94.4%	79.5%	87.5%	47.4%	93%	43%	NA		NA
	NA				NA			87.2%
100%	92.3%	96.9%	78.9%		NA			
11.2%	15.4%	41.8%	68.4%		NA		NA	46.8%
0	5.1%	18.8%	10.5%		3/88 (3.4%)		(Two lines or >) 1.4%.	2.2%

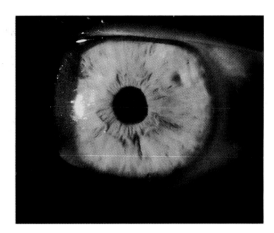

Fig. 9.2. LASIK after undercorrected radial keratotomy. (Courtesy of J. Guell, M.D.)

ally significant corneal haze. The mean change in spherical equivalent refraction from preoperative level at 6 months was 8.50 D in the lower-myopia group and 13.06 D in the higher-myopia group. Visual rehabilitation after surgery was rapid.

In this study, LASIK resulted in a stable refractive correction over 6 months, excellent visual acuity, no irregular astigmatism, and insignificant corneal scarring. Predictability of the outcome was better in patients with less than 12.0 D of myopia.

Evaluation of LASIK After Other Refractive Procedures

A total of 99 eyes that had LASIK after other refractive procedures, including penetrating keratoplasty, trauma surgery, phacoemulsification, radial keratotomy (Fig. 9.2), photorefractive keratectomy (PRK), or posterior vitrectomy with a 6-month follow-up were evaluated. The scattergram of intended versus achieved correction is shown in Fig. 9.3. The LASIK procedure showed efficacy, predictability, and safety and was concluded to be the procedure of choice for refractive correction after these procedures.

Evaluation of Regression

Guell, Muller, and Lohmann also studied the possible correlation of postoperative regression and epithelial hyperplasia after PRK and after LASIK. The results are displayed in Fig. 9.4.

Aesculap-Meditec MEL-60

Chansue et al.

Patient Selection and Counseling

This LASIK study was performed by Chansue in Bangkok, Thailand, with a follow-up period of 6 to 9 months. Prospective patients undergo a detailed ocular examination, including manifest and cyclo-

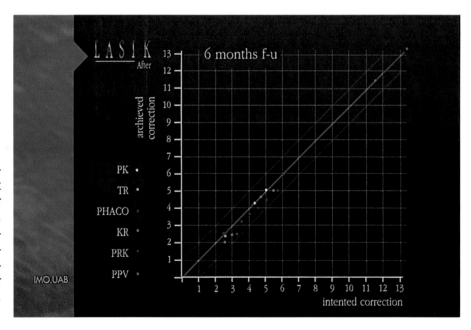

Fig. 9.3. Scattergram of intended vs. achieved correction at 6 months following LASIK after penetrating keratoplasty (PK), corneal trauma (TR), phacoemulsification (PHACO), radial keratotomy (KR), photorefractive keratectomy (PRK), or posterior vitrectomy (PPV). (Courtesy of J. Guell, M.D.)

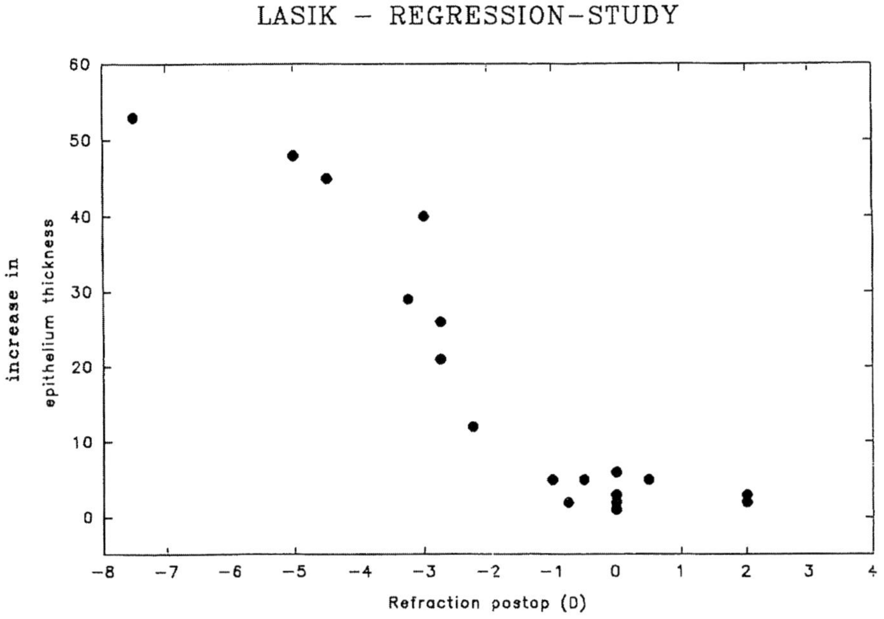

LASIK - REGRESSION-STUDY

Fig. 9.4. Correlation between regression after LASIK and epithelial hyperplasia, as measured by pachymetry. (Courtesy of J. Guell, M.D., and C. Lohmann, M.D.)

plegic refraction, keratometry, corneal topography, pachymetry, slit lamp examination, tonometry, and fundoscopy, including indirect ophthalmoscopy to detect any peripheral retinal degeneration. The patients are well counseled regarding the procedure: various types of refractive error are explained and spectacles mentioned as the safest means of achieving good vision. Alternatives are discussed, including contact lens wear and refractive surgery. The advantages and disadvantages of LASIK are compared with those of other keratorefractive procedures, and known side effects and complications are presented. Patients are encouraged to take their time in considering the risks and benefits of all alternatives and making an educated decision to best suit their individual needs.

Instrumentation
The setup is a semisterile laser suite. The microkeratome used is the Automatic Corneal Shaper; The laser is the Aesculap-Meditec MEL-60 argonfluoride excimer laser (Table 9.6). Other instruments used are shown in Table 9.7.

Preoperative Preparations
Photoablation alters the surface area of the stromal bed. In myopic cases, it reduces the surface area in the ablated zone. In effect, the flap has to squeeze itself into the reduced area and "microwrinkles" occur, causing the micro-irregular astigmatism seen

transiently after the surgery. Also, flap thickness probably affects the smoothness of the resulting postoperative corneal surface. A thinner flap will conform more readily to the modified shape of the stromal bed than a thicker one. On the other hand, a thicker flap may "hide" microwrinkles (created by the disparity of the surface areas of the flap and the stromal bed) better than a thinner one.

As in PRK, larger photoablation zones may result in a lower risk of disabling night glare. On the other

Table 9.6. Specifications for the Aesculap-Meditec MEL-60 Argon-Fluoride Excimer Laser

- A fluence of 250 mJ/cm^2 at a wavelength of 193 nm is generated.
- A scanning-slit delivery system with external masks for various types of correction is used. The masks also act as a suction fixation device to stabilize the globe.
- A contracting iris diaphragm mask is used for spherical myopic corrections.
- These are separate rotating masks for corrections of myopia and hyperopia, each with or without astigmatism.
- Laser fluence is calibrated using thin metal foil before the beginning of each case.

Table 9.7. Other Instruments Used for LASIK

- ALK-type corneal marker.
- Four-incision RK marker.
- Corneal cap spoon and a moist chamber for the corneal cap. Although a hinged corneal flap is intended, these become useful if the resection accidentally creates a complete cap.
- 8.5-mm applanation lens.
- Barraquer applanation tonometer.
- Solid-bladed wire speculum.
- 15-ml bottle of BSS with an irrigating cannula.
- Kelman-McPherson-type forceps.
- Absorptive sponges (preferably Merocel).

hand, larger zones result in deeper ablation. Multiple-zone ablation changes surface area less than a large, single-zone ablation. As a result, the corneal flap may assume the new shape with fewer microwrinkles.

Photoablation should be performed so that at least 250 μm of stroma remains under the flap. There is evidence that endothelial damage can occur when photoablation leaves less than 200 μm of cornea underneath.[18] Moreover, remaining stroma that is too thin may become ectatic and make the procedure inaccurate.

Patient Preparation

The patient arrives about 1 hr prior to the scheduled time and is reexamined at the slit lamp to ensure that the operative eye is healthy. The procedure is reviewed one last time before surgery begins. The patient is then premedicated with 1 drop of 4% pilocarpine, 0.3% tobramycin, and 0.4% benoxinate drops given every 5 min for at least 20 min. No oral medication is given.

Surgical Technique

Microkeratome Assembly and Excimer Laser Setting: Proper assembly of the microkeratome at the beginning of each case is the single most important step in LASIK. A new blade should be used for each patient. The microkeratome stop should be set so that the resection creates a 30° to 60° hinge for a 8.5-mm flap. The keratome head is then test run on the suction ring to ensure a smooth transition across the ring.

For surface photorefractive keratectomy, the MEL-60 is set so that it produces 1.0 to 2.0 D of overcorrection, depending on the size of the ablation zone. This is partly because the ablation algorithm of the MEL-60 depends on the optical model of photoablation and does not take into account the wound-healing response associated with surface PRK. In LASIK, however, this "fudge factor" does not need to be applied.

The author prefers to use a 6.0-mm single zone for corrections up to 5.5 D. From −6.0 D, double zones of 6.0 and 5.0 mm are used. In corrections of −9.0 D and above, triple zones of 6.0, 5,0, and 4.0 mm are used.

Microkeratome Resection: The surgical site is painted with Hibitane solution. A plastic drape is preferred to cloth, as the latter can give rise to foreign bodies in the interface. The speculum is placed, and the patient is instructed to fixate the eye at the light in the MEL-60 microscope. The corneal marker is then centered on the entrance pupil and used to mark the cornea and limbus. The suction ring is applied in turn, centered on the limbal mark. The cut diameter is verified with the 8.5-mm applanation lens. The eye is then quickly checked for an adequate intraocular pressure of 65 mm Hg or higher with the Barraquer tonometer. The microkeratome head is then engaged and electrically driven across the suction ring. When the microkeratome head automatically stops, the translation is reversed and the head is driven back across the ring. Suction is then released, and the microkeratome/suction ring complex is taken off the eye en bloc. The flap is flipped nasally, and a piece of absorptive sponge is used to lightly dry the stromal bed.

Photoablation: The patient is again instructed to fixate at the light. The laser mask is then set to 4.0 mm and centered on the entrance pupil. Once proper centration is obtained vacuum is applied and the mask is fixed to the globe. The ablation is then carried out as planned.

Repositioning of the Flap: After the completion of photoablation, a few drops of 0.3% tobramycin are placed on the exposed stroma, which is then copiously irrigated with balanced salt solution. The interface stroma is wiped with sponges, and the flap is flipped back onto the stromal bed. The cannula is subsequently used to float the flap up, which lets the flap settle back properly on to the bed and washes away any remaining debris or stray epithelial cells. The cornea is then left to dry for 5 min. During this time, the central epithelium is kept moist while the peripheral gutter is kept dry. After 5 min, proper adherence is tested with the tip of the forceps, pressing on the cornea just peripheral to the epithelial wound. Stress lines radiating into the flap are a sign of good adherence.

Closing the Eye: Another drop of 0.3% tobramycin is applied to the eye. The wire speculum is then carefully removed, with the patient gazing nasally. A "lid test" to ensure adequate adherence is then performed, pressing a cotton-tipped applicator on the upper lid and drawing it up to reveal the cornea. The eye is taped shut with strips of thin paper adhesive tape (Micropore). A piece of eyepad is placed loosely over the lids, and an eyeshield is secured over the eye by three strips of adhesive tape.

Postoperative Management: The patient is instructed not to tamper with the eyeshield and not to permit water or anything else to get inside it. There may be some tearing and discomfort. Pain is usually minimal and is controllable with oral acetaminophen.

When the patient returns the next morning, the shield and gauze pad are carefully removed and the uncorrected visual acuity is tested. Slit lamp examination is performed to check for proper adherence of the flap and a clean interface. The patient is then instructed to start using combination antibiotic/corticosteroid drops four times daily and to put the eyeshield on whenever he or she goes to sleep. The patient is seen again in 1 week, when the eye is checked again for a secure flap and a clear interface. The eyeshield and the eyedrops are discontinued. No eye rubbing or swimming is allowed for 3 more weeks. Routine follow-ups are scheduled at 1 month, 3 months, 6 months, 1 year, 18 months, and 2 years postoperatively, at which times uncorrected visual acuity testing, manifest refraction, and slit-lamp examination are performed.

Results

Patient Population: In this report, 100 consecutive cases of primary spherical correction in fully sighted eyes (correctable to at least 20/40 preoper-

atively), with follow-ups at 6 to 9 months were retrospectively analyzed. Data were collected from 70 patients who had LASIK performed between March and July 1995. Preoperative spherical equivalent ranged from -2 to -18.5 D. For analysis, patients were grouped as low, moderate, and high myopics with crossovers at -6 and -10 D, respectively.

In each group, the excimer laser was set to the spherical equivalent of the preoperative cycloplegic refraction. Because the controller unit allowed increments only in steps of 0.5 D, the data entry was rounded to the nearest lower 0.5 D marks.

Efficacy, Accuracy, and Safety: A summary of the results is shown in Table 9.5. At the last visit, 24/27 eyes (88.9%) in the high-myopia group had 20/40 or better uncorrected visual acuity. The same percentage fell within $\pm$ 1.0 D of emmetropia. In the moderate group, better results were noted: a total of 92.5% (37/40) in this group had visual acuity of 20/40 or better, and 95.0% (38/40) were within $\pm$ 1.0 D of emmetropia. The low-myopia group fared the best. All eyes in this group had visual acuity of 20/40 or better, and all were within $\pm$ 1.0 D of emmetropia. For 20/20 or better vision, 29/33 eyes (87.9%) in this group met this criterion, and 26/33 (78.8%) fell within $\pm$ 0.5 D of emmetropia. No eye had lost more than one line of best corrected visual acuity at the last visit.

Complications: Although no serious complications occurred in this series, several intraoperative and postoperative complications are possible, including an imperfect microkeratome cut. A good cut should make a large corneal flap of uniform thickness with a hinge of 30° to 60°. Improper assembly of the microkeratome can result in cuts that range from a jumpy transition across the suction ring, creating irregular flaps, to cuts that stop prematurely and leave inadequate room for a well-centered photoablation. Complete resection of the corneal cap as opposed to a hinged flap can result from incorrect determination of the cut diameter because of excessive fluid between the applanation lens and the cornea or loss of suction and fixation of the suction ring at the stop. The procedure can be continued in the same fashion as the original cap technique for ALK.

Displaced/lost cap or flap is a rare complication which can be determined by testing the flap for ade-

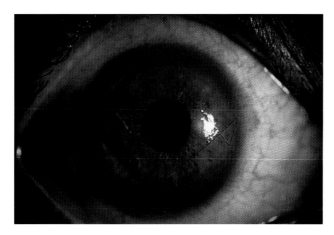

Fig. 9.5. A variation of the BRA suture. The 10-0 nylon suture is passed over the flap without going through it. (Courtesy of E. Chansue, M.D.)

quate adherence. This complication did not occur in the reported series. One patient outside the current report put her finger under the eyeshield the night after surgery and rubbed the flap off. She was seen the next morning, and the flap was cleaned and replaced. A variation of the BRA suture was utilized to secure the flap (Fig. 9.5).

Entry into the anterior chamber is a very serious complication. If the thickness plate is missing, the microkeratome can cut into the anterior chamber, damaging the iris and the crystalline lens in the process. This can be avoided by careful assembly of the microkeratome head. Infectious keratitis is one of the most dreaded complications in refractive surgery. Its incidence in LASIK is not known. It did not occur in this series and is likely to be very rare. A "dirty" interface occurred in a few cases when the hospital ran out of Merocel sponges. Brittle sponges give rise to interface foreign bodies which occasionally necessitate recleaning of the interface postoperatively. Epithelial ingrowth in the interface is a complication that may necessitate mechanical removal; it occurs approximately 2% of the time.

Transient micro-irregular astigmatism, inherent in all lamellar refractive surgery, manifests itself as "foggy" vision soon after surgery. Fortunately, this condition corrects itself as the cornea smooths out over time, and usually very little is left after the third month.

Under- and overcorrection was not uncommon in the nomogram development phase of LASIK.

However, an advantage of LASIK is that retreatment is very simple and fast. It is done by locating the edges and finding the plane under the existing flap with a Sinskey-type hook. Once located, the flap is easily flipped back, as in the primary surgery. The excimer laser is then used to correct the residual or consecutive refractive error, and the flap is repositioned as in the standard procedure. This is best done at 3 months after the original surgery, at which time refractive stability is achieved and the flap edges are still not too strongly adherent to the peripheral cornea.

Nidek EC-5000

Tsai et al.

Methods

In this study conducted in Taiwan by Tsai, the LASIK technique involved the use of Automatic Corneal Shaper to create a hinged 160-μm-thick flap to correct less than 10 D of myopia and a 130-μm flap to correct more than 10 D. The left eye flap was created first, followed by the right eye flap. The Nidek EC-5000 excimer laser was used for the stromal ablation. This laser system is reliable, allows setting by the surgeon based on the patient's condition, and can correct myopia and astigmatism at the same time. A disadvantage is that the working distance is too low.

Surgical Procedure: For myopia equal to or less than 6.0 D, a 5-mm-diameter optical zone with a 1-mm transition zone is ablated. The PRK program is used without change. For myopia of 6.0 to 10.0 D, the two ablation optical zones are 4.5 mm and 5 mm, with a 1-mm transition zone. The laser is set for 90–95% of the PRK program. For myopia of more than 15.0 D, three ablation optical zones and three passes are used. Depending on the amount of myopia and the pachymetry value, these were either 3.5, 4.0, 4.5, or 4.0 mm, 4.5 mm, and 5.0 mm. For these cases, the laser is set for 85–90% of the PRK program. Postoperatively, patients received 1 gtt of Maxitrol qid for 1 week, followed by 1 qtt of 1% FML qd for 1 month. Gentamicin solution is applied tid for 3 days.

Results

Low Myopia Group: There were 18 eyes (10 patients) in the group with myopia of −6.0 D or less and astigmatism of 3.0 D or less. Preoperatively, the mean spherical equivalent was -4.86 D $\pm$ 1.09, with a range of -2.13 to -6.38 D. One month postoperatively, the mean was 0.29 D $\pm$ 0.58 D, with a range of -0.5 to $+1.38$ D. Six months postoperatively, this had changed to a mean of -0.05 ± 0.52 D, with a range of -1.25 to $+0.75$ D.

At 6 months, 15/18 patients (83.3%) were within $\pm$ 0.5 D of the intended refraction, 94.4% were within $\pm$ 1.0 D, and 100% were within $\pm$ 2.0 D. A total of 38.9% of eyes had uncorrected visual acuity of 20/20 or better, 72.2% of 20/25 or better, 83.3% of 20/40 or better, and 94.4% of 20/60 or better. No eyes lost lines of best corrected acuity, most (16/18, 88.9%) remained the same, 5.6% gained one line, and 5.6% gained two lines at 6 months.

Moderate Myopia Group: Thirty-nine eyes of 25 patients had myopia of -6.0 to -10.0 D and astigmatism of 3.0 D or less. Preoperatively, the mean spherical equivalent was -8.61 D $\pm$ 1.38, with a range of -11.12 to -6.25 D. One month postoperatively, the mean was 0.04 ± 0.73 D, with a range of -1.75 to $+3.0$ D. Six months postoperatively, the mean was -0.31 ± 0.86 D, with a range of -3.38 to $+1.25$ D.

At 6 months, 26/39 patients (66.7%) were within $\pm$ 0.5 D of the intended refraction, 79.5% were within $\pm$ 1.0 D, and 92.3% were within $\pm$ 2.0 D. A total of 38.5% of eyes had uncorrected visual acuity of 20/20 or better, 51.3% of 20/25 or better, 82% of 20/40 or better, and 89.7% of 20/60 or better. One of the 39 eyes (2.5%) lost one line and one eye lost two lines of best corrected visual acuity. Three eyes (7.7%) gained one line, three eyes gained two lines, and 79.5% (88.9%) remained the same at 6 months.

High Myopia Group: Thirty-two eyes of 23 patients had myopia of -10.0 to -15.0 D and astigmatism of 3.0 D or less. Preoperatively, the mean spherical equivalent was -13.26 ± 1.60 D, with a range of -16.25 to -10.5 D. One month postoperatively, the mean was 0.62 ± 1.59 D, with a range of -1.5 to $+4.0$ D. Six months postoperatively, the mean was -0.23 ± 0.88 D, with a range of -3.0 to $+1.75$ D.

At 6 months, 5/32 of patients (46.9%) were within $\pm$ 0.5 D of the intended refraction, 87.5% were within $\pm$ 1.0 D, and 96.9% were within $\pm$ 2.0 D. Five of 32 (15.6%) eyes had uncorrected visual

acuity of 20/20 or better, 43.7% of 20/25 or better, 68.7% of 20/40 or better, and 90.6% of 20/60 or better. Thirty-seven percent maintained the same best corrected visual acuity, 9.4% gained one line, 34.4% gained two or more lines, 9.4% lost one line, and 9.4% lost two lines at 6 months.

Very High Myopia Group: A total of 19 eyes had myopia greater than -15.0 D and astigmatism of 3.0 D or less. Preoperatively, the mean spherical equivalent was -19.1 ± 1.9 D, with a range of -23.0 to -16.0 D. One month postoperatively, the mean was 0.75 ± 2.41 D, with a range of -2.75 to $+5.5$ D. Six months postoperatively, the mean was -0.25 ± 1.9 D, with a range of -2.4 to $+5.0$ D.

Eight of 19 eyes (42.1%) were within $\pm$ 0.5 D of the intended refraction, 47.4% were within $\pm$ 1.0 D, and 78.9% were within $\pm$ 2.0 D. One of 19 eyes (5.3%) had uncorrected visual acuity of 20/20 or better, 10.5% of 20/25 or better, 31.6% of 20/40 or better, and 52.6% of 20/60 or better. The same best corrected visual acuity was maintained by 21%; 21% gained one line, 47.4% gained two or more lines, and 10.5% lost one line at 6 months.

A summary of these results is shown in Table 9.5.

Summit Omnimed

Salah et al.

This was a retrospective study of 88 eyes of 63 patients who received excimer LASIK with the Automatic Corneal Shaper and the Summit Omnimed excimer laser under a hinged corneal flap without sutures.[19] The mean follow-up period was 5.2 months. The mean spherical equivalent of the manifest refraction before surgery was -8.24 D (range, -2.0 to -20.0 D), and after surgery it was $+0.22 \pm 1.42$ D.

Of the 40 eyes with a baseline refraction of -2.0 to -6.0 D, 63% had a refraction within $\pm$ 0.5 D of emmetropia. In eyes with a baseline refraction of -6.12 to -12.0 D, postoperative refraction was within $\pm$ 1.0 D in 65%. In eyes with a baseline refraction of -12.1 to -20.0 D, postoperative refraction was within $\pm$ 1.0 D in 43%. Overall, 72.8% of the eyes had a refraction within $\pm$ 1.0 D after surgery. Between 3 weeks and 5 months, the change in the mean spherical equivalent refraction was 0.61 D in the myopic direction. Uncorrected visual acuity after surgery was 20/20 or better in

36% and 20/40 or better in 71%. Three eyes (3.6%) lost two lines or more of spectacle-corrected acuity, two from progressive myopic maculopathy and one from irregular astigmatism. No eyes had vision-threatening complications.

The authors concluded that LASIK under a corneal flap can be effective in reducing myopia of 2.0 to 20.0 D with minimal complications. Current surgical algorithms need modification to improve predictability, and postoperative stability of refraction requires further study. A summary of the results is shown in Table 9.5.

VisX 20/20

Pérez-Santonja, Ismail and Alió

Patient Selection

Choosing a patient for LASIK must be done according to medical considerations as well as patient desires. Indications for LASIK include refusal to wear glasses, intolerance of contact lenses, anisometropia, and the firm desire of the patient to benefit from surgery for myopia. Potential hazards of this procedure should be explained to the patient.

Pérez-Santonja and coworkers advocate the use of LASIK for young patients with preserved accommodation and with myopia between -6.0 and -18.0 D, or for patients with a myopia between -18.0 and -23.0 D when phakic anterior chamber lenses are contraindicated. For older patients in whom accommodation has been lost, a clear lens extraction with a low-power posterior chamber intraocular lens (IOL) may be suggested.

Contraindications for LASIK include eyes that show any corneal pathology, such as corneal dystrophy or keratoconus. Eyes with corneal thickness less than 450 μm are excluded. Patients with glaucoma, cataracts, or any serious pathology of the retinal periphery or macula are also excluded. Any weak or degenerated retinal areas should be treated previously by laser therapy.

Patients first undergo a complete eye examination, with particular attention to keratometry, videokeratography, corneal thickness, and refraction. It is very important to be cautious in making subjective or objective measurements of refraction beyond -20.0 D. A trial contact lens can be used to determine the exact correction in myopia greater than -20.00 D.

Surgical Technique

The Automatic Corneal Shaper and the VisX 20/20 excimer laser are used. After verification of the appropriate informed consent, the patient changes into a clean jumpsuit, and one drop of pilocarpine 2% is instilled in the eye to be operated on. The patient is given either diazepam or another antianxiety agent; the dosage is individualized, but is typically comparable to 5 mg of diazepam. Before the patient enters the laser room, the excimer laser device is calibrated for proper ablations and the microkeratome system is tested. The suction ring must work properly and be closed all the way (for the largest diameter, usually between 7.2 and 8.5 mm), and the microkeratome had to be prepared with the 160-μm plate in place and the stop screw installed in the back position for the hinge flap technique.

In the operating room, the patient is prepared with Betadine sponges, taking care to prevent full-strength Betadine from coning in contact with the corneal surface. The patient is draped in a fashion that allows the surgeon to avoid contact with the eyelashes during surgery. The other eye is closed with an eyepad. A wire-type speculum is placed, and the patient's head is positioned so that the cornea is centered in the palpebral fissure.

In most cases, topical anesthetic is preferred. Topical anesthetic drops are placed approximately 2 min and 1 min prior to the procedure. Retrobulbar and peribulbar injections create additional levels of risk. They are also generally more uncomfortable for the patient than the procedure itself when done with topical anesthetic. At this point, surgery may be commenced.

For the first keratectomy, the cornea is marked with gentian violet using a corneal marker, which has 3- and 10.5-mm rings linked by a pararadial line. The suction ring, closed all the way, is centered around the outer marking line and the vacuum pump turned on. The intraocular pressure is checked using the Barraquer tonometer after drying the corneal surface. One must be sure that the intraocular pressure is above 65 mmHg. The 7.2-mm lens is inserted to ensure that the disc diameter is at least 7.2 mm. The corneal surface is moistened using BSS, and the microkeratome head is inserted into the dovetail on the suction ring. A footswitch is depressed until the stop screw hits the suction ring; then the footswitch is depressed in the reverse position, and the keratome head is removed from the ring. Then the suction ring is also removed. The hinged flap is lifted using a 23-g cannula or spatula and placed against the nasal sclera. The stromal bed is dried, and the cornea is prepared for the second keratectomy.

The second refractive keratectomy is performed using an excimer laser. The laser is programmed using the PRK algorithm, although some surgeons subtract 10% from the planned correction. A multizone approach is preferred because it reduces the ablation depth and achieves a smoother ablation profile. The surgeon should choose the largest multizone diameters in such a way that the remaining corneal thickness after surgery is greater than 380 μm. At present, the authors are using a triple ablation zone, with 50% of the correction done at the first zone, 30% at the second zone, and 20% at the third zone. The authors choose a 4.5-mm (first zone)–5.0 mm (second)–5.5 mm (third) or a 5 mm–5.5 mm–6 mm triple zone, depending on the intended correction and the preoperative corneal thickness, in such a way that the resulting central corneal thickness after surgery is greater than 380 μm.

After the excimer laser is programmed, the patient is asked to fixate on a He-Ne beam while the white illumination is decreased to provide a good centration. The time between the first keratectomy and laser ablation is minimized in an attempt to control the hydration. After ablation, the stromal bed and flap are irrigated with BSS and the flap is replaced to its original position. With the 23-g cannula, the interface is irrigated copiously. The flap is then centered and rotated for proper alignment by the pararadial mark. The keratectomy incision is dried with oxygen, air, or Weckcell sponges. After approximately 5 min, the flap is checked for adhesion by depressing the peripheral cornea and watching to make sure that the resulting indentation goes into the flap. When adhesion is ensured, an eyepatch is not necessary. Postoperatively, a steroid-antibiotic combination is instilled in the eye for 1 to 4 weeks.

Clinical Results

A total of 120 eyes with 8.0 to 20.0 D of myopia underwent LASIK (Table 9.5). The average follow-up period was 6 months. Postoperatively, 50% of eyes had uncorrected visual acuity of 20/40 or bet-

ter, and 60% were within ± 1.0 D of the intended correction. Pérez-Santonja and collaborators found that only phakic anterior chamber intraocular lenses were superior to LASIK in terms of the optical results.

Complications

Undercorrection and overcorrection are the most common complications. In this series undercorrection greater than −1.5 D and overcorrection greater than +2.5 D were present in 16% and 4% of the eyes, respectively. Undercorrection may be managed either by radial keratotomy or by elevating the flap and performing another laser ablation 3 to 6 months after surgery. The solution to an overcorrected LASIK is either hyperopic lamellar keratoplasty or laser thermokeratoplasty.

Interface dot remnants, although they do not affect visual acuity, must be avoided with careful cleaning during flap replacement. Epithelium in the interface is not a frequent condition after LASIK (1%) and usually was limited to the edge of the flap. Epithelium in the central cornea can be treated with the YAG laser focused either on the plaque or slightly deeper. The epithelium needs to be removed surgically with a blunt spatula when it covers too large an area to use the YAG laser. Epithelial implantation should be removed as soon as possible in such a way that the wound-healing process is minimized (Fig. 9.6). Flap displacement is managed by lifting the flap, cleaning the stromal bed, and reapplying the flap in place. Disc loss is possible

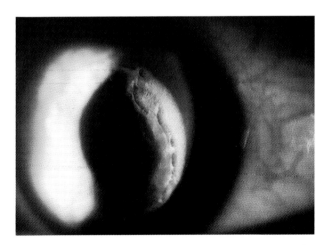

Fig. 9.6. Severe epithelial ingrowth 6 months after LASIK. (Courtesy of J.J. Perez-Santonja, M.D.)

after an inadvertent creation of a disc instead of a flap with the microkeratome. If the disc is lost, two options remain. One is to leave it off and allow the eye to reepithelialize and perhaps clear. The second option is to harvest donor tissue and rebuild the disc.

Irregular astigmatism was a rare complication (0.8%) after LASIK with a sutureless technique. Night disturbances were present in 23–30% of the eyes and could be decreased using larger ablation diameters or excluding patients with very large pupils. Peripheral melting of the flap edge was present in 1.2% of cases. This complication has not been previously reported.

At present, night halos, decentration of the laser ablation, and peripheral melting are the main concerns, although some of these complications may decrease with new excimer laser systems.

Nidek EC-5000, Chiron Technolas 116, VisX 20/20, Summit Apex Plus

Gimbel et al.

Methods

At the Gimbel Eye Centre Gimbel and associates began doing LASIK in April 1995 using the Automatic Corneal Shaper and the Nidek EC-5000 excimer laser. They chose this laser system primarily because of the focus adjustment of the slit illuminators, which allows excellent visualization of the interface when repositioning the corneal flap. Also, the variable magnification on the Nidek and other systems that have this feature is an advantage, allowing the use of low magnification for the microkeratome cut and high magnification for inspection of the interface. Gimbel and coworkers also used the Chiron Technolas 116, the VisX 20/20, and the Summit Apex Plus laser systems for LASIK.

In the first 10 months 189 procedures were performed. For the first 42 eyes the enhancement rate was 47%, but at this point it is 27%—still higher than one would expect after experience with PRK. During the learning period, the nomograms for LASIK with each laser were worked out. The enhancement rate should decrease with more experience. The approach was conservative, targeting undercorrection because of the ease of myopic LASIK enhancement surgery compared with hyperopic enhancement surgery.

The LASIK procedure was used initially primarily on high myopes of 10 D or more, but later also for corrections of lower myopes (5 D of myopia). Because of the excellent results with PRK using the Nidek laser, Gimbel and associates have been cautious in performing LASIK in the moderately myopic group, since the problems with LASIK occur at a deeper level (in the striae) than the superficial haze that may be encountered with PRK. With the scanning delivery system on the Nidek, a very low incidence of haze that reduced best corrected visual acuity in PRK patients was experienced.

Surgical Procedure: The microkeratome cut is made in the usual fashion. After repositioning, gentle irrigation under the flap is used to remove air bubbles and debris, and the flap is floated into position. The technique of repositioning the flap is still evolving. Gimbel and coworkers began gently wiping the flap with a moist sponge but found that this occasionally caused wrinkles in the flap. A cannula was tried to express fluid from the interface. Currently, a curved cyclodialysis spatula is used, as recommended by Roberto Zaldivar, M.D. (personal communication, 1996), to express moisture from under the flap. The fluid is wicked away from the edges with a moistened Merocel sponge. After about 5 min, when the striae confirm good adhesion, the speculum is removed. The eye is examined after approximately 30 min to ensure that the flap is still in a good position.

Intraoperative complications have been related to anatomical challenges from small orbits, loss of suction during the pass of the keratome, exposure problems causing the microkeratome to stop prematurely, and thin flaps which may be associated with a combination of very small and very steep corneas.

The retreatments for undercorrection have been straightforward. The corneal flap, previously marked at the slit lamp, is lifted with a Sinskey hook. The flap is turned, and an additional laser refractive cut is made in the bed. The flap is repositioned in the usual fashion. After retreatment, particular care is taken to ensure that no epithelial edge has encroached beneath the edge of the flap. Healing of a slightly wrinkled flap can cause astigmatism. With the improvement in surgical technique, this problem has been minimized. Just as the development of haze after PRK induces astigmatism, any microwrinkles in repositioning the flap can also lead to astigmatism in LASIK.

Results
The 6-month postoperative data are summarized in Table 9.5.

CONCLUSION

Compared with surface PRK, the LASIK procedure has the advantage of not disturbing Bowman's layer or the epithelium in the visual axis. As a result, epithelialization can be more rapid, reducing the risk of infiltrates, ulcerations, and haze. Enhancement procedures also carry a lower risk. The rapid visual recovery and minimal need for medication in the postoperative period make the procedure very attractive from both the surgeon's and patient's standpoints.

LASIK does introduce another instrument into the refractive surgical procedure, creating additional demands for quality control of the instrument and the disposable blades, as well as cleaning and assembly of the instrument. The additional instrumentation also requires manual skill development, a learning curve, and the potential for human error. The more involved surgical technique also leads to differences in the results achieved by different surgeons and different clinical experiences, all of which make standardization of the technique difficult. The greatest source of individual differences is the method of repositioning the flap to avoid debris, wrinkles, and warpage.

When encountering complications with LASIK, one is acutely aware that the cornea has been invaded at a deeper level than with PRK and that problems have greater significance than surface PRK problems because of the depth of the flap. The complications may include a partial, poor-quality, or thin cut; a washboard cut; a flap not sufficiently decentered nasally or decentered in the wrong direction; interface debris; epithelial ingrowth; wrinkles of the flap; a cap rather than a flap; and a lost cap or dislodgment of the cap after the patient has gone home.

The comparisons of LASIK with PRK are reminiscent of the ongoing comparisons of phacoemulsi-fication with manual extracapsular cataract extraction. Like phacoemulsification, LASIK technology will improve as microkeratome designs are modified, making the procedure safer and consistent in the full range of anatomical variations, such as narrow palpebral fissures, deep orbits, low intraocular pressure, and very small, very large, very steep, and very flat corneas. Laser optics are being modified to provide increased working distances, and manufacturers will be providing slit and oblique illumination to increase visualization and help avoid interface debris and flap wrinkles. New designs will also reduce the risks of metallic particulate matter and complications from instrument failure due to the quality control issues mentioned previously. Also, risks will diminish with greater individual and collective clinical experience, and management of complications will be refined.

LASIK is an exciting and challenging technique, and in time it will find its rightful place in our armamentarium of refractive surgery techniques. In considering the advantages of LASIK over our historical PRK experience, we must not forget that PRK is also evolving and the results are improving, with a reduced incidence of central islands, haze, and night vision problems because of new algorithms, scanning delivery systems, larger optical zones, and blend zones up to 9 mm.

REFERENCES

1. Barraquer JI. Queratoplastia refractiva. *Estudios Inform Oftal Inst. Barraquer* 1949;10:2–21.
2. Pallikaris IG, Papatzanaki ME, Stathi EZ, et al. Laser in situ keratomileusis. *Lasers Surg Med.* 1990;10:463–468.
3. Buratto L, Ferrari M, Rama P. Excimer laser intrastromal keratomileusis. *Am J Ophthalmol.* 1992;113:291–295.
4. American Academy of Ophthalmology. Epikeratoplasty. Ophthalmic procedure assessment. *Ophthalmology.* 1996;103:983–991.
5. Bas AM, Nano HD Jr. In situ myopic keratomileusis. Results in 30 eyes at 15 months. *Refract Corneal Surg.* 1991;7:223–231.
6. Arenas-Archila E, Sánchez-Thorin JC, Naranjo-Uribe JP, et al. Myopic keratomileusis in situ: a preliminary report. *J Cataract Refract Surg.* 1991;17:424–435.

7. Sher NA. Barak M, Daya S, et al. Excimer laser photorefractive keratectomy in high myopia. A multicenter study. *Arch Ophthalmol*. 1992;110:935–943.

8. Serdarevic O, Vinciguerra P, Bottoni F, et al. Excimer laser photorefractive keratectomy for the treatment of high myopia. *Invest Ophthalmol Vis. Sci*. 1992;33:763.

9. Ibrahim O, Waring GO, Salah T, El Maghraby A. Automated in situ keratomileusis for myopia. *J Refract Surg*. 1995;11:431–441.

10. Price FW, Whitson WE, Gonzales JS, Gonzales CR, Smith J. Automated lamellar keratomileusis in-situ for myopia. *J Refract Surg*. 1996;12:29–35.

11. Lyle WA, Jin GJC. Initial results of automated lamellar keratoplasty for correction of myopia: one year follow-up. *J Cataract Refract Surg*. 1996;22:31–43.

12. Casebeer JC, Slade SG. *A Comprehensive System for Refractive Surgery: ALK Course Manual*. January 1996.

13. Barraquer JI. Queratomileusis para la corrección de la miopía. *Arch Soc Amer Oftal Optom*. 1964;5:27–48.

14. Pallikaris IG, Siganos DS. Excimer laser in situ keratomileusis and photorefractive keratectomy for correction of high myopia. *J Refract Corneal Surg*. 1994;10:498–510.

15. Buratto L, Ferrari M, Genesi C. Keratomileusis for myopia with the excimer laser (Buratto technique): short-term results. *Refract Corneal Surg*. 1993;(suppl)9:S130–S133.

16. Slade SG, Brint SF. Excimer laser myopic keratomileusis. In: Rozakis GW, ed. *Refractive Lamellar Keratoplasty*. Thorofare, NJ: Slack; 1994:125–137.

17. Güell JL, Muller A. Laser in situ keratomileusis (LASIK) for myopia from −7 to −18 diopters. *J Refract Surg*. 1996;12:222–228.

18. Kim K, Jeon S, Edelhauser HF. Corneal endothelial permeability after deep excimer laser ablation. *Invest Ophthalmol Vis Sci*. 1996;37:S84.

19. Salah T, Waring GO III, El Maghraby A, et al. Excimer laser in situ keratomileusis under a corneal flap for myopia of 2 to 20 diopters. *Am J Ophthalmol*. 1996;121:143–155.

Prevention and Management of Complications of Lamellar Refractive Surgery

Lucio Buratto
Massimo Ferrari

INTRODUCTION

The complications which may occur during keratomileusis operations are highly correlated with the technique and the instruments used during the operation. The older procedures, such as the techniques of Barraquer,[1] Krumeich,[2,3] and Ruiz,[4-8] are now considered obsolete. They have in common refractive correction obtained by using a mechanical instrument capable of modifying the thickness and curvature of the primary lamella—for instance, the cryolathe in Barraquer's technique, the bench in Krumeich's technique and the microkeratome in Ruiz's technique (the classical in situ keratomileusis technique). The complications are specific to the technique and depend largely on the use of these instruments.

The introduction of the excimer laser (an advanced keratomileusis technique)[9-17] has radically changed the scenario of keratomileusis. It brings with it enormous benefits and advantages, significantly reducing the percentage and severity of a large proportion of the complications. The adjunct use of the excimer laser brought with it, admittedly with a lower incidence, factors, problems, and complications which were completely new to the operators accustomed to keratomileusis in its more traditional form. Each technique has its own distinctive characteristics and difficulties. If these are ignored or poorly evaluated, they can result in severe complications, particularly if the surgeon has little experience with lamellar corneal surgery.

In general, suitable training, good experience, and a great deal of careful attention, in addition to adequate theoretical and practical knowledge of the instruments and the techniques, are sufficient to prevent or avoid the majority of the complications which may arise during keratomileusis. Moreover most of the complications can be remedied if they are correctly interpreted.

TECHNIQUES OF KERATOMILEUSIS

The techniques of keratomileusis can be divided into two categories:

Older
   Barraquer's technique
   Krumeich's technique
   Ruiz's technique
Current or advanced
   Laser in situ keratomileusis (LASIK)
   Excimer laser intrastromal keratomileusis
      (ELISK) on the flap

Every technique, and every evolutionary and technological period, has its own instruments, methods, and complications. However, a detailed analysis of the complications of outdated procedure is unnecessary. Following is a brief overview of the problems observed with the historical techniques, followed by a detailed examination of the more recent methods.

COMPLICATIONS OF CLASSICAL TECHNIQUES WITH A MECHANICAL REFRACTIVE PROCEDURE

Operations using the techniques which involve a mechanical refractive procedure have the highest percentage of complications and the most serious complications. Intraoperative complications occur principally at two distinct times intraoperatively: during the cut with the microkeratome and during the refractive cut. In order to understand the correct function of the microkeratome, the surgeon must have extensive theoretical and practical knowledge. Lack of such knowledge has been and still is a decisive factor in most of the problems with the keratomileusis operation. The difficulty of assembling the instrument or the difficulty of obtaining adequate fixation of the corneal lamella during surgery cause a high percentage of complications.

The complications resulting from the microkeratome during the primary cut will be described in brief initially, and then more extensively later on because they are still valid today. The complications resulting from the mechanical refractive cut will be summarized briefly in Tables 10.1, 10.2, and 10.3 because they are now grouped with the older techniques which are no longer used.

Complications during the Cut with the Microkeratome

- Corneal perforation: This can occur during the primary cut (even during the refractive cut—however, only with Ruiz's in situ technique). It results in violent decompression of the eye, with severe anatomical and functional damage to the eye. It is caused by the absence or the wrong application of the plate in the head of the microkeratome or by a cut in abnormally thin corneas.
- Superficial keratotomy: This results from poor suction or poor adhesion between the ring and the sclerocorneal plane or because of a cut which is too rapid.
- Keratotomy of irregular thickness: This is due to poor adhesion between the suction ring and the tissue, loss or reduction of suction during the cut, or the use of a blunt blade.
- Incomplete keratotomy: This is caused by human or mechanical error, electrical failure of

the microkeratome, or stoppage of the progression.
- Decentered keratotomy: This is caused by incorrect centering of the suction ring on the pupillary center or poor adhesion of the ring on the sclerocorneal plane during the cutting phase.
- Keratotomy with an irregular surface: A cut surface with folds, grooves, or dentellation is most frequently caused by an irregular run of the microkeratome along the ring guides, hindered sliding of the microkeratome resulting from poor exposure of the eye, or poor positioning of the speculum due to obstructions by the connecting wires between the motor and the microkeratome.

COMPLICATIONS OF CURRENT OR ADVANCED TECHNIQUES

The arrival of the excimer laser, further technological evolution, and the sophisticated precision offered by photoablation of the corneal stroma for refractive surgery made an important contribution to improving the quality of this type of surgery, with a significant reduction in the percentage of complications. Elimination of the retention methods of the lamella, simplification of the instruments, and nontraumatic micron precision of the excimer laser mean that keratomileusis is not only an effective technique from a refractive point of view but, more important, it is the safest technique available today. Keratomileusis with the excimer laser for the intrastromal procedure to modify the refractive procedure is, at the time of writing, the most modern and most widely used keratomileusis procedure.

The refractive procedure can be done in two ways:

1. By performing the laser ablation on the stromal portion of the resected corneal disk (the ELISK on the flap technique).
2. By performing laser photoablation directly on the underlying intrastromal portions in situ, which are left exposed (LASIK or ELISK technique in situ) after a 360° resection of the corneal disk or a partial cut to form a corneal flap.

Table 10.1. Complications of Barraquer's Technique

Intraoperative Complications	Postoperative Complications	Comments
Small, shallow, or decentered primary cut compared to the expected parameters; the operation must be aborted due to the impossibility of performing the refractive cut. Loss of or damage to the primary corneal disk, either during the "freeze" phase (temperature insufficient to ensure freezing) or during the refractive procedure at the lathe (detachment from the lathe support), or through an error in calculating the parameters for the refractive procedure or incorrect assembly of the instrument. Superficial and/or decentered refractive cut due to an interruption of the freeze process or to incomplete and/or inadequate fixation of the corneal disk to the lathe support. Irregular refractive cut with altered thickness due to insufficient freezing of the corneal disk. Inability to perform the refractive cut because it has been impossible to freeze the corneal disk.	A slow healing process and slow histological, anatomical, and immunological restoration due to freezing of the lamella, which kills the keratocytes. This phenomenon is the cause of many of the frequent complications in the postoperative period, such as retarded reepithelialization, filamentous keratitis on a trophic base, impurities, and adhesions at the interface. Optical complications are linked to edema and hypotransparency of the corneal tissue secondary to freezing, which can persist for prolonged periods after surgery. Slow recovery of function linked to the slow cellular repopulation of the corneal disk. Significant percentage of postoperative astigmatism linked to irregularity of the stromal procedure on the corneal disk or to microtraction forces between the keratectomized, treated tissue and the host corneal bed.	This technique was the debut of keratomileusis as a lamellar technique. The necessity for and dependence on freezing of the lamella, and the use of a technically complex instrument such as the cryolathe, limited and hindered the initial development of ketatomileusis. Nevertheless, this first technique laid the foundation for the development of the current keratomileusis techniques.

Currently, the latter is the more widely used technique.

The complications most frequently observed with the corneal refractive procedures with the excimer laser can be classified as follows:

Preoperative
Intraoperative
    Related to the primary cut
    Related to the refractive cut
Postoperative
    Anatomical
    Optical

Preoperative Complications

As a Result of the Anesthesia

- Retrobulbar hemorrhage and/or bulbar perforation: basically caused by the retrobulbar or parabulbar injection. This type of injection should be avoided if possible. It should be used only when increased exposure of the eye is necessary to improve the use of the suction ring and facilitate the cut with the microkeratome.
- Chemosis of the conjunctival plane: normally linked to the parabulbar injection and therefore

Table 10.2. Complications of Krumeich's Technique

Intraoperative Complications	Postoperative Complications	Comments
The need to abort the operation because of a cut which is too small, too thin, or decentered. Destruction of or damage to the lamella: can be caused by incorrect assembly of the bench, incorrect evaluation of the zero value, incorrect positioning of the die, imperfect hold of the lamella on the surface of the die, or an unsuitable blade edge. The damage can be repaired only by using homoplastic tissue. A refractive cut which is irregular, decentered, or altered in thickness: caused by imperfect centering or positioning of the primary corneal limbus on the die of the bench, or imperfect hold between the dentellated retention ring and the underlying corneal lamella, and/or poor suction between the die and the lamella.	Unpredictability of the refractive result. The various technical phases of positioning and fixation of the flap can modify the diameter and thickness of the primary disk, with consequent changes in the expected refractive result. Another cause of this complication is the difficulty of interpreting the original nomograms.	The technique represents an important advance in the technique because it avoids freezing the tissue. For many years, the BKS instrument was widely used and extensively studied in operations of keratomileusis. Nevertheless, the number of corneal surgeons who routinely used the BKS 1000 for lamellar surgery was limited, probably by the technical and instrumental difficulties, which are significant even today.

not indicated for keratomileusis. It can result in a difficult support and poor adhesion between the suction ring and the conjunctival-scleral plane and complications during the cut with the microkeratome.

- Deepithelialization or damage to the epithelium: linked to excessive use of topical anesthesia. When such anesthesia is used, 3 drops are sufficient.

As a Result of the Application of the Surgical Drape and the Blepharostat

The surgical drape, when used correctly, must cover the edges of the eyelids and the eyelashes and provide adequate protection of the entire operating field. The initial contact of the steri-drape with the corneal epithelium (which is thinner and unstable due to the surface anesthetic, particularly if this is instilled more than once to obtain adequate topical anesthesia) can produce some areas of corneal-epithelial stress. Abrasions or epithelial stress can occur accidentally through contact with the blepharostat or other operating instruments.

As a Result of the Corneal Markings

Use of the epithelial pen or marker can cause the following problems:

- Dispersion of small, dry fragments of gentian violet, which can be deposited on the precorneal site and damage the interface during the cut.
- Small epithelial abrasions if the tip of the pen is dry or if the marker has flaws.

Table 10.3. Complications of Ruiz's Technique

Intraoperative Complications	Postoperative Complications	Comments
Difficulty performing two cuts which are superimposed and centered. Even minimal decentering between the two keratectomies produces distortion of the central optical zone, which can be clearly highlighted using corneal topography. This complication results in the formation of irregular astigmatism, which is proportional to the degree of the distortion itself, and altered visual function (glare, diplopia, reduction of the contrast sensitivity). Difficulty obtaining exact thicknesses and diameters with the mechanical cut of the microkeratome. Even the assembly of the microkeratome, with the plate different from that indicated for the correction of the specific myopic defect, can result in inadequate thickness of the keratectomized lamella. Also, incorrect interpretation of the numerical values reported on the nomograms, resulting in the incorrect choice of the plate, can produce an inadequate refractive result.	Irregular astigmatism, which appears to be the most frequent and the most dreaded complication of this technique. It is the result of imperfect centering of the second keratectomy and therefore of the two superimposed optical zones. One type of irregular astigmatism, which is located more anteriorly, results from imperfect adhesion of the superficial lenticle to the deeper one (because of its thinness) or from traction induced by the suture.	This apparently simple technique, which has been streamlined by the advent of sophisticated, complex operating instruments, nevertheless involves considerable technical and procedural difficulties. The more or less constant and complete use of the microkeratome, the need for the double keratectomy, and the significant percentage of complications such as irregular astigmatism have limited and restrained the use of this technique by refractive surgeons. Nevertheless, it was a major contribution in the establishment of the in situ techniques as we know them today.

Intraoperative Complications

Linked to the Primary Cut (Common to All Techniques)

Corneal Perforation (Fig. 10.1)

- Caused by total absence or abnormal assembly of the plate in the microkeratome. It may also occur during keratectomy in a cornea which is irregular in thickness or is too thin.
- Produces rapid decompression of the eye, with serious damage to the eye.

- Can be prevented by careful control of the exact position of the plate in the head of the microkeratome; use of a reliable microkeratome, with safe insertion of the plate and a stable hold; and accurate, precise presurgical pachymetry.
- What to do: As soon as liquid is observed, stop suction immediately. Remove the ring and the microkeratome; evaluate the extent of damage; suture the cornea; refill the anterior chamber; and try to repair the damage to the anterior and posterior segments as much as possible.

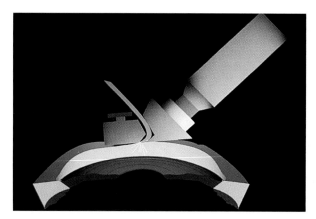

Fig. 10.1. Corneal perforation with resulting decompression of the cornea and the anterior chamber: side view.

Keratotomy Which Is Too Superficial (Fig. 10.2)

- Due to the wrong plate; insufficient adhesion of the suction ring to the sclerocorneal plane; or excessively rapid progression of the cut along the ring guides.

- Produces a corneal lamella with a thickness different from the expected one.

- Can be prevented by ensuring that the plate inserted corresponds to the one calculated by the preoperative programs; ensuring that the holes in the pneumatic ring are open and free from impurities or debris; ensuring that the conjunctival plane is free from edema or irregu-

Fig. 10.2. Keratectomy with thickness of the entire cut reduced: side view.

larities which may interfere with good adhesion of the ring (blebs following filtration surgery, etc.); limiting the speed of the microkeratome during the keratectomy; and avoiding excessive use of anesthetic eyedrops (which can cause epithelial edema or abrasions and promote detachment of the epithelium during the use of the microkeratome).

- What to do: Perform an in situ photoablation with the excimer laser if the cut has sufficiently exposed the central stroma. Otherwise, reposition the cut tissue (with or without sutures) and repeat the surgery after 4–6 months.

Complications During LASIK (During the Photorefractive Cut)

- Decentered ablation due to incorrect centering of the laser on the anterior stromal portions of the cornea.

- Incorrect ablation due to errors in setting the laser during preparation. This mistake can involve both the diameter of the optical zone and the dioptric value to be corrected, and the axis of the astigmatism in the event of an astigmatic ablation.

- Lesions of the flap: mechanical alterations, contamination of the flap due to debris, etc., in the phase prior to or following laser treatment. It is advisable to avoid even minimal movement or manipulation of the flap to prevent even minor trauma. Lesions to the flap can occur during ablation with LASIK if a corneal flap is present. If not suitably protected, the portion of the flap which remains attached to the underlying bed can be damaged by laser photoablation of the stromal bed. This occurs particularly if the optical zone is wide or in astigmatic treatments where the ablation is extended to the peripheral portions of the corneal cut. This problem can be avoided by protecting the flap at the site of the hinge.

- Faulty laser: insufficient supply of liquid nitrogen from the cylinder to the cavity; poor maintenance (hypotransparency of the mirrors); or electrical blackout, which precludes laser treatment. The procedure can be continued by performing the refractive cut in situ using a microkeratome.

Complications During ELISK on the Disk

- Decentered ablation due to off-center positioning of the lamella under the diaphragm of the laser during the refractive procedure.
- Loss and lesions of the corneal disc: These can be limited or avoided by placing the corneal disc on a Teflon support and covering it with a sterile glass during transport in the operating environment.
- Incorrect ablation: Ablation on the epithelial portion instead of the stromal part of the disc. A photorefractive keratectomy (PRK) preceded by a lamellar keratectomy would be the result. In ablation on a flap which has not been flattened correctly, the outcome is an inadequate refractive and functional result.
- Faulty laser: The lamella can be replaced and then redetached once the laser has been repaired; the cut is then completed and the treated lamella replaced. Alternatively, if the lamella is thick (about 270–300 μm) and suitable instruments are available, it is possible to resort to an in situ procedure, either with a workbench and the relative dies or with the cryolathe.

Keratectomy of Irregular Thickness
(Figs. 10.3, 10.4)

- Due to irregularity, damage, or debris present on the guides of the suction ring; poor suction during the cut; insufficient cutting capacity of

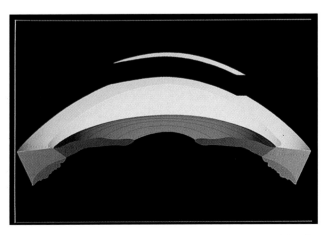

Fig. 10.3. Keratectomy with thickness reduced in the final part of the cut: side view.

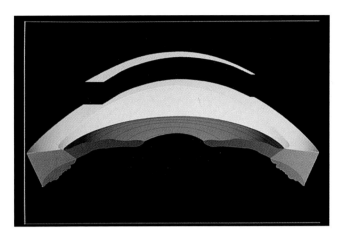

Fig. 10.4. Keratectomy with greater thickness in the final part of the cut: side view.

the blade; or lateral sliding of the microkeratome during the cutting phase.
- Produce a lamella of nonuniform thickness over the entire cutting area.
- Can be prevented by examining and cleaning the guides of the suction ring and the microkeratome; avoiding conditions which can reduce the correct suction; changing the blade with every operation; and examining the blade edge under a microscope before every operation.
- What to do: Replace the flap and repeat the operation after 6 months with a deeper keratectomy than the previous one.

Incomplete Primary Keratectomy
(Figs. 10.5, 10.6)

- Due to an electrical blackout, incorrect use of the foot pedal, stoppage of the microkeratome, incorrect setting of the stop point of the microkeratome, interruption of the progression of the guides, motor failure, insufficient movement of the blade holder, the pneumatic ring, or obstruction by the eyelids, blepharostat, or other object along the cutting path.
- Produces an incomplete lamella compared to the 360° resection or a flap different from that planned. The interruption can occur inside or outside the optical zone.
- Can be prevented by doing the following before the operation: check the assembly and func-

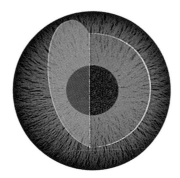

Fig. 10.5. Incomplete keratectomy with the incision interrupted in the optical zone: view from above.

tioning of the microkeratome, the situation of the sliding guides, the state of the conjunctiva and the holes of the pneumatic ring, the exposure of the eye and the position of the blepharostat.

- What to do: If the resection has exceeded the optical zone by at least a couple of millimeters, continue for at least another 1 ml with a manual lamellar keratectomy using a Beaver blade or a Crescent knife; then perform an in situ ablation. If the resection has not exceeded the optical zone, replace the lenticle (with or without sutures) and repeat the surgery after 6 months.

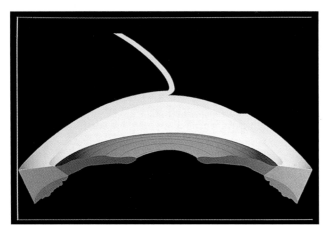

Fig. 10.6. Incomplete keratectomy with incision interrupted in the optical zone: side view.

Decentered Keratectomy (Figs. 10.7 to 10.10)

- Due to poor patient compliance during surgery, surgeon error in centering the precorneal optical axis, or incorrect placement of the suction ring to the corneal apex.
- Produces problems in performing an ablation on an optical zone of sufficient size. Avoid performing the refractive procedure at the center of the cut; it produces poor refractive and functional results, irregular astigmatism, and functional disorders (diplopia, glare, etc.).
- Can be prevented by asking the patient to stare at the reference target point of the microscope during the initial centering of the optical axis. Correctly center the virtual precorneal pupillary center with the marker and correctly center the suction ring on the corneal apex.
- What to do: Perform an in situ laser ablation, centering it well on the prepullary stromal bed (and not on the cut area). If the decentering is marked, replace the cut lamella and repeat the procedure after 6 months.

Keratectomy With an Irregular Surface (Fig. 10.11)

- Due to irregularity of the blade edge, variable progression of the microkeratome along the guides of the ring, hindrances during the cutting phase (reduced eye exposure, the blepharostat, etc.), or lateral sliding of the microkeratome along the ring guides.
- Produces a cut surface of unsuitable smoothness and uniformity.
- Can be prevented by checking the blade edge and replacing it after every operation, checking the correct assembly of the microkeratome and the ring, checking the conjunctival plane, and performing a smooth cut. Ensure that there are no obstructions along the path of the microkeratome (eyelids, blepharostat, sheet, etc.); moisten the cornea and the guides of the ring prior to cutting with the microkeratome.
- What to do: Replace the flap (with or without sutures) and repeat the operation after 6 months; perform a homoplastic keratomileusis[18]; or try to smooth the surface of the flap and the stromal bed using an excimer laser.

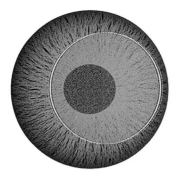

Fig. 10.7. Decentered keratectomy.

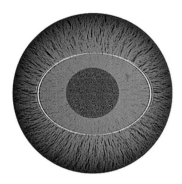

Fig. 10.8. Keratectomy of abnormal shape: oval.

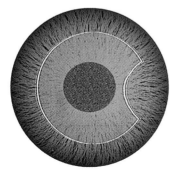

Fig. 10.9. Keratectomy of abnormal shape: incomplete.

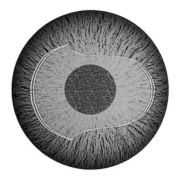

Fig. 10.10. Keratectomy of abnormal shape: pearshaped.

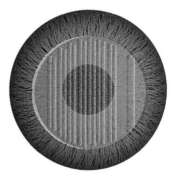

Fig. 10.11. Keratectomy with jagged, irregular incision surface.

A 360° Cut of the Lamella with a Flap Technique (Figs. 10.12, 10.13)

- Due to poor assembly or inadequate calibration of the microkeratome's stop mechanism; poor functioning of the stop mechanism; or use of a ring which does not allow sufficient exposition of the cornea.
- Produces a 360° keratectomy instead of creating a flap.
- Can be prevented by checking the assembly of the microkeratome's stop mechanism very carefully prior to surgery.
- What to do: As an in situ ablation is planned, the cut lamella is usually too thin for an on-the-

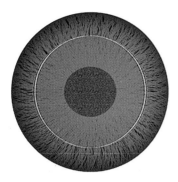

Fig. 10.12. Full-circle (360°) ring keratectomy as opposed to a flap: view from above.

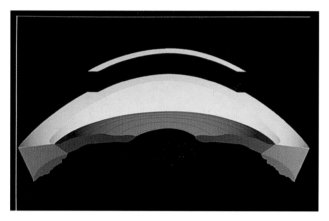

Fig. 10.13. Full circle (360°) ring keratectomy as opposed to a flap: side view.

flap technique, so LASIK is performed according to the refractive program set. Then the keratectomized limbus is repositioned in its original position. The dehydration of the surfaces is completed for the sutureless technique or an external retention suture is placed on the lenticle. An antitorque suture on such a thin lenticle can result in folds and distortions which are difficult to manage in the postoperative period.

Incorrect Execution of the Refractive Ablation

- Due to decentering of the photoablation, errors in the astigmatic ablation, incorrect setting of the data in the laser's software, or insufficient

drying of the area subjected to the laser treatment.

- Produces poor clinical-functional results or irregular astigmatism, depending on the specific case.
- Can be prevented by careful, accurate control of both the centering of the refractive procedure and the insertion of the data into the computer.
- What to do: For hypo- and hypercorrection, proceed as described later. In the event of severe irregular astigmatism and/or marked functional disturbances, perform a homoplastic keratomileusis. In particularly serious situations, penetrating keratoplasy is a potential technique if the problem cannot be resolved by homoplastic lamellar keratoplasty.[19,20]

Postoperative Complications

Anatomical Complications
Epithelial Ingrowth or Impurities at the Interface (Figs. 10.14, 10.15)

- Due to the involuntary introduction of epithelial cells into the stroma during the cut with the microkeratome, manipulations of the interstromal surfaces, introduction of instruments at the interface, folding of the lenticle on itself during the operation, or inaccurate irrigation and cleansing of the surfaces involved. Infection can also occur.[21]
- Produces areas of hypotransparency, with consequent irregular astigmatism and decreased vision.

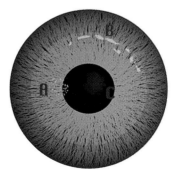

Fig. 10.14. Epithelialization: (a) Epithelial cysts through migration. (b) Multiple peripheral epithelializations. (c) Central epithelialization.

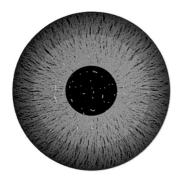

Fig. 10.15. Debris at the interface.

- Can be prevented by being careful when treating the interstromal surfaces.
- What to do: Remove the epithelial cells using the Nd:YAG laser or intrastromal (ISL) laser only if the epithelial cells are limited in extension and poorly developed or if they are creating astigmatism or hypovision. If the cellular accumulation is extensive, a surgical technique is preferred. This involves lifting the flap, cleaning the interface, replacing the flap, and suturing.

Loss or Displacement of the Flap (Fig. 10.16)

- Due to incorrect calibration of the stop mechanism for the progression of the cut, which creates a flap poorly connected to the underlying stroma; insufficient interstromal dehydration and resulting poor adhesion between the surfaces; incorrect repositioning of the flap at the end of the operation; or eye rubbing by the patient in the immediate postoperative period.

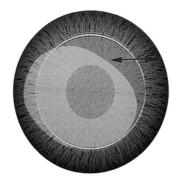

Fig. 10.16. Displacement of the flap from its primary bed.

- Produces epithelialization of the interface, an incorrect refractive result, and functional disorders.
- Can be prevented by careful calibration of the stop and careful dehydration of the surfaces using filtered compressed air if necessary; a retention suture should be placed if necessary.
- What to do: Remove the epithelial cells from both stromal surfaces, i.e., from the limbal and in situ ones—and affix a retention suture; leave the patient without a flap. The postoperative situation has a course similar to that of PRK, but with greater haze and a poorer refractive result. Substitution of the flap with a homoplastic one should also be considered following total removal of the epithelium.

Optical Complications
Undercorrection

- Due to spontaneous regression or inaccurate presurgical refractive evaluation, unstable ametropia, incorrect interpretation of the nomograms, or incorrect setting of the laser's software.
- Produces errors in the calculation of the expected refraction, patient dissatisfaction, and the need for another operation.
- Can be prevented by careful selection and evaluation of the preoperative refraction, correct interpretation and setting of the laser software, and correct postoperative therapy.
- What to do: Repeat the in situ treatment, either lifting the lamella or repeating the lamellar cut with the microkeratome; or use surface techniques (RK or PRK).

Overcorrection

- Due to incorrect calculation of the preoperative refraction or incorrect setting of the parameters in the laser software.
- Produces errors in the expected refractive result, patient dissatisfaction, and the need for another operation.
- Can be prevented by careful evaluation of the preoperative refraction and correct setting of the laser software at the time of the operation.
- What to do: In situ hyperopia treatment using an excimer laser after lifting the lenticle, or

holmium laser thermal keratoplasty (LTK) or hyperopic PRK.

Regular or Irregular Astigmatism

- Due to surface irregularities, decentered primary cut or refractive procedure, or persistence of the preexisting astigmatic situation; incorrect marking of the axis for the astigmatic treatment; abnormal position of the patient's head; or incorrect preoperative topography.

- Produces poor functional recovery, double vision, and reduction of contrast sensitivity.

- Can be prevented by identifying the correct astigmatic axis and performing the treatment on this axis; avoiding decentering; and accurately programming the correction of the preexisting astigmatism.

- What to do: For regular astigmatism, it is possible to perform an astigmatic keratotomy, an astigmatic PRK, an astigmatic LASIK, or an astigmatic LTK. For irregular astigmatism, try to smooth the corneal surface by applying a contact lens. Lift the flap and reposition it to smooth out any irregularities. Perform a smoothing laser ablation of the interstromal surfaces or a deep homoplastic keratoplasty.

CONCLUSIONS

The continual technical, instrumental, and surgical innovations in the field of keratomileusis have made a significant contribution to reducing the complications reported over the years by various authors. The operation is therefore not only safer, it also provides simpler solutions to the problems which may occur both during the operation and in the postoperative period.

The use of the laser not only eliminates many possible complications but also helps to solve any problems linked to the many contingent factors in refractive surgery.

It is obvious that for a successful keratomileusis operation, the surgeon and his team must have accurate, in-depth theoretical and practical training.

Even though the action of the microkeratome is greatly facilitated by automation and by simplification of the instruments, its use depends on the centration and precise calibration by the surgeon, who must recognize not only the value of this instrument but also its limitations.

Ignoring these concepts can result in complications which not only affect the immediate outcome of surgery but are also difficult to manage and resolve in the long term.

REFERENCES

1. Barraquer JL. *Tecnica Quirurgica General ed Cirugia Refractive de la Cornea*. Bogotá: Instituto Barraquer De America; 1989;277–366.

2. Swinger CA, Barker BA. Prospective evaluation of myopic keratomileusis. *Ophthalmology*. 1984;91:785–792.

3. Courderc JL, Lozano Mouri F. Freeze or no freeze myopic keratomileusis: which is the best? *Eur J Implant Ref Surg*. 1989;1:157–177.

4. Ruiz LA, Rowsey IJ. Situ keratomileusis. *Invest Ophthalmol Vis Sci*. 1988;29(suppl):392.

5. Price FW, Whitson WE, Gonzales JS, Celedon RG. Smith J. Automated lamellar keratomileusis in situ for myopia. *J Refract Surg*. 1996;12:29–35.

6. Arenas-Archila E, Sanchez Thorin JC, Naranjo Uribe JP, Hernandez Lozano A. Myopic keratomileusis in situ: a preliminary report. *J Cataract Refract Surg*. 1991;17:424–435.

7. Gomes M. Keratomileusis in situ using manual dissection of corneal flap for high myopia. *J Refract Corneal Surg*. 1994;10:255–257.

8. Ibrahim O, Waring GO, Salah T, Maghraby AE. Automated in situ keratomileusis for myopia. *J Refract Surg*. 1995;11:431–441.

9. Buratto L. Intrastromal photoablation with excimer laser for the treatment of high myopia. Presented at the First Italian Meeting on Excimer Laser, January 1990.

10. Buratto L, Ferrari M. The excimer laser in myopic keratomileusis. Presented at the First International Congress on the Myopic Keratomileusis, Mestre (Venice), June 1990.

11. Buratto L, Ferrari M, Genisi C. Intrastromal keratomileusis by excimer laser (193 nm): clinical results with 1 year follow up. Presented at the First Annual Congress of the Summit International Laser User Group. Geneve, Sept. 1991.

12. Buratto L, Ferrari M, Rama P. Excimer laser intrastromal keratomileusis. *Am J Ophthalmol*. 1992;113:291–295.

13. Buratto L, Ferrari M. Excimer laser intrastromal keratomileusis: case reports. *J Cataract Refract Surg.* 1992;18:37–41.

14. Buratto L, Ferrari M. Intrastromal keratomileusis with excimer laser (Buratto's technique): long term clinical results. Presented at the International Meeting on Cataract and Refractive Surgery, San Diego CA. April 1992.

15. Buratto L, Genisi C, Ferrari M. Intrastromal keratomileusis with excimer laser (Buratto's technique): short term clinical results. Presented at the Second Annual Congress of the Summit International Laser User Group. Montreux, September 1992.

16. Bas AM, Onnis R. Excimer laser in situ keratomileusis for myopia. *J Refract Surg.* 1995;11(suppl): 229–233.

17. Kremer FB, Dufek M. Excimer Laser in situ keratomileusis. *J Refract Surg.* 1995;11:244–247.

18. Villasenor RA. Homoplastic keratomileusis for myopia. *Refract Corneal Surg.* 1985;25:515–525.

19. Haimovici R, Culbertson WW. Optical lamellar keratoplasty using the Barraquer microkeratome. *Refract Corneal Surg.* 1991;7:42–45.

20. Hanna KD, David T, Besson J, Pouliquen Y. Lamellar keratoplasty with the Barraquer microkeratome. *Refract Corneal Surg.* 1991;7:177–181.

21. Nascimento EG, Carvalmo MJ, De Freitas D, Campos M. Nocardial keratitis following myopic keratomileusis. *J Refract Surg.* 1995;11:210–211.

11

Phakic Myopic Intraocular Lenses

Georges Baïkoff

INTRODUCTION

During the introduction of intraocular lenses (IOLs) for the correction of aphakia in the 1950s, the IOL pioneers, Strampelli, Barraquer and Choyce,[1-3] also developed the concept of correction of myopia by implantation of an anterior chamber lens in a phakic eye. At that time, apart from Sato's[4] publications on radial keratotomy, no corneal refractive surgery existed. The design and rigidity of the first-generation anterior chamber lenses unfortunately led to serious complications involving corneal decompensation and increased intraocular pressure. Since the initial anterior chamber lenses were designed, cataract surgery evolved with the use of extracapsular extraction and then phacoemulsification. Posterior chamber lenses were then developed, generally replacing anterior chamber lenses in the correction of aphakia. Most of the anterior chamber lenses were abandoned because of the high rate of complications. Nevertheless, some types of flexible anterior chamber lenses, particularly the Kelman implant, have remained safe.[5]

An alternative to the IOL correction of myopia was developed by José Barraquer.[6] The development of corneal lamellar refractive surgery began with Barraquer's technique of freeze keratomileusis. Over time, lamellar surgery has been simplified with the introduction of nonfreeze keratomileusis[7] and then with automated lamellar keratoplasty (ALK) involving semiautomation of corneal cutting. Recent ALK results from multicenter clinical trials unfortunately show lack of accuracy and loss of refractive effect[8,9] over time, particularly in patients corrected for large degrees of myopia. Correction of very high myopia with ALK requires extensive thinning of the cornea, sometimes with only 200 μm or

less of posterior corneal stroma remaining. This amount of thinning increases the risk of corneal ectasia and of induced keratoconus, particularly with increased intraocular pressure. In addition, the optical quality can be deficient in terms of contrast sensitivity due to problems related to the interface. Corneal complications such as epithelial downgrowth can occur because of the absence of sutures. Most recently, lamellar refractive surgery has been combined with laser corneal ablation. Despite the increased accuracy of this technique compared to that of ALK, laser in situ keratomileusis (LASIK) is still a lamellar refractive surgical procedure; therefore, the problems of excessive weakening of the posterior cornea and of optical effects linked to the interface remain.

Over the past decade, several surgeons worldwide[10-13] have reintroduced and refined phakic IOLs. IOL implantation can potentially correct any degree of myopia, depending on the power of the implant. Both phakic IOL implantation and clear lens extraction respect totally corneal architecture. Neither the central optical zone nor the corneal positive asphericity is compromised. The phakic myopic implants offer several potential advantages over clear lens extraction. Compared with clear lens extraction, myopic implantation is reversible, preserves accommodation, and reduces the risk of retinal complications. The concept of reversibility is important. Apart from myopic phakic implantation, only intracorneal rings[14] offer this possibility. The relationship between positive corneal asphericity and optimal visual function is still not defined. Nevertheless, myopic phakic implantation and intracorneal ring insertion are the only techniques that respect positive corneal asphericity. It should be emphasized, though, that intracorneal rings currently correct only low amounts of myopia and probably will not correct large amounts in the future.

CURRENTLY AVAILABLE PHAKIC MYOPIC IOLS

Iris-Fixated Implants: The Fechner-Worst Implant

The Fechner-Worst implant was developed as a modification of the lobster claw lens used for aphakia (Fig. 11.1). Initially the lens was biconvex, but recently it has been modified. Currently, the anterior face is convex and the posterior face is concave (Fig. 11.2). The diameter of the optical zone is about 5 mm, allowing thinning of the optical edges. During insertion, the anterior chamber must be filled with a viscoelastic agent. The lens is held with a special forceps, and the iris is pinched at the 9:00 and 3:00 o'clock positions with the claws of the haptic. Iridectomy should be performed routinely to prevent pupillary blockage.

Anterior Chamber Implant: The Baïkoff Implant

The design of the Baïkoff implant is based on that of the Kelman lens for correction of aphakia. In the Baïkoff lens, however, there is a negative optical part. Initially, this lens was designed with an angulation of 25° and relatively thick optical edges. Because of potential endothelial lesions observed with this first-generation lens, angulation was reduced and the optical edges were thinned. These modifications substantially increase the clearance

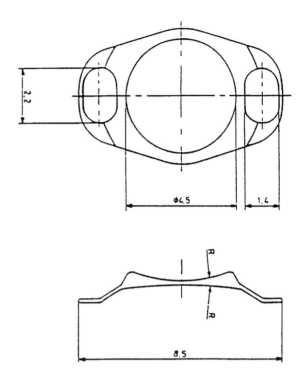

Fig. 11.2. The biconcave Fechner-Worst iris claw lens. (Courtesy of P.U. Fechner, Germany)

between the endothelium and the implant edges (Figs. 11.3, 11.4). Recent modifications also include the incorporation of an anterior convex surface and a posterior concave surface.

The diameter of the optic is about 5 mm. The surgical technique for the insertion of this lens is the same as that for secondary implantation of an anterior chamber lens in an aphakic eye. An incision, with or without a corneal tunnel, is performed; the

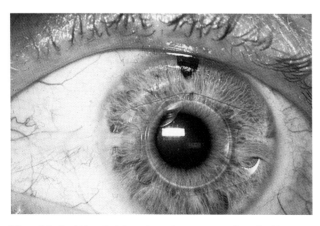

Fig. 11.1. Worst iris claw in a myopic phakic eye. (Courtesy of Jan Worst, the Netherlands)

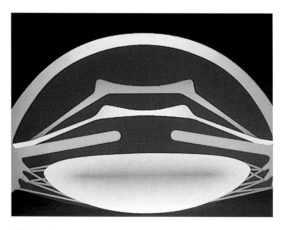

Fig. 11.3. Comparison of two generations of Baïkoff angle-fixated lenses. The first design (high vaulted) has been abandoned.

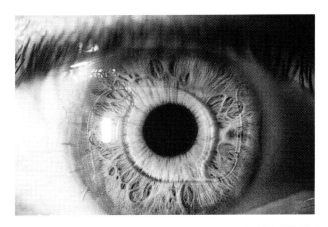

Fig. 11.4. Anterior chamber phakic myopic IOL (ZB5M) (G. Baïkoff).

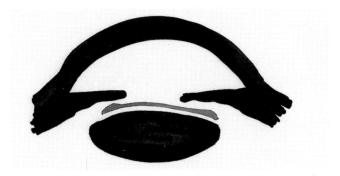

Fig. 11.5. Posterior chamber myopic phakic IOL.

anterior chamber is filled with a viscoelastic agent; and the lens is introduced into the anterior chamber. The suture is placed even in the presence of a corneal tunnel to ensure tight closure and prevent postoperative flat chambers.

Horizontal insertion is preferable to vertical insertion because of the curvature of the implant. The IOL must be placed in its definitive position since the shape of the footplates prevents rotation in the anterior chamber. The surface of the lens is fluorinated to reduce adhesion of endothelial cells to the polymethylmethacrylate (PMMA) material.

Posterior Chamber Implants: Fyodorov and Fechner Implants

Fyodorov was the first to design a posterior chamber lens for myopic correction. The initial lens was collar button-shaped and centered on the pupil. The design was modified subsequently and the implant currently is placed completely in the posterior chamber, floating between the anterior surface of the lens and the posterior surface of the iris (Figs. 11.5 to 11.7).

The Fyodorov implant currently is made of Collamere (a copolymer of collagene and HEMA). The Fechner implant, a modification of the Fyodorov implant, is made of silicone. Haptic designs of both implants had been undergoing multiple modifications. In inserting the lens, the pupil is dilated and viscoelastic substance is placed in the anterior chamber. Because of the flexibility of the material, the implant can be bent or rolled through a self-sealing corneal incision 3 to 4 mm in width.

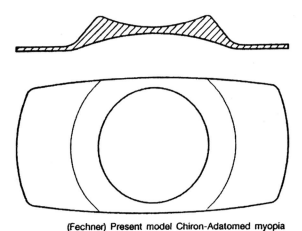

(Fechner) Present model Chiron-Adatomed myopia

Fig. 11.6. Fechner silicone posterior chamber IOL.

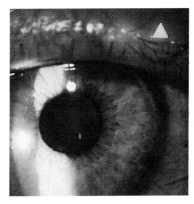

Fig. 11.7. The anterior segment after implantation of a silicone posterior chamber phakic myopic IOL.(Courtesy of Antonio Marinho, Portugal)

The implant is placed in front of the anterior lens surface. Miosis of the pupil is then induced. The diameter of the implant is determined by the dimension of the posterior chamber. Iridectomy is required because of the risk of pupillary blockage.

IMPLANT POWER AND SIZE DETERMINATION

The power of the implant is determined by the patient's refraction. Calculation tables had been established by Van der Heidje[15] for the Fechner-Worst implant, taking into consideration the subjective refraction, the keratometry, and the depth of the anterior chamber. Chiron-Domilens has established similar tables for the Baïkoff implant. Calculation of the appropriate lens power to achieve emmetropia is quite simple. For a spectacle correction of -8 to -10 D, an implant of the same power is used. For a spectacle correction between -11 and -15 D, 1 D in absolute value is subtracted; that is, for a myope of -15 D in spectacle correction, a -14 D implant is used. For a spectacle correction from -16 to -18 D, 2 D are subtracted for the calculation of the implant power, and for a spectacle correction of -20 or more, 3 D are subtracted. A similar system for calculation of implant power is used for posterior chamber implants. Measurement of axial length is unnecessary, since all myopic implants compensate for ametropia in the same way as contact lenses.

One of the advantages of the Worst implant[16] is the use of a single-diameter implant. The Baïkoff implant[17] exists in three sizes for every power (12.5, 13.0, and 13.5 mm). The appropriate diameter of the Baïkoff implant currently is determined by calculating white to white and adding $+0.5$ mm. The 12.5-mm implants are used most often. The appropriate diameter will probably be determined more accurately in the future using ultrasound measurements of the anterior chamber. Recently, Alleman (personal communication) has demonstrated the feasibility of using ultrasonic biometry of the anterior segment to calculate the internal diameter of the anterior chamber from scleral spur to scleral spur with increased precision (Fig. 11.8).

The posterior chamber implants of Fyodorov and Fechner appear to require more accurate measurement of the diameter of the posterior chamber.

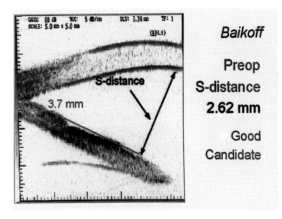

Fig. 11.8. Ultrasonic biometry analysis of the anterior chamber to define safety distances and good candidates for anterior chamber myopic phakic IOL implantation. (Courtesy of N. Alleman, São Paulo, Brazil)

Marinho (personal communication) has suggested oversizing the posterior chamber implant to increase the distance from the crystalline lens.

RESULTS

Visual Results

The visual results of myopic implants are excellent (Table 11.1), considering the high degree of myopia corrected. The average uncorrected visual acuity in studies with both the Fechner-Worst implants and the Baïkoff implant is about 20/40, and the best corrected visual acuity is about 20/30.[16,18–21] The studies have demonstrated an increase in best corrected visual acuity postoperatively compared to the preoperative best corrected visual acuity. The usual increase in best corrected visual acuity is one to two lines. The mean spherical equivalent refractions reported in these series are: Menezo (Worst lens), -0.50 to -0.75 D with an initial mean myopia of -14.50 D; Landez (Worst lens), -0.93 D for an initial mean refraction of -14.50 D; Baïkoff, -1 D for an initial mean refraction of -12.47 D; Marinho (Fechner lens), -0.47 D for an initial mean myopia of -17.3 D. It should be emphasized that in the Chiron-Domilens Baïkoff series, the targeted spherical equivalent refraction was -1 D. In that series the attained spherical equivalent refraction deviates from the intended goal by only -0.4 D. In the

Table 11.1. Refractive Outcome of Myopic Phakic IOLs

Type of IOL Series (Ref.)	No. of Eyes	Months of Follow-up, Mean (Range)	Preop Myopia Mean (Range)	Within % ± 1.0 D	Within % ± 2.0 D
Anterior Chamber					
Baïkoff ZB5M Baïkoff[20] (1995)	91	12 (12)	−12.47 D (−8 to −15 D)	74.7%	97.8%
Baïkoff ZB5M Perez-Santonja (1995)	255	(12–48)	(−10 to −26 D)	86%	
Iris-Fixated					
Worst-Fechner Fechner[10] (1989)	62	12 (2–14)	(−6.5 to −28 D)	63%	
Worst-Fechner Fechner [19] (1991)	109	25 (13–51)	(−5 to −31 D)	69%	
Worst-Fechner Landesz[16] (1993)	34	20 (3–60)	−14.40 D (−7 to −30 D)	58.8%	76.4%
Worst-Fechner Perez-Santonja (1996)	32	18 (6–30)	(−10 to −33 D)	76%	
Posterior Chamber					
Fechner-Fyodorov Marinho[21] (1996)	38	(3–24)	−17.3 D (−7 to −28 D)	71%	90%

Landez series (Worst lens), 81% of eyes corrected for less than −20 D of myopia are within 1 D of the desired refraction. In the Baïkoff series, 70–80% of the patients are within 1 D, and in the Marinho series (Fechner lens), 71% are within 1 D. The absence of induced postoperative hyperopia is very important. The Baïkoff series demonstrated no change in uncorrected near visual acuity postoperatively. Phakic IOLs do not cause loss of best corrected visual acuity from induced irregular astigmatism or interface opacification that can occur after corneal lamellar surgery.

Endothelium

Corneal endothelial protection is very important in phakic myopic IOL implantation. Initial myopic anterior chamber implantation by Strampelli, Barraquer, and Choyce failed because of frequent corneal decompensation at 3 to 5 years postoperatively. In recent prospective studies of Landez (Worst lens) done on 35 eyes, no corneal decompensation occurred. Landez reported 5.6% endothelial cell loss at 6 months and 8.9% loss at 1 year. Menezo reported similar results, with 3.32% cell loss at 6 months, 5.5% at 1 year, and 7.6% at 2 years (Table 11.2).

In the Chiron-Domilens multicenter study of the Baïkoff second-generation lens, central endothelial cell loss was 3.30% at 6 months, 4.47% at 1 year, 5.60% at 2 years, and 5.52% at 3 years. Peripheral endothelial cell loss was 3.2% at 6 months, 4.22% at 1 year, 4.36% at 2 years, and 3.88% at 3 years. These results are not statistically significant, since they are within the error of specular microscopy and demonstrate that the current generation of myopic phakic IOLs causes no more endothelial cell loss than conventional cataract surgery. It should be

Table 11.2. Endothelial Cell Loss After Implantation of Myopic Phakic IOL: Percent of Postoperative Cell Loss

Type of Lens	Reference	Follow-up (Years)		
		1	2	3
Baïkoff	Baïkoff[20]	4.47%	5.60%	5.52%
Worst	Menezo[18]	5.50%	7.60%	—

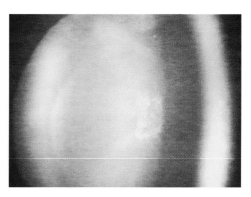

Fig. 11.9. Subcapsular lens opacification after silicone posterior chambe implant in a myopic phakic eye. (Courtesy of P.U. Fechner, Germany)

emphasized that myopic IOL implantation depends on surgical skill, and increased endothelial cell loss may be observed, as in the first series of the Fechner lenses, because of surgical trauma. Lens design is also critical for endothelial cell protection. The first-generation Baïkoff lens was modified because of endothelial cell lesions seen in the periphery and provoked by touch of the lens edges.[22,23] The second-generation Baïkoff lens has not caused significant endothelial cell loss during up to 3 years of follow-up. Myopic IOL implantation should not be considered if corneal dystrophies exist, if the anterior depth is less than 3 mm, if the corneal diameter is too large or too small, or if there is any other pathology of the anterior segment.

Cataract

There are no reported cases of cataracts induced by implantation of either the Baïkoff anterior chamber implant or the Worst iris-fixated implant. However, Fechner et al.[24] reported that with the posterior chamber silicone implant, anterior subcapsular opacities occurred in 8 of 45 eyes that had clear or almost clear crystalline lenses preoperatively (Fig. 11.9). The reason for cataract formation is not yet known. It is not clear whether these cataracts are linked to surgical trauma or to a toxic effect of the posterior chamber implant. New materials are under investigation. Zaldivar[25] did not report any cataract formation after implantation of the first-generation Fyodorov posterior chamber implant (Staar) in 80 eyes. The average follow-up period, however, was less than 1 year.

At present, posterior chamber implantation for the correction of myopia should be avoided in younger patients. In middle-aged or elderly patients, if there is cataract formation, the myopic implant could be removed and cataract extraction

could be performed, with implantation of an IOL to correct aphakia. Posterior chamber myopic lenses can be easily removed. The Baïkoff angle-supported anterior chamber lens can also be removed easily, except in a few cases in which synechiae form in the area of the footplates. Synechia formation is exceedingly rare and usually occurs with implantation of oversized intraocular lenses. Removal of the Worst iris-fixated lens is much more difficult and can lead to tearing of the iris.

Retinal Detachment

Retinal detachment has been reported following myopic IOL implantation in phakic eyes. Alio and collaborators[26] observed three retinal detachments, one of which was in their own series. One retinal detachment was reported in a Chiron-Domilens series of 133 eyes with implants.[20] Marinho[21] (Fechner posterior lens) documented one retinal detachment in 35 eyes. No retinal detachments were reported either in the Landez et al.[16] or Menezo et al.[18] series (Worst lens). Retinal detachment in high myopes is a problem that remains controversial. Refractive surgery should never be proposed in a high myope without careful examination of the peripheral retina and knowledge of the absence of dangerous lesions.

If peripheral retinal pathology is noted but is not extensive, it should be treated prophylactically. Only after healing following treatment should any refractive surgery be proposed. Extensive retinal pathology is a contraindication to refractive surgery in high myopes. Unfortunately, no good studies today have directly compared the frequency of retinal detachment after myopic IOL implantation in phakic eyes with that in patients after clear lens extraction or after lamellar refractive surgery. Studies of clear lens extraction on high myopes have documented a very low rate of retinal detachment[27], a rate that is much lower than after cataract surgery in high myopes. The studies of lamellar refractive surgery have not assessed the complication rate of retinal detachment.

Halos

Nocturnal halos can be observed in patients following myopic phakic IOL implantation because of the 4.5- to 5-mm diameter of the optical zones. Halos were noted in 20–30% of cases in the series of Landez (Worst lens), Baïkoff, Zaldivar, and Marinho (posterior implant). In a Chiron-Domilens multicenter trial of 133 cases with the Baïkoff IOL halos necessitated explantation in one case. In the Marinho study of 38 posterior chamber IOLs, two implants were removed because of halos. All studies to date have reported decreasing halos over time. Current modifications of the Baïkoff IOL include design changes in the edges of the implant to reduce diffraction and enlargement of the optical zone. It is well known that glare and halos are observed after both lamellar and laser corneal refractive surgery, particularly if the optical zone is too small or decentered. It should be emphasized that myopic implants allow preservation of normal corneal asphericity in the whole optical zone. Therefore, patients with myopic implants, unlike some patients who have undergone corneal refractive surgery, do not experience increased myopia at night.

IOL Rotation and Dislocation

The Baïkoff angle-supported implant can rotate if the IOL is too small. If rotation is limited to 20° or 30° and if, after 6 months, the new position remains stable, the lens is considered to be in a satisfactory position. If, however, rotation is significant and continues, a larger implant is needed. In the Chiron-Domilens multicenter trial of the Baïkoff IOL, rotation was noted in about 6% of cases. Exchange of the IOL was considered only in 1.5% of cases. Rotation or dislocation of the Fechner-Worst IOL can occur when the iris claw is not attached sufficiently to the iris. Cases have been reported by

Risco and Cameron[28] and by Menezo et al.[18] If iris fixation of a Fechner-Worst IOL is done incorrectly, the pupil may be deformed. No cases of ovalization of the pupil were reported by Landez and Menezo. In the multicenter trial of the Baïkoff IOL, very small pupillary ovalizations were observed in about 20% of cases (Fig. 11.10). Substantial ovalization was reported in 3% of cases. In a large amount of pupillary deformation occurs, the IOL can be removed to obtain a round pupil. Pupillary ovalization can occur because of either oversized lenses or a chronic irritation in the irido-corneal angle resulting from touch of the PMMA bridge linking the two footplates.[29] Current modifications of footplate and haptic designs will probably reduce the risk of pupillary ovalization. In addition, more accurate preoperative measurements of the anterior chamber will decrease the risk of pupillary deformation. Decentration also can occur with posterior chamber IOLs. Over the past 2 years, five different designs have been tested by Zaldivar to decrease the risk of decentration. Definitive results have not been published. Marinho has reported removal of one posterior chamber IOL in a series of 38 implants because of malpositioning.

Inflammatory Reactions

Some cases of postoperative uveitis have been reported in all published series of myopic implants. All cases of uveitis resolved following topical or systemic corticosteroid treatment. No inflammatory

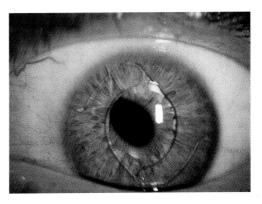

Fig. 11.10. Pupil ovalization observed after implantation of an anterior chamber myopic phakic IOL (G. Baïkoff).

reactions have led to loss of best corrected visual acuity. Perez Santonja et al.,[30] Alio et al.,[31] and Leroux Lesjardins et al.[32] performed photometrical studies of the aqueous humor after myopic IOL implantation. During the first postoperative year, a slight rise in cells and flare was reported with both angle-supported implants and iris-fixated implants. Subclinical cells and flare have been more significant with the Worst implant than with the Baïkoff one. Leroux Lesjardins[32] demonstrated that 3 years after IOL implantation with the angle-supported IOL, cell and flare meter readings were normal.

Ocular Hypertension and Glaucoma

There have been no reported cases of chronic glaucoma induced by myopic IOL implantation with either the angle-supported, iris claw, or posterior chamber implants. Irido-corneal angle trauma during surgery or uveal irritation by a foreign material of the implant may lead to ocular hypertension. Nevertheless, after long-term follow-up, no ocular hypertension has been noted. In patients with iris-fixated or posterior chamber implants, an iridectomy must be performed, since pupillary blockage was reported in early cases without iridectomy. Iridectomy is not necessary with the Baïkoff anterior chamber implant since there is no risk of pupillary blockage. If the surgeon decides to perform an iridectomy with the Baïkoff implant, the iris opening should not be performed in the basal position to prevent the implant footplate from entering the opening if there is slight rotation of the IOL.

CONCLUSION

High myopes can be very visually disabled. A surgical solution must be proposed for high myopes who cannot tolerate contact lenses and cannot see adequately with glasses. Myopic IOL implantation in a phakic eye is currently a treatment for patients with high myopia. Radial keratotomy can achieve satisfactory results in patients with low myopia. Current techniques of photorefractive keratotomy achieve the best results with low and moderate myopia. ALK can correct high degrees of myopia but the results are imprecise and unstable, particularly because of weakening of the posterior plan. Initial results with LASIK appear promising, but longer follow-up and more investigation are necessary.

Myopic IOL implantation in phakic eyes can be an alternative for the treatment of high myopia.[33] Specular microscopy to assess corneal endothelial density is necessary annually, and the implant should be removed if endothelial cell loss is 50% or greater. An advantage of myopic IOL implantation in a young patient is preservation of accommodation and reversibility of the procedure. Clear lens extraction should be reserved for patients with myopia of more than 20 D or for patients with lower degrees of high myopia who are over 40 years of age. Highly myopic patients who have worn contact lenses probably will prefer visual function after myopic IOL implantation rather than after corneal refractive surgery. Highly myopic patients who have worn glasses rather than contact lenses probably will be less disappointed by the optical imperfections of corneal remodeling surgery.

REFERENCES

1. Strampelli B. Anterior chamber lenses. *Arch Ophthalmol.* 1961;66:12–17.
2. Barraquer J. Anterior chamber plastic lenses. Results of and conclusions from five years experience. *Trans Ophthalmol Soc UK.* 1959;70:393–424.
3. Choyce DP. *Intraocular Lenses and Implants. The Correction of Myopia.* London: HK Lewis; 1964:153–155.
4. Sato T. Posterior incision of cornea. *Am J Ophthalmol.* 1950;33:943–948.
5. Auffarth GU, Wesendahl TA, Brown SJ, Apple DJ. Are there acceptable anterior chamber intraocular lenses for clinical use in the 1990's? An analysis of 4104 explanted anterior chamber intraocular lenses. *Ophthalmology.* 1994;101:1913–1922.
6. Barraquer JJ. Queratomileusis para la correcion de la miopia. *Arch Soc Am Oftal Optom.* 1964;5:27–48.
7. Swinger CA, Krumeich J, Cassiday D. A new device for viable refractive keratoplasty. *Invest Ophthalmol Vis Sci.* 1985;26:151.
8. Laroche L, Gautier L, Thrist J C1, et al. Nonfreeze myopic keratomyleusis for myopia in 158 eyes. *J Refract Corneal Surg.* 1994;10:400–412.
9. Price FW, Whitson WE, Gonzalez JS, et al. Automated lamellar keratomileusis in situ for myopia. *J Refract Surg.* 1996;12:29.
10. Fechner PU, Van Der Heijde GL, Worst JGF. The correction of myopia by lens implantation into phakic eyes. *Am J Ophthalmol.* 1989;107:659.

11. Joly P, Baïkoff G, Bonnet P. Mise en place d'un implant négatif de chambre antérieure chez des sujets phakes. *Bull Soc Ophtalmol.* 1989;5:727–730.

12. Baïkoff G, Joly P. Comparison of minus power I.O.L.s and myopic epikeratoplasty in phakic eyes. *Refract Corneal Surg.* 1990;6:252–260.

13. Fyodorov SN, Zuvey UL. Analysis of long term clinical and functional results of intraocular correction of high myopia. *Ophthalmosurgery.* 1990;2:3–6.

14. Nose W, Neves RA, Schanzlin D, Belfort R. Intrastromal corneal ring. One year results of first implants.

15. Van Der Heijde GL. Some optical aspects of implantation of an IOL in a myopic eye. *Eur J Implant Ref Surg.* 1989;1:41–43.

16. Landesz, Worst JGF, Siertsema JV. Negative implant. A retrospective study. *Doc Ophthalmol.* 1993;83:261–270.

17. Baïkoff G. Phakic anterior chamber IOL. *Intern Ophthalmol Clin.* 1991;31:75–86.

18. Menezo JL, Cesneros A, Hueso JR. Long-term results of surgical treatment of high myopia with Worst-Fechner intraocular lenses. *J Cataract Refract Surg.* 1995;21:93–98.

19. Fechner PU, Strobel J, Wichmann N. Correction of myopia by implantation of a concave Worst iris claw lens into phakic eyes. *Refract Corneal Surg.* 1991;7:286–298.

20. Baïkoff G. Anterior chamber phakic IOLs. In: Elander R, Rich L, Robin J, eds. *Textbook of Refractive Surgery.* Philadelphia, PA: WB Saunders Co; in press.

21. Marinho A, Neves MC, Into MC, Vaz F. Posterior chamber silicone intraocular implant in phakic eyes. A two year follow-up. *Refract Corneal Surg.* In press.

22. Mimouni F, Colin J, Koffi V, Bonnet P. Damage to the corneal endothelium from anterior chamber intraocular lenses in phakic myopic eyes. *Refract Corneal Surg.* 1991;7:277–281.

23. Saragoussi JJ, Cotinat J, Renard G, Saldovelli M, Abenhaim A, Pouliquen Y. Damage to the corneal endothelium by minus power. *Refract Corneal Surg.* 1991;7:282–285.

24. Fechner PU, Haigis W, Wichmann W. Posterior chamber myopia lenses in phakic eyes. *J Cataract Refract Surg.* 1996;22:178–182.

25. Zaldivar R. ISRS, Atlanta, GA, October 26–28, 1995.

26. Alio L, Ruiz-Moreno JM, Artola A. Retinal detachment as a potential hazard in surgical correction of severe myopia with phakic anterior chamber lenses. *Am J Ophthalmol.* 1993;115:145–148.

27. Colin J, Robinet A. Clear lensectomy and implantation of low-power posterior chamber intraocular lens for the correction of high myopia. *Ophthalmology.* 1994;101:107–112.

28. Risco JM, Cameron JA. Dislocation of a phakic intraocular lens. *Am J Ophthalmol.* 1994;118:666–667.

29. Saragoussi JJ, Othenin-Girard Ph, Pouliquen YM. Ocular damage after implantation of over-sized minus power anterior chamber intraocular lens in myopic phakic eyes. Case report. *Refract Corneal Surg.* 1993;9:105–109.

30. Perez-Santonja JJ, Hernandez JL, Benitez del Castillo JM. Fluorophotometry in myopic phakic eyes with anterior chamber intraocular lenses to correct severe myopia. *Am J Ophthalmol.* 1994;118:316–321.

31. Alio JF, Delahoz F, Ismail MM. Subclinial inflammatory reaction induced by phakic anterior chamber lenses for the correction of high myopia. *Ocular Imunol Inflammation.* 1993;1:219–223.

32. Leroux lesjardins S, Heligon JP, Ozdemir N. Tolérance à moyen terme des implants myopiques de chambre intérieure dans le traitement chirurgical de la myopie forte. *J Fr Ophthalmol.* 1995;18:45–49.

33. Drews RC. Risk benefit analysis of anterior chamber intraocular lenses for the correction of myopia in phakic patients. *Eur J Implant Ref Surg.* 1991;3:171–194.

12

Clear Lens Extraction

Joseph Colin
Anne Robinet

INTRODUCTION

The removal of the clear crystalline lens in patients with high myopia remains one of the most controversial current refractive surgical procedures. Clear lens extraction (CLE) is technically easy to perform, and with subsequent implantation of a low-power or negative intraocular lens (IOL), it is effective.

CLE provides rapid, predictable, and refractively stable visual rehabilitation. In the rare case where there is a refractive surprise, the implant can be removed and replaced, usually easily and safely. Furthermore, the quality of visual rehabilitation is superb, with no irregular astigmatism and excellent optical results. However, CLE is an invasive procedure that may result in severe vision loss. The primary risk with this procedure is the increased potential for retinal detachment.

Several authors have claimed that the optical benefits of CLE are usually outweighed by the severity of the risks and the availability of safer alternatives. Advances in phacoemulsification, small incision surgery, posterior chamber IOLs, and viscoelastics have reduced the risks of cataract surgery. These developments have led us to reconsider this surgical option and to question the current risks versus the potential benefits for patients.

CLE may be considered for high myopia and hyperopia, in bilateral cases, or in anisometropia with relative amblyopia.

CLE FOR MYOPIA

Historical Background

A century ago, Fukala[1,2] began to treat high myopia by removing the clear lens. However, although acceptable refractive results were obtained, severe intra- and postoperative complications were common. The modern era of lens implant surgery for myopia began with the work of Barraquer[3] but was marked by the occurrence of frequent inflammatory and corneal complications Verzella[4-7] reported the results of CLE in several hundred eyes with more than -14 D of myopia. He stressed the need for careful pre- and postoperative retinal evaluation and treatment. The refractive results were not very accurate due to the limited range of available lens implant powers. Verzella reported a 0.7% incidence of retinal detachment. However, the technique remained controversial because of the high risk of retinal detachment in long eyes after cataract surgery.[8]

Indications

Selection of patients for CLE depends on the degree of ametropia, age, retinal examination, vitreous status, intraocular pressure (IOP), and visual acuity.[9-11] Patients are usually selected on the basis of preoperative myopia of more than 12 D, a best corrected visual acuity of 20/100 or better, and intolerance of contact lenses. Informed consent with a perfect understanding of the potential risks must be obtained from all patients prior to surgery. CLE is discussed with patients older than 35 years, when contact lens tolerance decreases and prebyopia begins. At this age also, nuclear sclerosis and lens opacities are more frequent.

CLE may be a secondary procedure after complications following implantation of phakic myopic IOLs. For example, if progressive endothelial cell loss occurs after implantation, the IOL must be explanted. The refractive status may be restored by removing the clear lens through the same incision, with minimal additional corneal damage.

Contraindications

Patients with a history of retinal detachment in one eye must not be selected for CLE. Elevated IOP is a relative contraindication because of the difficulty of checking visual fields and the optic disc in highly myopic eyes and the risk of increasing the IOP after surgery.

Argon Laser Retinal Treatment

Indications: In patients with lattice degeneration, retinal tear, or hole, we perform argon laser photocoagulation before CLE. Focal treatment is used for small lesions, and circumferential treatment is used for diffuse degeneration.[12,13]

Procedure: The argon green laser is commonly used. Retinal photocoagulation is performed 2 months before lens surgery, using 100- to 200-mW, 500-μm, 0.1-sec retinal spots. Three rows of nearly confluent burns are placed immediately around focal lesions. When circumferential laser photocoagulation is required, four sessions are necessary to obtain the 360° retinal treatment. Radial extensions are performed anteriorly to the ora serrata in the horizontal and vertical meridians.

Surgical Procedure

Anesthesia: Surgery may be performed under general anesthesia to maintain a very quiet eye or under local anesthesia with careful injections in very long eyes.

Incision: After conjunctival peritomy, a scleral tunnel is created along the steepest meridian to try

to decrease the astigmatism often associated with high myopia. A viscoelastic substance is injected into the usually deep anterior chamber.

Capsulorhexis: A large capsulorhexis (5.5 to 6.0 mm) is indicated to prevent the constriction syndrome of the anterior capsule, which may tear the retinal periphery.

Removal of the Lens: Hydrodissection is important to facilitate rotation of the nucleus and removal of the lens. Due to the softness of the nucleus, lens extraction can be accomplished in most cases primarily with irrigation and aspiration. In patients with a harder nucleus, low-power phacoemulsification must be performed. In such cases, a divide-and-conquer technique may be used, and the four quadrants are aspirated without cracking.

Choice of the IOL: Because of the available powers, polymethylmethacrylate (PMMA) IOLs are currently used in all cases. The diameter of the optic may be 5.5 or 7 mm to obtain better visualization of the retina, according to different retinal surgeons. If the calculation of the IOL's power gives a zero value, it is preferable to implant an IOL rather than let the eye remain aphakic. The IOL may act as a diaphragm between the anterior and posterior segments to stabilize the vitreous.

Pharmacia, Chiron, Allergan, and Alcon have negative-power IOLs up to −10 D with increments of 1 D. Powers beyond those available commercially in the United States can be obtained by special order. Silicone IOLs, if powers are available, should not be implanted in highly myopic eyes. Acrylics may be a better material for implantation to retain all the advantages of the small-incision surgery.

The formation of moisture droplets on the posterior surface of a silicone IOL during a posterior segment fluid–air exchange procedure has been reported (J. Knaub, personal communication). The major concern was that the view of the fundus was impaired, requiring the surgical procedure to be discontinued. Francese and collaborators showed that visualization could be quickly restored by applying a viscoelastic substance to the posterior IOL surface.[14]

D.J. Apple reported on irreversible silicone oil adhesion to silicone IOLs and concluded that implantation of silicone IOLs should be reconsidered in patients with severe vitreal-retinal problems or for those at risk for such problems (oral presentation, annual meeting of the American Academy of Ophthalmology, Atlanta, October 1995).

Calculation of the Power: IOL power calculations are discussed in Chapter 13. Careful, repeated measurements of the axial length must be performed to avoid errors induced by myopic staphylomas. The targeted postoperative refraction error must be low myopia (−1 or −2 D) to allow the patient to maintain comfortable uncorrected near vision after the postoperative loss of accommodation.

In case of weak zonulae, a capsular bag PMMA ring (Morcher, Inc., Germany) may be implanted to maintain the bag and to stretch the posterior capsule. This ring prevents retraction of the anterior capsule and may delay opacification of the posterior capsule. (Fig. 12.1)

Cleaning of the posterior and anterior capsules must be as complete as possible to remove the epithelial cells responsible for early posterior capsule opacification in young eyes. (Fig. 12.2)

Two or three sutures are usually necessary to close the incision even if it is self-sealing.

Intraoperative Complications

CLE via phacoemulsification is easier and induces fewer complications than cataract surgery in highly myopic eyes with dense nuclei and weak zonules

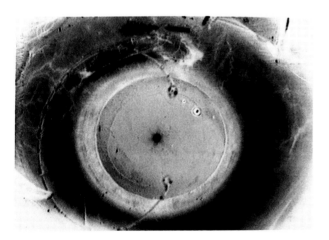

Fig. 12.1. Capsular bag PMMA ring that prevents retraction of the anterior capsule.

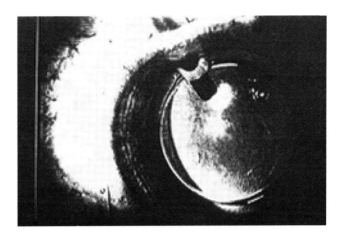

Fig. 12.2. Intraocular lens after clear lens extraction for high myopia.

(G. Baïkoff, oral communication, annual meeting of the Society of Cataract and Refractive Surgery, Seattle, June 1996). In Baïkoff's comparative study and about 450 eyes, the incidence of capsular tears, zonular dehiscences, and vitreous loss was very low after CLE. In young myopic eyes under local anesthesia, positive pressure may occur during surgery, leading in some cases to iris prolapse.

Postoperative Management

Early refraction is needed, usually 7 days following surgery, to check the accuracy of the IOL power calculation. If a refractive error is found, the IOL may be easily explanted and replaced with a new lens. Postoperative medication includes topical antibiotics and dexamethasone three times a day for 2 weeks. A retinal examination is performed 1 month after surgery and afterward once a year. If the posterior capsule must be opened, the retina is checked before and 1 month after capsulotomy.

Results

In the authors' study of CLE, 52 eyes of 30 patients underwent surgery from January 1990 to January 1991.[15,16] The mean preoperative spherical equivalent was −16.9 ± 3.26 D; the axial length was greater than 29 mm in 64% of eyes, and 15.3% of the IOLs used were minus powered. Twenty-eight patients were followed for a minimum of 4 years. Two patients were lost to follow-up. The results are discussed below.

Refractive Results

Spherical Equivalent: Thirty one eyes (63.2%) were within 1.0 D of emmetropia, and 45 eyes (91.8%) were within 2.0 D of emmetropia. These results are identical to those found at the 1-year evaluation. The mean spherical equivalent was −0.92 ± 0.86 D. Four eyes experienced a myopic shift between 0.50 D and 1.0 D. Among these eyes, two were myopic and two were hyperopic 1 year after surgery. No eye had a refractive change of more than 1.0 D.

Visual Results: The distance best corrected visual acuity was 20/40 (decimal score = 0.53) at 4 years compared with 20/35 (0.57) preoperatively and 20/33 (0.61) at 1 year. In eyes with an open capsule it was 0.62, and in eyes with an intact capsule it was 0.48.

The percentage of eyes achieving best corrected visual acuity of 20/40 or better was 75% preoperatively, 88.5% at 1 year, and 65.3% at 4 years. At the last evaluation, the percentage was 83.3% in eyes with posterior capsulotomies but only 54.8% in eyes with intact posterior capsules.

Two eyes (4.1%) had a decrease in best corrected visual acuity of more than two lines (one after a macular complication and one following retinal detachment).

Mean uncorrected visual acuity was 20/80 (0.25) compared with 20/66 (0.30) at 1 year. This value was 20/63 (0.34) in eyes with an open posterior capsule and 20/100 (0.20) in eyes with an intact capsule. A total of 65.3% of the eyes achieved 20/100 or better compared with 84.6% at 1 year (83.3% in eyes with an open capsule and 54.8% in eyes with an intact capsule).

Endothelial Cell Loss: Of the 16 eyes with preoperative and 1-year postoperative specular microscopy, the average endothelial cell loss was 66 cells/-mm^2 or 2.2% (2935 ± 208 versus 2869 ± 228).

Retinal Complications: At 9 months postoperatively, subfoveal choroidal neovascularization developed in one eye. The best corrected distance visual acuity, which had been 20/50 (preoperatively as well as postoperatively before this complication developed) decreased to 20/200, and the near vision with correction decreased from J2 to J4. Review of postoperative complications indicated that no new

cases of macular complication occurred during the 4-year follow-up period.

One case of a retinal detachment was observed 18 months after surgery in a 30-year-old female with a preoperative myopia of −20 D and an axial length of 31 mm. Her posterior capsule was intact; her peripheral retina had been treated preoperatively. The retinal tear occurred in an area outside the quadrant which was treated. Three surgical procedures were necessary to reattach the retina. The final visual corrected acuity was 20/200 because of chronic macular edema. The fellow eye, which was also treated by CLE for myopia, showed no signs of retinal peripheric degeneration.

Argon Laser Retinal Treatment: Before surgery, 19 eyes had undergone focal coagulation, 12 eyes had undergone circumferential photocoagulation, and 21 eyes had had no treatment. During the 1-year postoperative period, an additional seven focal treatments and two additional circumferential treatments were performed. At 4 years, one eye which had not received a preoperative argon laser treatment required a focal treatment for lattice degeneration.

Posterior Vitrous Detachment (PVD): Preoperatively, the incidence of PVD was 57.7%; the proportion was greater in older eyes. During the first postoperative year, two new cases of PVD were detected and two additional new cases were found at the 4-year evaluation. No additional complications occurred in these four eyes.

Posterior Capsule Opacification: Polishing of the posterior capsule under topical anesthesia may be considered if the opacification is related mainly to epithelial cellular proliferation. The procedure is particularly easy if a small-diameter optic IOL has been implanted. The YAG capsulotomy is postponed until it is absolutely necessary. A small, precise capsulotomy of less than 3 mm is recommended.

Nd:YAG Capsulotomies: During the 4-year follow-up period, 18 eyes (36.7%) required neodymium: YAG capsulotomy for posterior capsule opacification. The mean time was 19.6 months ± 6.9 months (range, 9 to 33 months). No early complications arose as a result of the capsulotomy procedure. Three eyes with too small capsulotomies needed secondary enlargement. IOP was less than 20 mm Hg in all eyes during the entire follow-up period.

Comparison of Published Results

During the past few years, CLE has been increasingly used for the treatment of high refractive errors, either for myopia or hyperopia. The major risks of intraocular surgery are obvious, especially retinal detachment, cystoid macular edema, and endophthalmitis. There is no question that the risk of visual loss from intraocular surgery is greater than from refractive corneal surgery. However, the risk in corneal surgery is not insignificant. In addition, most of the visual side effects, variable visual acuity, and star bursting effects are obviated by leaving the cornea intact. However, the potential risk of severe loss of vision remain the major concern of this surgical option.

Barraquer et al.[17] performed a retrospective study evaluating the incidence of retinal detachment following CLE in myopic patients (165 eyes). Prophylactic treatment with the argon laser was performed in 10 eyes. The surgical techniques included intracapsular cataract extraction (ICCE) and manual extracapsular cataract extraction (ECCE); only 15% of the patients received an IOL. The authors found an incidence of 7.3% of retinal detachment an average of 30.7 ± 26.6 months post-operatively, 50% occurring during the first 2 years after surgery. The retina was reattached in 75% of the cases. An association between retinal detachments and YAG capsulotomies was found in this series.

J. C. Javitt[18] has estimated the risk of severe visual loss after CLE. If both eyes are operated on, the risk of a bad outcome in either eye is 9.2% for moderate visual impairment and 6.6% for severe impairment or blindness, assuming independence of eyes.

Lyle and Jin[19] evaluated CLE in highly myopic eyes via phacoemulsification. The visual results were comparable to those of the authors, although the rate of Nd:YAG capsulotomies was high in their series, no complications were associated with this procedure and no retinal detachments were reported. (Table 12.1)

Centurion and co-workers[20] reported on 35 highly myopic eyes which underwent ECCE and IOL implantation. All eyes had prophylactic treatment of the peripheral retina prior to lens surgery. There was no report of retinal detachment after 7 years of follow-up. YAG capsulotomy was performed in 66% of the eyes. Myopia was reduced to ± 2.0 D of the intended correction in 20% of the eyes and to ± 1.0 D in 54% of the eyes (Table 12.1). The authors concluded that CLE with preoperative prophylactic retinal treatment is safe and effective in the correction of high myopia.

Table 12.1. Different Reports of CLE for High Myopia

	Lyle[19] (1994)	Centurion[20] (1996)	Colin[15] (1994)	Colin[16] (1995)
No. of eyes	31	54	52	48
Mean follow-up (mo)	21.7		12	48
Percent of eyes within ± 1 D of emmetropia	68	74	63.2	57.1
Percent of eyes within ± 2 D of emmetropia	90		91.2	89.7
Percent of BCVA ≥ 20/100				
With Yag			98	82
Without Yag				62
Percent of BCVA ≥ 20/40	77		38.4	
Percent of retinal detachment	0	0	0	1.9
Percent of YAG capsulotomies	58	66	7.6	36.7
Percent of eyes losing two lines			1.9	4.1

The authors' series, using modern cataract surgery technique for CLE and prophylactic retinal treatment, confirms the accurate refractive results obtained at 1 year and stability of the mean spherical equivalent. The incidence of retinal detachment was 1.9% at 4 years; in Barraquer' report,[17] the incidence was 3.7% 2 years after surgery and 5.4% at 4 years. Capsulotomy was not associated with retinal detachment in the authors' study.

The primary concern with this operative procedure is the inevitable vitreal-retinal degeneration, with subsequent retinal detachment.[21–23] The incidence of retinal detachment in myopic patients undergoing CLE is higher than in the emmetropic population; the results vary widely with the surgical technique and the definition of high myopia.[24–26]

The major question is: Is the 1.9% risk of retinal detachment at 4 years acceptable? The normal lifetime myopia risk of retinal detachment with no surgery is 2.4%, or 0.06% yearly.[27] This is 40 times the risk in the emmetropic eye without surgery. More large series with long follow-up periods are necessary to confirm the results with our small series.

Long, continuous follow-up in evaluating the outcomes of CLE for high myopia is absolutely necessary before considering this surgical procedure as a routine option for refractive surgery, especially since in most cases the surgery is bilateral.

CLE FOR HYPEROPIA

There have been only a few published reports of the results of CLE for the treatment of high hyperopia (Table 12.2). The retinal risks following lensectomy are smaller than those following surgery in myopic eyes.

Siganos and collaborators[28] reported on 3-year results of CLE and IOL implantation in normally sighted, highly hyperopic eyes. Hyperopes aged 35 or more usually need presbyopic correction that adds more diopters to the already existing plus correction, translated in turn into more spherical and chromatic aberrations, more constricted visual fields, and a further decrease in image quality.

The results were excellent in terms of accuracy, safety, and rapid stability of refraction (Table 12.2).

Table 12.2. Reports of CLE for Hyperopia

	Lyle[19] (1994)	Siganos[28] (1995)
No. of eyes	6	17
Mean follow-up (mo)	19	
Percent of eyes within ± 1 D of emmetropia	100	100
Percent of BCVA ≥ 20/40	100	100
Percent of YAG capsulotomies	33	17.6
Percent of eyes losing two lines	0	0
Percent of retinal detachment	0	0

The SRK II formula was used to calculate the IOL power, which was aimed at −1.5 D. The mean IOL power was 31.8 ± 0.6 D. The IOL used was a 6-mm optic biconvex single-piece PMMA (Coburn, Model 68UV).

The mean spherical equivalent for distance was +9.61 ± 0.46 D (+6.75 to + 13.75 D). The mean uncorrected visual acuity improved from counting fingers (CF) preoperatively to 0.84 (range, 0.7 to 1.0) at 3 years.

Care should be taken to exclude nanophthalmic eyes that are small, with a relatively big crystalline lens and high hyperopia. These eyes are at high risk of developing serious complications, including choroidal effusion, angle closure glaucoma, and retinal detachment.[29]

Lyle and Jin[19] have reported excellent visual rehabilitation in seven hyperopic eyes with a mean preoperative refraction of +6.52 (range, +4.25 to +7.87 D) (Table 12.2). J.T. Holladay and J.P. Gills have reported the efficacy and safety of implanting two IOLs in high hyperopes to provide adequate power; however, longer follow-up will be necessary (see Chapter 13).

CONCLUSION AND FUTURE DEVELOPMENTS

The main advantages of CLE are accuracy, stability, ease, absence of irregular astigmatism, and no need for expensive equipment. The complications of CLE are much less than those of cataract surgery in myopic eyes with harder nuclei. There are three disadvantages: the procedure is invasive; there is constant loss of accommodation; and the risk of retinal detachment is great in high myopes.

With modern cataract surgical techniques and with surveillance by a retinal specialist before and after surgery, CLE for the correction of high refractive errors represents an alternative with acceptable risks to corneal procedures and to other intraocular implant procedures. Future developments include possible use of multifocal IOLs to restoration of pseudoaccommodation but with a risk of decreased contrast sensitivity in eyes with poor retinal function, and the prevention of secondary cataract to avoid opening of the posterior capsule, which is a known risk factor for retinal detachment.[30]

REFERENCES

1. Fulkala V. Operative behandlung der hochstgradigen myopie durch apakie. *Graefe's Arch Ophthalmolol.* 1890;36:230.

2. Fukala V. Bietrag sur hochgradigen Myopie. *Ber Dtsch Ophtal Ges.* 1896;25:265.

3. Barraquer J. *La extraccion intracapsular del cristalino: Ponencia oficial del XL Congreso de la Sociedad Hispanoamericana de Grande Espana, 1962.* Barcelona, Spain: Graficas Typus; 1961:39.

4. Verzella F. Microsurgery of the lens in high myopia for optical purposes. *Cataract.* 1984;1:8–12.

5. Verzella F. *High Myopia: Microsurgical Extracapsular Extraction of the Lens for Optical Purposes.* Bologna: Lens Editions; 1983:15–28.

6. Verzella F. Microsurgery of the lens in high myopia for optical purposes. *Cataract.* 1984;1:8–12.

7. Verzella F. High myopia: refractive lensectomy and posterior chamber implants. *Cataract.* 1985;2:25–27.

8. Golderg MF. Clear lens extraction for axial myopia: an appraisal. *Ophthalmology.* 1987;94:571–82.

9. Buratto L. Considerations on clear lens extraction in high myopia. *Eur J Implant Refract Surg.* 1991;3:221–226.

10. Neumann AC, McCarty GR. Lensectomy for the treatment of myopia. In: Thompson FB, ed. *Myopia Surgery: Anterior and Posterior Segments.* New York: Macmillan Publishing; 1990:101–27.

11. Praeger DL. Five years' follow-up in the surgical management of cataracts in high myopia treated with the Kelman phacoemulsification technique. *Ophthalmology.* 1979;86:2024–2033.

12. Kanski JJ, Daniel R. Prophylaxis of retinal detachment. *Am J Ophthalmol.* 1975;79:197–205.

13. Zweng HC, Little HL, Hammond AH. Complications on argon laser photocoagulation. *Trans Am Acad Ophthalmol Otolaryngol.* 1974;78:194–204.

14. Francese JE, Christ FR, Buchen SV, et al. Moisture droplet formation on the posterior surface of intraocular lenses during fluid/air exchange. *J Cataract Refract Surg.* 1995;21:685–689.

15. Colin J, Robinet A. Clear lensectomy and implantation of low-power posterior chamber intraocular lens for the correction of high myopia. *Ophthalmology.* 1994;101:107–112.

16. Colin J, Robinet A. Clear lensectomy and implantation of low-power posterior chamber IOL for the correction of high myopia: 4 year follow-up. Presented at the annual meeting of the American Academy of Ophthalmology, Atlanta, October 1995.

17. Barraquer C, Cavelier C, Mejia LF. Incidence of retinal detachment following clear lens extraction in myopic patients. *Arch Ophthalmol.* 1994;112:336–339.

18. Javitt JC. Clear lens extraction for high myopia. Is this an idea whose time has come? *Arch Ophthalmol.* 1994;112:321–323.

19. Lyle WA, Jin GJC. Clear lens extraction for the correction of high refractive error. *J Cataract Refract Surg.* 1994;20:273–276.

20. Centurion V, Caballero JC, Medeiros OA, et al. Clear lens extraction and high myopia. *J Ref Corneal Surg.* In press.

21. Badr LA, Hussain HM, Jabak M, Wagoner MD. Extracapsular cataract extraction with or without posterior chamber intraocular lenses in eyes with cataract and high myopia. *Ophthalmology.* 1995;102:1139–1143.

22. Percival SPB, Setty SS. Sight-threatening pathology related to high myopia after posterior chamber lens implantation: a prospective study. *Eur J Implant Ref Surg.* 1993;5:95–98.

23. Werblin TP. Should we consider clear lens extraction for routine refractive surgery? *Refract Corneal Surg.* 1992;8:480–481.

24. Nielson NE, Naeser K. Epidemiology of retinal detachment following extracapsular cataract extraction: a follow-up study with an analysis of risk factors. *J Cataract Refract Surg.* 1993;19:675–680.

25. Arnold PN. Incidence of retinal detachment. Letter to the editor. *J Cataract Refract Surg.* 1994;20:363–364.

26. Lindstrom RL. Cataract surgery and lens implantation. Editorial overview. *Curr Opinion Ophthalmol.* 1993;4:1–2.

27. Lindstrom RL. Retinal detachment in axial myopia. *Dev Ophthalmol.* 1987;14:37–41.

28. Siganos DS, Pallikaris IG, Siganos CS. Clear lensectomy and intraocular lens implantation in normally sighted highly hyperopic eyes. Three year follow-up. *Eur J Implant Ref Surg.* 1995;7:128–133.

29. Osher RH. Comment on clear lens extraction and intraocular lens implantation in normally sighted hyperopia eyes. *J Refract Corneal Surg.* 1994;10:122–124.

30. Javitt JC, Tielsch JM, Canner JK, et al. National outcomes of cataract extraction; increased risk of retinal complications associated with Nd:YAG laser capsulotomy. *Ophthalmology.* 1992;99:1487–1498.

13

Intraocular Lens Power Calculations for Cataract and Refractive Surgery

Jack T. Holladay

IOL CALCULATIONS REQUIRING AXIAL LENGTH

Theoretical Formulas

The theoretical formula for intraocular lens (IOL) power calculations has not changed in almost 30 years since the original description by Fyodorov in 1967.[1,2] Although several investigators have presented the theoretical formula in different forms, there are no significant differences except for slight variations in the choice of retinal thickness and corneal index of refraction. There are six variables in the formula: (1) corneal power (K), (2) axial length (AL), (3) intraocular lens (IOL) power, (4) effective lens position (ELP), (5) desired refraction ($DPostRx$), and (6) vertex distance (V). Normally, IOL power is chosen as the dependent variable and the equation is solved for using the other five variables, where distances are given in millimeters and refractive powers in diopters:

$$IOL = \frac{1336}{AL - ELP} - \frac{1336}{\dfrac{1336}{\dfrac{1000}{\dfrac{1000}{DPostRx} - V} + K} - ELP}$$

The only variable that cannot be chosen or measured preoperatively is ELP. The improvements in IOL power calculations over the past 30 years are a result of improving the predictability of ELP. Figure 13.1 illustrates the physical locations of the variables.

The term *effective lens position* was adopted by the Food and Drug Administration in 1995 to describe the position of the lens in the eye, since the term *anterior chamber depth* is not anatomically accurate for lenses in the posterior chamber and can lead to confusion for the clinician. The ELP for IOLs before 1980 was a constant of 4 mm for every lens in every patient (first-generation theoretical formula). This value worked well in most patients because the majority of lenses implanted were iris clip fixation, in which the principal plane averages approximately 4 mm posterior to the corneal vertex. In 1981, Binkhorst improved the prediction of ELP by using a single-variable predictor, the axial length, as a scaling factor for ELP (second-generation theoretical formula).[3] If the patient's axial length was 10% greater than normal (23.45 mm), he increased the ELP by 10%. The average value of ELP was increased to 4.5 mm because the preferred location of an implant was in the ciliary sulcus, approximately 0.5 mm deeper than the iris plane. Also, most lenses were convex-plano, similar to the shape of the iris-supported lenses. The average ELP in 1996 increased to 5.25 mm. This increased distance occurred primarily for two reasons: the majority of implanted IOLs are biconvex, moving the principal plane of the lens even deeper into the eye, and the desired location for the lens is in the capsular bag, which is 0.25 mm deeper than the ciliary sulcus.

In 1988, we proved[4] that using a two-variable predictor, axial length and keratometry, could significantly improve the prediction of ELP, particularly in unusual eyes (third-generation theoretical formula).

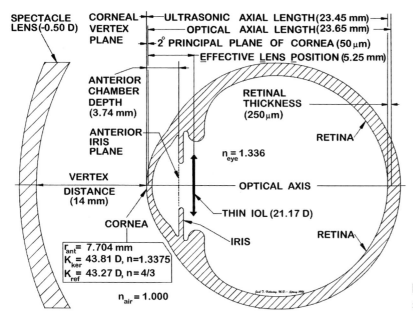

Fig. 13.1. Standardized pseudophakic schematic eye.

The original Holladay 1 formula was based on the geometrical relationships of the anterior segment. Although several investigators have modified the original Holladay two-variable prediction formula, no comprehensive studies have shown any significant improvement using only these two variables.

In 1995, Olsen and collaborators. published a four-variable predictor that used axial length, keratometry, preoperative anterior chamber depth, and lens thickness.[5] Their results did show improvement over the current two-variable prediction formulas. The explanation is very simple. The more information we have about the anterior segment, the better we can predict the ELP. This explanation is a well-known theorem in prediction theory, where the more variables that can be measured in describing an event, the more precisely one can predict the outcome.

In a recent study,[6] Holladay and collaborators discovered that the anterior and posterior segments of the human eye are often not proportional in size, causing significant error in the prediction of the ELP in extremely short eyes (<20 mm). Even in eyes shorter than 20 mm, the anterior segment was completely normal in the majority of cases. Because the axial lengths were so short, the two-variable prediction formulas severely underestimated the ELP, explaining part of the large hyperopic prediction errors with current two-variable prediction formu-

las. After recognizing this problem, Holladay and coworkers began to take additional measurements on extremely short and extremely long eyes to determine if the prediction of ELP could be improved by knowing more about the anterior segment. Table 13.1 shows the clinical conditions that illustrate the independence of the anterior segment and the axial length.

Data was gathered data from 35 investigators around the world. Several additional measurements of the eye were taken, but only seven preoperative variables (axial length, corneal power, horizontal corneal diameter, anterior chamber depth, lens thickness, preoperative refraction, and age) were found to be useful in significantly improving the prediction of ELP in eyes ranging from 15 to 35 mm.

The improved prediction of ELP is not totally due to the formula but is also a function of the technical skills of the surgeons who are consistently implanting the lenses in the capsular bag. A 20 D IOL that is 0.5 mm axially displaced from the predicted ELP will result in approximately a 1.0 D error in the stabilized postoperative refraction. However, when using piggyback lenses totaling 60 D, the same axial displacement of 0.5 mm will cause a 3 D refractive surprise; the error is directly proportional to the power of the implanted lens. This direct relationship to lens power explains why the problem is much less

Table 13.1. Clinical Conditions Demonstrating the Independence of Anterior Segment and Axial Length

Anterior Segment Size	Axial Length		
	Short	**Normal**	**Long**
Small	Small eye Nanophthalmos	Microcornea	Microcornea + axial myopia
Normal	Axial hyperopia	Normal	Axial myopia
Large	Megalocornea + Axial hyperopia	Megalocornea	Large eye Buphthalmos + axial myopia

evident in extremely long eyes, since the implanted IOL is either low plus or minus to achieve emmetropia following cataract extraction.

The Holladay 2 formula and the interim results of the 35 investigators were presented at the annual meeting of the Society of Cataract and Refractive Surgery, June, 1996 in Seattle. A-scan manufacturers and software programs that implement the new formula became available in the fall of 1996. Once these additional measurements become routine among clinicians, a new flurry of prediction formulas using seven or more variables will emerge, similar to the activity following Holladay two-variable prediction formula in 1988.[4] The standard of care will reach a new level of prediction accuracy for extremely unusual eyes, just as it has for normal eyes. Calculations on patients with axial lengths between 22 and 25 mm with corneal powers between 42 and 46 D will do well with current third-generation formulas (Holladay 1,[4] SRK/T,[7] and Hoffer Q[8]). In cases outside this range, the Holladay 2 formula should be used to ensure accuracy.

Normal Cornea with No Previous Keratorefractive Surgery

CLE for High Myopia and Hyperopia

The intraocular power calculations for clear lens extraction (CLE) are no different from the calculations when a cataract is present. The patients are usually much younger, however, and the loss of accommodation should be discussed thoroughly. The actual desired postoperative refraction should also be discussed, since a small degree of myopia (−0.50 D) may be desirable to someone with no accommodation to reduce the dependence on spectacles.

This procedure is usually reserved for patients who are outside the range of other forms of refractive surgery. Consequently, the measurements of axial length, keratometry, etc., are usually quite different from those in the typical cataract patient because of the degree of refractive error. In most cases of high myopia, the axial lengths are extremely long (>26 mm). In cases of high hyperopia, the axial lengths are very short (<21 mm).

In patients with myopia exceeding 20 D, removing the clear lens often results in postoperative refractions near emmetropia with no implant. The exact result depends on the power of the cornea and the axial length. The recommended lens powers usually range from −10 D to + 10 D in the majority of these cases. The correct axial length measurement is very difficult to obtain in these cases because of the abnormal anatomy of the posterior pole. Staphylomas are often present in these eyes, and the macula is often not at the location in the posterior pole where the A-scan measures the axial length. In these cases, it is recommended that a B-scan be performed to locate the macula (fovea) and recheck the measurement determined by the A-scan. There have been 3 to 4 D surprises because the macula was on the edge of the staphyloma, and the A-scan measured to the deepest part of the staphyloma. Such an error results in a hyperopic surprise because the distance to the macula is much less than the distance to the center of the staphyloma. The third-generation theoretical formulas yield excellent results if the axial length measurement is accurate and stable.

In patients with hyperopia exceeding +8 D, axial lengths are often less than 21 mm and require lens powers that exceed the normal range (>34 D). In these cases, piggyback lenses are necessary to achieve emmetropia.[6] The only formula available at this time in these eyes is the Holladay 2. If the required lens power is less than or equal to 34 D, then the piggyback lenses are not required and third-generation theoretical formulas may be used.

Piggyback IOLs to Achieve Powers Above 34 D

In patients with axial lengths shorter than 21 mm, measurements should be calculated using the Holladay 2 Formula. In these cases, the size of the anterior segment is unrelated to the axial length.[6] In many of these cases, the anterior segment is normal in size and only the posterior segment is abnormally short. In a few cases, however, the anterior segment is small in proportion to the axial length (nanophthalmos). The differences in the size of the anterior segment in these cases can cause an average of 5 D hyperopic error with third-generation formulas because they predict the depth of the anterior chamber to be very small. Using the newer formula can reduce the prediction error in these eyes to less than 1 D.

Accurate measurements of axial length and corneal power are especially important in these cases because any error is magnified by the extreme dioptric powers of the IOLs. Placement of both lenses in the bag with the haptics aligned is essential. Inadvertently placing one lens in the bag and the other in the sulcus can cause a 4 D refractive surprise.

Patients with Previous Keratorefractive Surgery

Background

The number of patients who have had keratorefractive surgery (radial keratotomy [RK], photorefractive keratectomy [PRK], or laser-assisted in-situ keratomileusis [LASIK]) has been steadily increasing over the past 20 years. With the advent of the excimer laser, these numbers are predicted to increase dramatically. Determining their corneal power accurately is difficult and usually is the determining factor in the accuracy of the predicted refraction following cataract surgery. Providing this group of patients the same accuracy with IOL power calculations available to our standard cataract patients presents an especially difficult challenge for the clinician.

Preoperative Evaluation

Corneal evaluation   At present, far more patients have had RK than PRK and LASIK combined. Also, our long-term follow-up of RK patients is much greater. The long-term studies of RK patients reveals that some have hyperopic shifts in their refraction and develop progressive against-the-rule astigmatism.[9] The long-term refractive changes in PRK and LASIK are unknown, except for the regression effect following attempted PRK corrections exceeding 8 D. No matter which procedure the patient has had, the stability or instability of the refraction must be determined. This determination includes daily fluctuations from morning to night, as well as long-term changes over the past few years. Each of these factors must be used in determining the desired postoperative target refraction and in preparing the patient for the visual changes and realistic expectations following the procedure.

In all of these cases, biomicroscopy, retinoscopy, corneal topography, and endothelial cell counts are recommended. These first three tests are primarily directed at evaluating the amount of irregular astigmatism. This determination is extremely important preoperatively because the irregular astigmatism may be contributing to the reduced vision as well as to the cataract. The irregular astigmatism may also be the limiting factor in the patient's vision following cataract surgery. The endothelial cell count is necessary to recognize any patients with low cell counts from the previous surgery that may be at higher risk for corneal decompensation or prolonged visual recovery.

The potential acuity meter (PAM), super pinhole, and hard trial contact lens method are often helpful as secondary tests in determining the respective contribution to reduced vision by the cataract and the corneal irregular astigmatism. The patient should also be informed that only the glare from the cataract will be eliminated; any glare from the keratorefractive procedure will essentially remain unchanged.

Methods of determining corneal power   Accurately determining the central corneal refractive power is the most important and most difficult part of the IOL calculation process. The explanation is quite simple. Current instruments for measuring corneal power make too many incorrect assumptions with corneas that have irregular astigmatism. The cornea can no longer be compared to a sphere centrally, the posterior radius of the cornea is no longer 1.2 mm steeper than the anterior corneal radius, and so on. Because of these limitations, the calculated method and the trial hard contact lens method are most accurate, followed by corneal topography, automated keratometry, and finally manual keratometry.

Calculation method For the calculation method, three parameters must be known: the K-readings and refraction before the keratorefractive procedure and the stabilized refraction after the keratorefractive procedure. It is important that the stabilized postoperative refraction be measured before any myopic shifts from nuclear sclerotic cataracts occur. It is also possible for posterior subcapsular cataracts to cause an apparent myopic shift similar to capsular opacification, where the patient wants more minus in the refraction to make the letters appear smaller and darker. The concept we described in 1989 subtracts the change in refraction due to the keratorefractive procedure at the corneal plane from the original K-readings before the procedure to arrive at a calculated postoperative K-reading.[10] This method is usually the most accurate because the preoperative K values and refraction are usually accurate to ± 0.25 D. An example calculation to illustrate the calculation method is as follows:

Mean preoperative K = 42.50 at 90° and 41.50 at 180° = 42.00 D

Preoperative refraction = $-10.00 + 1.00 \times 90°$, vertex = 14 mm

Postoperative refraction = $-0.25 + 1.00 \times 90°$, vertex = 14 mm

Step 1. Calculate the spheroequivalent refraction for refractions at the corneal plane (SEQ_c) from the spheroequivalent refractions at the spectacle plane (SEQ_s) at a given vertex, where
a. SEQ = sphere + 0.5 (cylinder)
b. $SEQ_c = \dfrac{1000}{1000/SEQ_s - \text{Vertex(mm)}}$

Calculation for *preoperative* spheroequivalent refraction at the corneal plane:
a. $SEQ_R = -10.00 + 0.5 \cdot (1.00) = -9.50$ D

b. $SEQ_c = \dfrac{1000}{1000/-9.50 - 14} = -8.38$D

Calculation for *postoperative* spheroequivalent refraction at the corneal plane:
a. $SEQ_R = -0.25 + 0.5 \cdot (1.00) = +0.25$ D
b. $SEQ_c = \dfrac{1000}{1000/+0.25 - 14} = +0.25$ D

Step 2. Calculate the change in refraction at the corneal plane.

Change in refraction = preoperative SEQ_C − postoperative SEQ_C
Change in refraction = $-8.38 - (+.025) = -8.68$ D

Step 3. Determine the calculated postoperative corneal refractive power.

Mean postoperative K = mean preoperative K − change in refraction at corneal plane
Mean postoperative K = 42.00 − 8.68 = 33.32 D

This value is the calculated central power of the cornea following the keratorefractive procedure. For IOL programs requiring two K-readings, this value would be entered twice.

Trial hard contact lens method The trial hard contact lens method requires a plano hard contact lens with a known base curve and a patient whose cataract does not prevent refraction to approximately $\pm$ 0.50 D. This tolerance usually requires a visual acuity of better than 20/80. The patient's spheroequivalent refraction is determined by normal refraction. The refraction is then repeated with the hard contact lens in place. If the spheroequivalent refraction does not change with the contact lens, then the patient's cornea must have the same power as the base curve of the plano contact lens. If the patient has a *myopic shift* in the refraction with the contact lens, then the base curve of the contact lens is *stronger* than the cornea by the amount of the shift. If there is a *hyperopic shift* in the refraction with the contact lens, then the base curve of the contact lens is *weaker* than the cornea by the amount of the shift.

In the following example, the patient has a current spheroequivalent refraction of +0.25 D. With a plano hard contact lens with a base curve of 35.00 D placed on the cornea, the spherical refraction changes to −2.00 D. Since the patient had a myopic shift with the contact lens, the cornea must be weaker than the base curve of the contact by 2.25 D. Therefore, the cornea must be 32.75 D (35.00 − 2.25), which is slightly different than the value obtained by the calculation method. In equation form, we have the following:

SEQ refraction *without* hard contact lens = +0.25 D

Base curve of plano hard contact lens = 35.00 D

SEQ refraction *with* hard contact lens = −2.00 D

Change in refraction = −2.00 − (+0.25) = −2.25 D (myopic shift)

Mean corneal power =
base curve of plano HCL + change in refraction

= 35.00 + −2.25

= 32.75 D

Note that this method is limited by the accuracy of the refractions which may be limited by the cataract.

Corneal topography   Current corneal topography units measure more than 5000 points over the entire cornea and more than 1000 points within the central 3 mm. This additional information provides greater accuracy in determining the power of corneas with irregular astigmatism compared to keratometers. The computer in topography units allows the measurement to account for the Stiles-Crawford effect, actual pupil size, and so on. These algorithms allow very accurate determination of the *anterior* surface of the cornea.[11] They provide no information, however, about the posterior surface of the cornea. In order to determine the total power of the cornea accurately, the power of both surfaces must be known.

In normal corneas that have not undergone keratorefractive surgery, the posterior radius of curvature of the cornea averages 1.2 mm less than the anterior surface. In a person with an anterior corneal radius of 7.5 mm using the Standardized Keratometric Index of Refraction of 1.3375, the corneal power would be 45.00 D. Several studies have shown that this power overestimates the total power of the cornea by approximately 0.56 D. Hence, most IOL calculations today used a net index of refraction of 1.3333 (4/3) and the anterior

radius of the cornea to calculate the net power of the cornea. Using this lower value, the total power of a cornea with an anterior radius of 7.5 mm would be 44.44 D. This index of refraction has provided excellent results in normal corneas for IOL calculations.

Following keratorefractive surgery, the assumptions that the central cornea can be approximated by a sphere (no significant irregular astigmatism or asphericity) and that the posterior corneal radius of curvature is 1.2 mm less than the anterior radius are no longer true. Corneal topography instruments can account for the changes in the anterior surface but are unable to account for any differences in the relationship to the posterior radius of curvature. In RK, the mechanism of having a peripheral bulge and central flattening apparently causes similar changes in both the anterior and posterior radius of curvature, so that using the net index of refraction for the cornea (4/3) usually gives fairly accurate results, particularly for optical zones larger than 4 to 5 mm. In RKs with optical zones of 3 mm or less, the accuracy of the predicted corneal power diminishes. Whether this inaccuracy is due to the additional central irregularity with small optical zones or to the difference in the relationship between the front and back radii of the cornea is unknown. Studies measuring the posterior radius of the cornea in these patients will be necessary to answer this question.

In PRK and LASIK, the inaccuracy of these instruments in measuring the net corneal power is almost entirely due to the change in the relationship of the radii of the front and back of the cornea, since the irregular astigmatism in the central 3-mm zone is usually minimal. In these two procedures, the anterior surface of the cornea is flattened, with little or no effect on the posterior radius. Using a net index of refraction (4/3) will overestimate the power of cornea by 14% of the change induced by the PRK or LASIK, i.e., if patient had a 7 D change in the refraction at the corneal plane from a PRK or LASIK procedure with a spherical preoperative *K* value of 44 D, the actual power of the cornea is 37 D and the topography units will give 38 D. If a 14 D change in the refraction has occurred at the corneal plane, the topography units will overestimate the power of the cornea by 2 D.

In summary, the corneal topography units do not provide accurate central corneal power following

PRK, LASIK, and in RKs with optical zones of 3 mm or less. In RKs with larger optical zones, the topography units become more reliable. The calculation method and hard contact lens trial are always more reliable.

Automated keratometry Automated keratometers are usually more accurate than manual keratometers in corneas with small optical zone ($\leq$ 3 mm) RKs because they sample a smaller central area of the cornea (nominally 2.6 mm). In addition, the automated instruments often have additional eccentric fixation targets that provide more information about the paracentral cornea. When a measurement error on an RK cornea is made, the instrument almost always gives a central corneal power that is greater than the true refractive power of the cornea. This error occurs because the samples at 2.6 mm are very close to the paracentral knee of the RK. The smaller the optical zone and the greater the number of RK incisions, the greater the probability and magnitude of the error. Most of the automated instruments have reliability factors that are given for each measurement, helping the clinician determine the reliability in the measurement.

Automated keratometry measurements following LASIK or PRK yield accurate measurements of the front radius of the cornea because the transition areas are far outside the 2.6-mm zone that is measured. The measurements are still not accurate, however, because the assumed *net* index of refraction (4/3) is no longer appropriate for the new relationship of the front and back radii of the cornea after PRK or LASIK, just as with the topographic instruments. The *change* in central corneal power, as measured by the keratometer from PRK or LASIK, must be increased by 14% to determine the actual refractive change at the plane of the cornea. Hence, the automated keratometer will overestimate the power of the cornea proportional to the amount of PRK or LASIK performed.

Manual keratometry Manual keratometers are the least accurate in measuring central corneal power following keratorefractive procedures because the area that they measure is usually larger than automated at 3.2 mm in diameter. Therefore, measurements in this area are extremely unreliable for RK corneas with optical zones $\leq$ 4 mm. The one

advantage of the manual keratometer is that the examiner is able to see the reflected mires and the amount of irregularity present. Seeing the mires does not help achieve a better measurement, but it does allow the observer to discount the measurement as unreliable.

The manual keratometer has the same problem with PRK and LASIK as topographers and automated keratometers and is therefore no less accurate. The manual keratometer overestimates the change in the central refractive power of the cornea by 14% following PRK and LASIK.

Choosing the Desired Postoperative Refraction Target Determining the desired postoperative refractive target is no different than in other patients with cataracts in which the refractive status and the presence of a cataract in the other eye are the major determining factors. A complete discussion of avoiding refractive problems with cataract surgery is beyond the scope of this text and is thoroughly covered in the reference given.[12] A short discussion of the major factors follows.

If the patient has *binocular cataracts,* the decision is much easier because the refractive status of both eyes can be changed. The most important decision is whether the patient prefers to be myopic and read without glasses or nearly emmetropic and drive without glasses. In some cases, the surgeon and patient may choose an intermediate distance (-1.00 D) as the best compromise. Targeting for monovision is certainly acceptable, provided the patient has successfully utilized monovision in the past. Trying to produce monovision in a patient who has never experienced this condition may cause intolerable anisometropia and require further surgery.

Monocular cataracts allow fewer choices for the desired postoperative refraction because the refractive status of the other eye is fixed. The general rule is that the operative eye must be within 2 D of the nonoperative eye in order to avoid intolerable anisometropia. In most cases this means matching the other eye or targeting for up to 2 D nearer emmetropia. For example, if the nonoperative eye is -5.00 D, then the target would be -3.00 D for the operative eye. If the patient is successfully wearing a contact lens in the nonoperative eye or has already demonstrated the ability to accept monovision, then an exception can be made to the general rule. It should always be stressed, however, that should the patient be unable to continue wearing a contact lens, the necessary glasses for binocular correction may be intolerable and additional refractive surgery may be required.

Special Limitations of IOL Power Calculation Formulas As discussed previously, the third-generation formulas (Holladay 1, Hoffer Q, and the SRK/T) and the new Holladay 2 are much more accurate than previous formulas the more unusual the eye. Older formulas such as the SRK1, SRK2, and Binkhorst 1 should not be used in these cases. None of these formulas will give the desired result if the central corneal power is measured incorrectly. The resulting errors are almost always in the hyperopic direction following keratorefractive surgery because the measured corneal powers are usually greater than the true refractive power of the cornea.

To further complicate matters, the newer formulas often use keratometry as one of the predictors to estimate the effective lens position (*ELP*) of the IOL. In patients who have had keratorefractive surgery, the corneal power is usually much flatter than normal and certainly flatter than before the keratorefractive procedure. In short, a patient with a 38 D cornea without keratorefractive surgery would not be expected to be similar to a patient with a 38 D cornea with keratorefractive surgery. Newer IOL calculation programs are now being developed to handle these situations and will improve our predictability in these cases.

Intraoperative Evaluation
Intraoperative Visualization and Corneal Protection Intraoperative visualization is usually more difficult in the patient with previous RK than in the normal cataract patient and is somewhat similar to severe arcus senilis or other conditions that cause peripheral corneal haze. The surgeon should be prepared for this additional difficulty by making sure that the patient is lined up to visualize the cataract through the optical zone. This usually means lining the microscope perpendicular to the center of the cornea so that the surgeon is looking directly through the optical zone at the center of the cataract. When removing the peripheral cortex, the eye can be rotated so that visualization of the periphery is through the central optical zone. It is also prudent to coat the endothelium with viscoelastic to

minimize any endothelial cell loss, since the keratorefractive procedure may have caused some prior loss.

Intraoperative Autorefractor/Retinoscopy Large refractive surprises can be avoided by using intraoperative retinoscopy or hand-held autorefractors. These refractions should not be relied on, however, for fine tuning the IOL power, since there are many factors at surgery that may change in the postoperative period. Factors such as the pressure from the lid speculum, axial position of the IOL, intraocular pressure, and so on may cause the intraoperative refraction to be different than the final stabilized postoperative refraction. If the intraoperative refraction is within 2 D of the target refraction, no lens exchanges should be considered unless intraoperative keratometry can also be performed.

Postoperative Evaluation
Refraction on the first postoperative day On the first day after cataract surgery, patients who previously have had RK usually have a hyperopic shift similar to that occurring on the first postoperative day following the RK. This phenomenon is primarily due to the transient corneal edema that usually exaggerates the RK effect. These patients also exhibit the same daily fluctuations during the early postoperative period after their cataract surgery as they did after the RK. Usually this daily shift is in a myopic direction during the day due to the regression of corneal edema after awakening in the morning.[13] Because the refractive changes are expected and vary significantly among patients, no lens exchange should be contemplated until after the first postoperative week or until after the refraction has stabilized, whichever is longer.

Very few results of cataract surgery following PRK and LASIK are available. In the few cases operations have been performed, the hyperopic shift on the first day and daily fluctuations appear to be much less, similar to those occurring in the early postoperative period following these procedures. In most cases, the stability of the cornea makes these cases no different than those of patients that have not had keratorefractive surgery.

Long-term results Long-term results of cataract surgery following RK are very good. The long-term hyperopic shifts and development of against-the-

---

rule astigmatism over time following cataract surgery should be the same as in the long-term studies following RK. The problems with glare and starburst patterns are usually minimal because the patient has had to adjust to these unwanted optical images following the initial RK. If the patient's primary complaints before cataract surgery are glare and starbursts, it should be made clear that only the glare due to the cataract will be removed by surgery. The symptoms due to the RK will remain unchanged.

Long-term results following PRK and LASIK are nonexistent. Since there are no signs of hyperopic drifts or development of against-the-rule astigmatism in the 5-year studies following PRK, one would not expect to see these changes. However, the early studies following RK did not suggest any of these long-term changes either. Only time will tell whether central haze, irregular astigmatism, or other problems will develop in the future.

IOL CALCULATIONS USING *K* VALUES AND PREOPERATIVE REFRACTION

Formula and Rationale for Using Preoperative Refraction vs. Axial Length

In a standard cataract removal with IOL implantation, the preoperative refraction is not very helpful in calculating the power of the implant because the crystalline lens will be removed, so dioptric power is being removed and then replaced. In cases where no power is being removed from the eye, such as a secondary implant in aphakia, piggyback IOL in pseudophakia, or a minus IOL in the anterior chamber of a phakic patient, the necessary IOL power for a desired postoperative refraction can be calculated from the corneal power and preoperative refraction—the axial length is not necessary. The formula for calculating the necessary IOL power is as follows:[14]

$$IOL = \frac{1336}{\dfrac{1336}{\dfrac{1000}{\dfrac{1000}{PreRx} - V} + K} - ELP} - \frac{1336}{\dfrac{1336}{\dfrac{1000}{\dfrac{1000}{DPostRx} - V} + K} - ELP}$$

where *ELP* = expected lens position in millimeters (distance from the corneal vertex to the principal

plane of intraocular lens), *IOL* = intraocular lens power in diopters, *K* = net corneal power in diopters, *PreRx* = preoperative refraction in diopters, *DPostRx* = desired postoperative refraction in diopters, and *V* = vertex distance in millimeters of refraction.

Cases Involving Calculation from Preoperative Refraction

As mentioned above, the appropriate cases for using preoperative refraction and corneal power include (1) secondary implant in aphakia, (2) secondary piggyback IOL in pseudophakia, and (3) a minus anterior chamber IOL in a highly myopic phakic patient. In each of these cases, no dioptric power is being removed from the eye, so the problem is simply to find the IOL at a given distance behind the cornea *ELP* that is equivalent to the spectacle lens at a given vertex distance in front of the cornea. If emmetropia is not desired, then an additional term, the desired postoperative refraction (*DPostRx*), must be included. The formulas for calculating the predicted refraction and the back-calculation of the effective lens position *ELP* are given in the reference and will not be repeated here.[14]

Example: Secondary Implant for Aphakia

The patient is 72 years old, and is aphakic in the right eye and pseudophakic in the left eye. The right eye can no longer tolerate an aphakic contact lens. The capsule in the right eye is intact, and a posterior chamber IOL is desired. The patient is −0.50 D in the left eye and would like to be the same in the right eye.

Mean keratometric *K* = 45.00 D
Aphakic refraction = +12.00 sphere at vertex of 14 mm
Manufacturer's anterior chamber depth (ACD) lens constant = 5.25 mm
Desired postoperative refraction = −0.50 D

Each of these values can be substituted in the refraction formula above except for the manufacturer's ACD and the measured *K*-reading. The labeled values on IOL boxes are primarily for lenses implanted in the bag. Since this lens is intended for the sulcus, 0.25 mm should be subtracted from 5.25 mm to arrive at the equivalent constant for the sulcus. The *ELP* is therefore 5.00 mm. The *K*-reading must be converted from the measured keratometric *K*-reading (n = 1.3375) to the net *K*-reading (n = 4/3) for the reasons described previously in the discussion of corneal topography. The conversion is performed by multiplying the measured *K*-reading by the following fraction:

$$\text{Fraction} = \frac{(4/3) - 1}{1.3375 - 1} = \frac{1/3}{0.3375} = 0.98765$$

Mean refractive *K* = mean keratometric
K · fraction
Mean refractive *K* = 45.00 · 0.98765 = 44.44 D

Using the mean refractive *K*, aphakic refraction, vertex distance, *ELP* for the sulcus, and the desired postoperative refraction, the patient needs a 22.90 D IOL. A 23 D IOL would yield a predicted refraction of −0.57 D.[14]

Example: Secondary Piggy-Back IOL for Pseudophakia

In patients with a significant residual refractive error following the primary IOL implant, it is often easier surgically and more predictable optically to leave the primary implant in place and calculate the secondary piggyback IOL power to achieve the desired refraction. This method does not require knowledge of the power of the primary implant or the axial length. The method is particularly important in cases where the primary implant is thought to be mislabeled. The formula works for plus or minus lenses, but negative lenses are just now becoming available.

The patient is 55 years old, had a refractive surprise after the primary cataract surgery, and was left with a +5.00 D spherical refraction in the right eye. There is no cataract in the left eye, and he is plano. The surgeon and the patient both desire him to be −0.50 D, which was the target for the primary implant. The refractive surprise is believed to be due to a mislabeled IOL, which is centered in the bag and would be very difficult to remove. The secondary piggyback IOL will be placed in the sulcus. This is very important, since trying to place the second lens in the bag several weeks after the primary surgery is very difficult. More important, it may displace the primary lens posteriorly, reducing its effective power and leaving the patient with a hyper-

opic error. Placing the lens in the sulcus minimizes this posterior displacement.

Mean keratometric *K* = 45.00 D
Pseudophakik refraction = +5.00 sphere at a vertex of 14 mm
Manufacturer's ACD lens constant = 5.25 mm
Desired postoperative refraction = −0.50 D

Using the same style of lens and constant as in the previous example and modifying the *K*-reading to net power, the formula yields a +8.64 D IOL for a −0.50 D target. The nearest available lens is +9.0 D, which would result in −0.76 D. In these cases, extreme care should be taken to ensure that the two lenses are well centered with respect to one another. Decentration of either lens can result in poor image quality and can be the limiting factor in the patient's vision.

Example: Primary Minus Anterior Chamber IOL in a Phakic Patient with High Myopia

The calculation of a minus IOL in the anterior chamber is no different than the aphakic calculation of an anterior chamber lens, except that the power of the lens is negative. In the past, these lenses were reserved for high myopia that could not be corrected by RK or PRK. Since most of these lenses fixate in the anterior chamber angle, iritis and glaucoma are concerns. Nevertheless, several successful procedures have been performed with good refractive results. Because successful LASIK procedures have been performed in myopias of up to −20.00 D, these lenses may be reserved for myopia exceeding this power in the future. Interestingly, the power of the negative anterior chamber implant is very close to the spectacle refraction for normal vertex distances.

Mean keratometric *K* = 45.00 D
Phakic refraction = −20.00 sphere at a vertex of 14 mm
Manufacturer's ACD lens constant = 3.50 mm
Desired postoperative refraction = −0.50 D

Using an *ELP* of 3.50 and modifying the *K*-reading to net corneal power yields a −18.49 D for a desired refraction of −0.50 D. If a −19.00 D lens is used, the patient will have a predicted postoperative refraction of −0.10 D.

REFERENCES

1. Fedorov SN, Kolina AI, Kolinko AI. Estimation of optical power of the intraocular lens. *Vestnk Oftalmol.* 1967;80(4):27–31.

2. Fritz KJ. Intraocular lens power formulas. *Am J Ophthalmol.* 1981;91:414–415.

3. Binkhorst RD. *Intraocular Lens Power Calculation Manual. A Guide to the Author's TI 58/59 IOL Power Module*, 2nd ed. New York: Richard D Binkhorst; 1981.

4. Holladay JT, Prager TC, Chandler TY, Musgrove KH, Lewis JW, Ruiz RS. A three-part system for refining intraocular lens power calculations. *J Cataract Refract Surg.* 1988;14:17–24.

5. Olsen T, Corydon L, Gimbel H. Intraocular lens power calculation with an improved anterior chamber depth prediction algorithm. *J Cataract Refract Surg.* 1995;21:313–319.

6. Holladay JT, Gills JP, Leidlein J, Cherchio M. Achieving emmetropia in extremely short eyes with two piggy-back posterior chamber intraocular lenses. *Ophthalmology.* 1996;103:1118–1123.

7. Retzlaff JA, Sanders DR, Kraff MC. Development of the SRK/T intraocular lens implant power calculation formula. *J Cataract Refract Surg.* 1990;16:333–340.

8. Hoffer KJ. The Hoffer Q formula: a comparison of theoretic and regression formulas. *J Cataract Refract Surg.* 1993;19:700–712.

9. Holladay JT, Lynn M, Waring GO, Gemmill M, Keehn GC, Fielding B. The relationship of visual acuity, refractive error and pupil size after radial keratotomy. *Arch Ophthalmol.* 1991;109:70–76.

10. Holladay JT. IOL calculations following RK. *Refract Corneal Surg J.* 1989;5:203.

11. Lowe RF, Clark BA. Posterior corneal curvature. *Br J Ophthalmol.* 1973;57:464–470.

12. Holladay JT, Rubin ML. Avoiding refractive problems in cataract surgery. *Survey Ophthalmol.* 1988; 32:357–360.

13. Holladay JT. Management of hyperopic shift after RK. *Refract Corneal Surg J.* 1992;8:325.

14. Holladay JT. Refractive power calculations for intraocular lenses in the phakic eye. *Am J Ophthalmol.* 1993;116:63–66.

14

Astigmatic Keratotomy

Vance Thompson

INTRODUCTION

Astigmatism was first corrected optically by Airy in 1827.[1] Donders later described the cylindrical correction of astigmatism in his well-known treatise.[2] The first attempts to describe and perform the surgical correction of astigmatism came in the second half of the 1800s by such notables as Snellen, Bates and others.[3,4] As an ophthalmology student, Lans performed animal experiments documenting that transverse corneal incisions could flatten the steep axis of astigmatism and that heating the cornea (today known as *thermokeratoplasty*) could steepen the flat axis.[5]

Today's refractive surgeon must keep these well-described basic principles in mind. Also, when planning a refractive surgery, the surgeon needs to keep in mind not only the astigmatic correction but also how it will affect, or not affect, the spherical equivalent component of the refractive error. Thus, astigmatic surgery has become much more than astigmatic keratotomy. This chapter will review current thoughts on correcting congenital (and refractive surgery–induced) astigmatism, with constant attention to how the patient's overall spherical equivalent will be affected.

PREOPERATIVE EVALUATION WHEN CONSIDERING ASTIGMATIC SURGERY

The workup starts with the nurse or technician taking a brief history and documenting the patient's goals and expectations. A medication review, both systemic and ocular, is performed, and the patient's allergies and medical problems are discussed. Particular emphasis is placed on making sure that there are no medical problems that would impair wound healing, such as collagen vascular disease or uncontrolled diabetes.

Visual acuity with and without current correction is determined. The dominant eye is tested, and the results are documented. In general, the nondominant eye is operated on first. The keratometer, invented by Helmholtz in 1856, is still a widely used instrument in refractive surgery and an important part of any refractive surgery evaluation.[6] The numbers defined as the steep and flat axes of cylinder are important, along with a qualitative assessment of the keratometric mires to help rule out irregular astigmatism. Corneal topography is the mainstay of any astigmatic (or any other refractive procedure) workup and is utilized for a number of reasons. First, corneal topography is helpful in assessing the anterior corneal curvature for any evidence of irregular astigmatism.[7] The main pathological topographic abnormality that must be ruled out is keratoconus. Clinical forms (i.e., reduced best corrected vision or abnormal keratometer readings) of keratoconus are not difficult to recognize, and the surgeon should recommend that the patient not have refractive surgery. But preclinical forms of keratoconus (so-called forme fruste keratoconus) may be undetected on routine exam (20/20 best corrected vision, normal keratometry, normal slit lamp exam) and can produce an unusual refractive surgical result[8] (Fig. 14.1). The author recommends that patients with preclinical keratoconus not undergo refractive surgery because of the risk of unpredictable results.

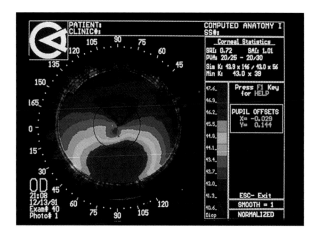

Fig. 14.1. This patient has 20/20 spectacle-corrected vision, normal central keratometry, and a normal slit lamp exam. Computed topography shows inferior temporal steepening consistent with preclinical keratoconus.

The majority of decisions made in astigmatic surgery are based on the manifest refraction. Soft contact lens wearers need to refrain from using lenses for at least 3 days before one can rely on the manifest refraction results. Gas-permeable, or hard, contact lens wearers should avoid using lenses for at least 2 weeks. For any patient, stability (both refractive and topographic) needs to be documented. In a rigid contact lens wearer, stability can be defined as two refractions at least a week apart that are not changing. Typically, rigid contact lens wearers are not told to remove their lenses prior to their initial consultation. If they are good candidates with appropriate expectations, they are asked to leave off their lenses for 2½ weeks prior to their scheduled surgery date. The manifest refraction is checked 1 week after the lenses are out and again a couple of days before surgery. If it is stable (i.e., less than 0.5 D change in power and less than 5° change in axis), the procedure is performed on the scheduled date. If the refraction has changed by more than these parameters, the procedure is postponed another week (or until the refraction stabilizes). In some patients, gas-permeable contact lenses need to be kept off the cornea for up to 6 weeks before surgery can be performed because of changing refraction. Allowing the refraction to stabilize is just as important in astigmatic surgery as in any other form of refractive surgery.

Cycloplegic refraction should be determined in all patients considering refractive surgery. This is taken into account when making decisions on surgical correction of the spherical component of the refraction. The astigmatic correction is based on the manifest refraction which has been refined, both power and axis, with a Jackson cross cylinder. Consideration is also given to topography when choosing the axis of astigmatic correction. In general, decisions are based on the manifest refraction for astigmatic axis correction, but if the refractive axis and the topographic axis differ by more than 10°, the topographic axis is favored.

Thorough slit lamp and funduscopic exams are performed on all patients. Tests such as the Schirmer test and corneal sensitivity determination are not routinely performed unless clinically indicated.

DISCUSSION BEFORE ASTIGMATIC SURGERY

Following thorough refractive, topographic, and eye health exams, a discussion on alternatives, risks, and expectations occurs. Optical alternatives, namely glasses and/or contact lenses, should be a part of every discussion about a refractive procedure. Surgical options for correcting astigmatism depend largely on the spherical equivalent component of the refraction. For example, a patient with astigmatism combined with mild to moderate myopia should have a choice between radial keratotomy (RK) combined with astigmatic keratotomy (AK), excimer laser photorefractive keratectomy (PRK) combined with AK, or a toric PRK correction of both myopia and astigmatism. A patient with astigmatism combined with hyperopia would be given options such as AK combined with a soft contact lens after complete healing, holmium laser thermokeratoplasty (LTK), hyperopic PRK with potential toric ablation of the astigmatic component, or AK with a refractive intraocular lens. During a discussion of options, it is acceptable for the surgeon to be candid about his or her opinion on the best options for that particular case. It is imperative that options (and their inherent risks) be discussed and documented to achieve proper informed consent.

Probably one of the most important matters to discuss preoperatively is the patient's expectations.

These expectations are often greater than the results that can be achieved. It is a rare patient who is unwilling to accept the limitations of astigmatism-reducing surgery as long as he or she is well informed and educated. It is important to explain to patients that this is one of the more unpredictable areas of refractive surgery, that undercorrection is the goal and that enhancement surgery may be needed. The time frame is also important to discuss, since this varies with the procedure. Additional incisional astigmatic corneal surgery should not be performed until the first procedure has taken nearly full affect and stabilized. This may take a month or two. For toric PRK procedures there can be changes up to a year postoperatively. Toric PRKs should not be enhanced until they have stabilized, which is at least 6 months postoperatively and typically longer. AKs combined with PRK should usually not be enhanced before 6 months postoperatively. Occasionally, the AK can be enhanced sooner if the time is more than 4 months postoperatively and the astigmatism axis is unchanged. But if the astigmatism axis has shifted after PRK/AK, a stable refraction that is at least 6 months old (and preferably longer) should be obtained. These are issues that the patient should not encounter for the first time in the postoperative period when vision is blurry and the patient asks about it. These situations are easily handled if these matters are discussed preoperatively.

OPTIONS FOR CORRECTING ASTIGMATISM

Modern refractive surgery offers many options for astigmatic correction. The main differentiating feature when deciding which procedure is best for which refractive error is the spherical equivalent. The options offered to an astigmatic patient with a plano spherical equivalent are different from those offered to a patient with a myopic spherical equivalent. The options for a patient with a hyperopic spherical equivalent with astigmatism are different from either of the other two. So it is always important to consider the spherical equivalent when considering the best approach to astigmatic correction.

ASTIGMATIC KERATOTOMY

The most common method for correcting astigmatism is AK. The goal of AK is to flatten the steep

cylinder axis. In general, this flattening is accompanied by a steepening of the flat axis. This process (relating the amount of flattening of the steep axis to the amount of steeping of the flat axis) is known as *coupling*.[9]

When evaluating AK nomograms, the surgeon needs to decide whether to utilize straight transverse incisions or arcuate incisions.[10] This decision is not critical when correcting small degrees of cylinder. In general, you can consider a 2-mm straight transverse incision equal to a 30° arcuate keratotomy. A 3-mm straight transverse incision is considered equal to a 45° arcuate keratotomy. For longer straight transverse corneal incisions, the similarities to arcuate corneal incisions begin to lessen.

It is important to understand that transverse corneal incisions made perpendicular to the visual axis will increase the circumference of the globe in that axis selectively (thus flattening only that axis). By contrast, a radial incision made in the cornea will increase the circumference of the whole peripheral corneal, accompanied by a flattening of the whole central corneal (i.e., a hyperopic shift in the spherical equivalent). So as long as an AK is made perpendicular to the visual axis (at all of its points), it should not change the overall flattening of the cornea and thus should not change the spherical equivalent.[11]

When considering long, straight, transverse corneal incisions, one needs to consider the distance from the incision to the center of the visual axis. In Fig. 14.2A, note that the distance from the center of the long, straight, transverse corneal incision to the center of the visual axis is less than the distance from the distal aspects of the incision to the center of the visual axis. Thus the whole incision is not perpendicular to the center of the visual axis. Since the outer aspects of these long transverse incisions are farther from the central cornea, they begin to exert some radial influences. In other words, long, straight, transverse incisions can flatten the overall corneal curvature (because of the radial influences occurring at the outer aspects of the incision) and thus cause a hyperopic shift. Unfortunately, one cannot always predict how much of a shift will occur. The amount of overall corneal flattening (i.e., hyperopic shift) that occurs when one attempts to correct large amounts of cylinder with straight transverse incisions can be quite variable.[12]

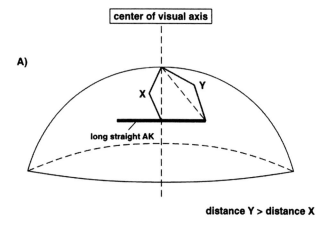

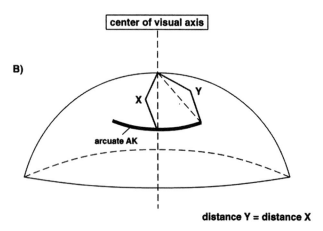

Fig. 14.2. (*A*) In a long, straight, transverse keratotomy, the distance from the center of the incision to the center of the visual axis is less than the distance from the outer aspects of the incision to the same center. (*B*) In an arcuate keratotomy, which follows the circumference of the cornea, all aspects of the incision are the same distance from the center of the pupil.

For this reason, the author favors arcuate keratotomy for the incisional approach to astigmatic correction. It does not matter how long the incisions are because all aspects of the incision will always be perpendicular to (and thus the same distance from) the center of the cornea (Fig. 14.2B). Thus all the influences will be on flattening the steep axis, and there will be no change in the spherical equivalent because there no radial influences are exerted. The surgeon needs to be wary because even an arcuate keratotomy can change the overall spherical equivalent somewhat, since the human hand does not always make a perfect arc with the incision. Usually the spherical equivalent will not change much; if it does, it will usually involve far less of a change in spherical equivalent compared to the change produced by long, straight, transverse incisions. This is why the best candidates for AK correction of astigmatism also have a myopic spherical equivalent. For small amounts of myopia in association with astigmatism, the astigmatic surgery may be all the patient needs, since the result will probably be a mild flattening effect of the overall cornea. In these patients (i.e., those with astigmatism and mild myopia), it is prudent to do the AK and observe any changes in the myopic component of the refraction before deciding whether or not to perform any myopia-reducing surgery. For more significant myopia, the patient may benefit from RK or excimer laser PRK in combination with the astigmatism-reducing surgery. The nomogram that the author utilizes for AK (see below) works for astigmatism in many different settings (i.e., AK alone or in combination with RK or PRK).

Another important factor when considering AK is the distance it will be from the center of the pupil. It is important to keep in mind that the optical zone size is a diameter measurement which is twice the distance of the distance of the incision from the center of the pupil (which is a radius measurement). For example, if an AK incision is placed at a 5.0 mm optical zone, it is only 2.5 mm from the center of the pupil. Two immediate concerns arise when placing AK incisions at small optical zones. First, there is always a zone of irregularity around any incision made in the cornea[13] (Fig. 14.3). If this zone gets too close to the pupil, irregular astigmatism can result in vision of poor quality. These symptoms can be even more pronounced in low light conditions such as nighttime (i.e., when the entrance pupil is more dilated). The other consideration when performing AK is to remember that there is always the risk of overcorrecting the cylinder, resulting in excessive flattening in the axis of the AK. If this occurs and the patient chooses to have the overcorrection repaired, a compression suture (to steepen the excessively flattened axis) is an option. If the original AK is at a 5-mm optical zone (again, only

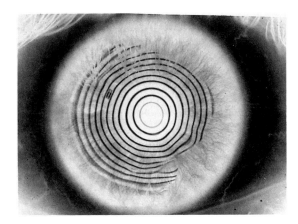

Fig. 14.3. Photokeratoscopic view of astigmatic keratotomy incisions (one inferonasal and the other superotemporal) 1 year postoperatively showing the zone of irregular astigmatism around them.

2.5 mm from the center of the cornea), the compression suture will be dangerously close the center of the visual axis. The suture can then become a source of bothersome visual symptoms. This situation is best avoided.

For this reason, it is preferable to perform all incisional astigmatism work at a large optical zone. Typically, the arcuate keratotomy is placed at a 7-mm optical zone. This provides a safe distance from the center of the pupil to the incision itself, not allowing any incisional irregular astigmatism to affect the quality of vision. It also keeps the incision a safe distance from the pupil in case a compression suture needs to be placed. Finally, it keeps the AK out of the zone of a 6.5-mm or smaller PRK.

Surgical Planning: The Arc-T Nomogram

As with any incisional corneal procedure, an accurate nomogram is of the utmost importance when performing AK. A quality nomogram should allow for two variables: the amount of intended astigmatic correction and the age of the patient.

Lindstrom was one of the first investigators to study and report the effect of age as a variable (i.e., increasing surgical effect from equal-length AKs with increasing age).[14] His studies led to the development of the arc-T nomogram.[15] Others refined this nomogram subsequently.[16] It is a relatively accurate nomogram based on a philosophy of arcuate corneal incisions placed at a large optical zone

of 7 mm. No astigmatism nomogram will ever be perfect because of patient-to-patient variables. Whatever nomogram is utilized, it is prudent to aim for undercorrection. One study found that by following the original arc-T nomogram, the median error in prediction was 0.25 D of undercorrection and 64% of eyes were undercorrected. This study also found that male patients achieved significantly more correction than female patients. These results led to a revision of the arc-T nomogram and to improvement in the accuracy of astigmatism-reducing surgery.[16] Even with improvements in nomograms, however, a titratable philosophy is as important in AK as in any refractive procedure because of the variable responses among patients. Patients also take comfort in the idea that their surgeon's philosophy is that it is better to enhance an undercorrection than back up an overcorrection.

Surgical Technique

Preparation for performing AK includes having the preoperative plan and corneal topography posted in the operating area within easy view. It is helpful to have the topography available so that it can serve as a double check to make sure that the astigmatic work is performed in the correct axis. Preoperatively, the patient receives 3 drops each of topical anesthesia and antibiotic. Prior to positioning the patient under the microscope, it is helpful to place a reference mark at the limbus of the operative eye with the patient in the upright position (Fig. 14.4). This mark is useful because when the patient lies down, ocular torsion can occur and lead to an inaccurate placement of the AK (since the goal is to correct the axis of cylinder when the patient is in the upright position).[17] After the patient is positioned under the microscope, the nonoperative eye is patched so that the patient knows which eye to fixate with. A lid speculum is placed while the patient is fixating on the fixation light. A Mendez ruler is positioned so that the 90° axis marker lines up with the 6:00 mark at the inferior limbus (Fig. 14.5). An arc-T marker is then utilized to place guiding marks in the steep axis of astigmatism (Fig. 14.6). Sterile dye can be used on AK marks for visualization. A drop of topical anesthetic is then put on the cornea to rinse off any excess dye, since it can cause keratitis postoperatively and be a source of tenderness and light sensitivity. The impression or mark left on

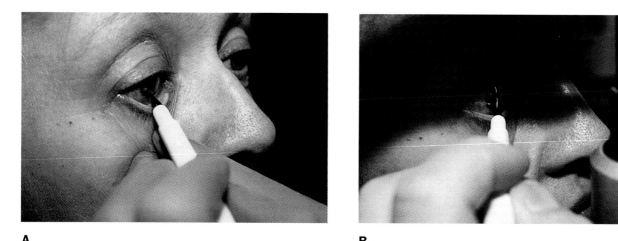

A   **B**

Fig. 14.4. (*A*) A reference mark can be made at the 6:00 position with a sterile marking pen to ensure accurate orientation of the 90° axis when the patient lies down. (*B*) This mark can also be placed by utilizing the slit lamp as a guide to mark the 6:00 position.

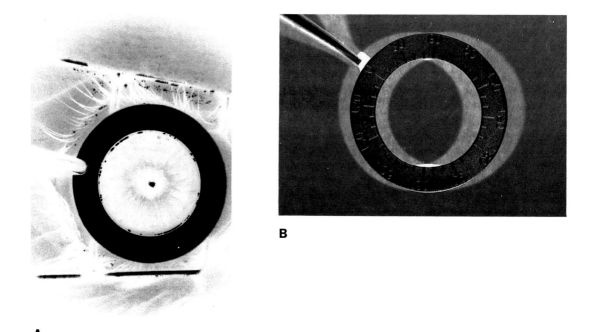

B

A

Fig. 14.5. (*A*) A Mendez ruler is positioned so that 90° lines up with the mark made at the limbus at the 6:00 position. (*B*) Due to glare from the microscope light, which obscures details, a Mendez ruler's axis degrees are shown.

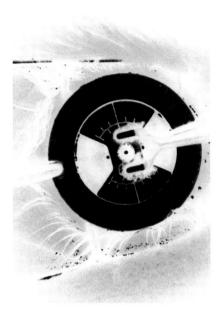

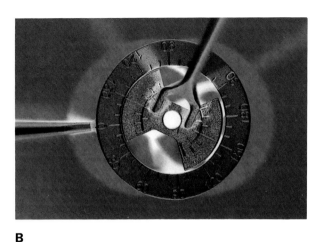

B

A

Fig. 14.6. (*A*) The arc-T marker is lined up in the steep axis of astigmatism, and a mark is made to guide the procedure. (*B*) Due to glare from the microscope light, which obscures details, a Mendez ruler with an arc-T marker is shown for detail.

the corneal surface by the arc-T marker (Fig. 14.7) provides a template from which the exact degrees of arcuate keratotomy can be determined based on the preoperative nomogram decision (Fig. 14.8). The arc-T marker places the marks at the 7-mm optical zone.

After making the markings for AK placement, the corneal thickness is measured. This should be performed at the incision site (Fig. 14.9). The diamond blade is set at .01 mm less than the pachymetry measurement (e.g., a thickness of 566 μm and a diamond setting of 556 μm). A front-cutting diamond

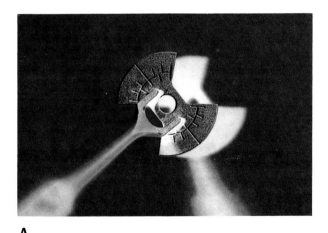

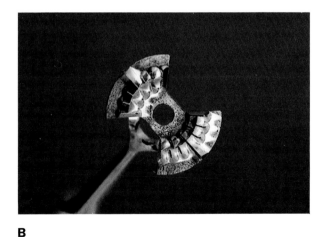

A   B

Fig. 14.7. (*A*) Surgeon's view of an arc-T marker. (*B*) Underside of an arc-T marker that makes the imprint on the corneal surface (see also Fig. 14.8).

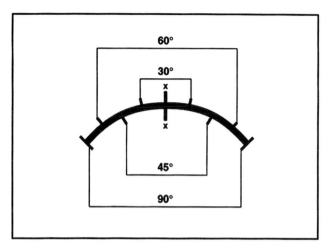

Fig. 14.8. Schematic of the mark made by the arc-T marker utilized to perform an AK an accurate length (in degrees) based on the preoperative nomogram decision.

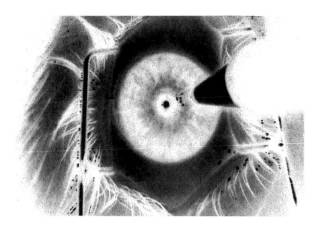

Fig. 14.9. Corneal thickness measurements are taken right at the AK site.

is used so that the blade can be "pushed" and visualized at all times during the incision (Fig. 14.10). A .12 forceps is used during the AK to stabilize the globe while performing the procedure. If an RK is to be performed, it is not unusual (with a reliable patient) to not fixate the globe during the procedure and rely on patient fixation. But while performing a transverse, or arcuate, incision, it is more difficult for the patient to hold fixation compared to a radial incision. Thus it is recommended that the surgeon fixate the globe. It is important to fixate about 1 mm posterior to the limbus (where Tenon's capsule inserts with the conjunctiva into the limbus) to provide for a more solid fixation (compared to fixating more posteriorly where the conjunctiva is looser, which provides for a more unstable attachment).[18] While making the incision, it is important to watch closely for any sign of fluid, which indicates a micro- or macroperforation.

If any sign of fluid occurs while making the incision, the blade is withdrawn from the cornea and the source investigated. Sometimes it is fluid that has accumulated in the fornices and has come onto the corneal surface because of pressure from the blade. Another source of fluid can be the blade itself. The tip may have accumulated any fluid from a wet corneal surface or the blade may have been rinsed off with sterile water and the excess water not dried with a microsponge prior to its use (Fig. 14.11). The other cause of fluid noted while making

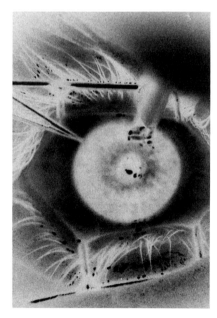

Fig. 14.10. A front-cutting diamond blade is used (in a "pushing" fashion) during the AK so that it can be visualized while making the incision. Note also that a .12 forceps is used at all times during the AK for stabilization of the globe while performing the procedure.

the incision is a true perforation, with resultant aqueous escaping from the anterior chamber. If it is a true perforation and it is small, pressure on the corneal surface may not cause fluid to continue to

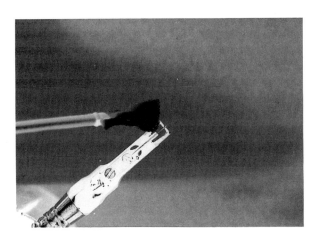

Fig. 14.11. (A) Fluid can accumulate around the diamond and its footplate and can be the source of a false sign of a microperforation. (B) A microsponge can be used to carefully dry up this excess moisture prior to performing the AK. Note that the microsponge is moistened slightly prior to drying the excess fluid, which minimizes damage to the previous diamond tip. (C) The diamond blade has been dried and is ready for use.

escape. If pressure is not causing more leakage, then the procedure can often be completed safely. If pressure is causing fluid to exude from the anterior chamber, then it is best to stop, allow the incision to heal, and repeat the surgery at a later date. Most full-thickness incisions are self-sealing and will not require suturing. If fluid is escaping from the incision without pressure on the cornea, then a suture should be placed. Perforations are more rare with AK than with RK. But also, with AK, it seems that a perforation has an increased chance of needing a suture compared to an RK incision, which appears to be self-sealing the majority of the time. A compression suture in an AK can be placed if necessary because the risk of visually significant irregular astigmatism is less with an AK compared to suturing an RK incision. With modern incisional surgery, utilizing accurate pachymeters and diamond blade calibrating microscopes, perforations should be extremely rare with attention to detail.

After completion of the AK, myopia surgery is done is planned. Whether performing RK or PRK, it makes sense to perform the AK first. When performing RK, if the AK is 45° or less, it is fine to situate the AK between the RK incisions. For larger AKs (i.e., 60° or more), consideration should be given to "jumping" the AK with the RK so that there is more room on either side of the AK in case a decision is made to extend the AK (Fig. 14.12). It is also important to not cross or intersect the RK incisions with an AK because of the problems that can result due to poor wound healing from unstable corneal tissue at the intersection.[19,20]

When performing AK prior to PRK, it is helpful to leave an island of epithelium just inside the AK prior to the excimer laser ablation. If all the epithelium is removed just inside the AK, there can be delayed reepithelialization because new epithelium can have difficulty crossing over the AK. This island of epithelium left just inside the AK can serve as a source of new epithelial cells in the early post-PRK healing period. Since the majority of excimer ablations occur at a 6-mm zone, the small amount of epithelium left just inside an AK placed at a 7-mm optical zone is typically insignificant.

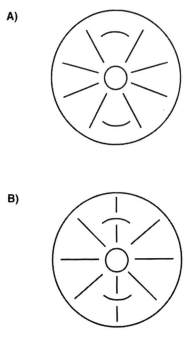

Fig. 14.12. (A) When combining an eight-incision RK with a relatively short AK (< 45°), the AK can be situated between the radial incisions. (B) When combining longer AKs (≥ 60°) with an eight-incision RK, it is helpful to have the radial incisions "jump" the AKs to leave room if a decision is made at a later date to extend the astigmatism incisions.

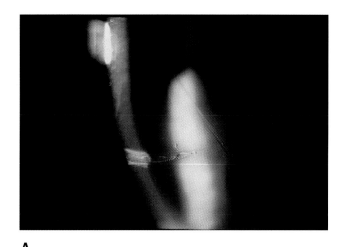 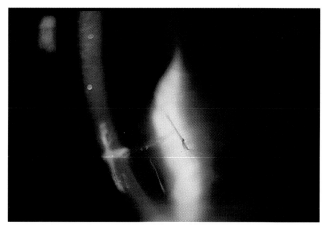

A   **B**

Fig. 14.13. (*A*) Excessive epithelial plug formation can be a cause of long-term excessive flattening in the axis of the AK and resultant overcorrected astigmatism. (*B*) An epithelial plug can be cleaned out of an incision and a suture(s) placed in the AK to reverse excessive flattening and overcorrected astigmatism.

Healing After AK

During the first couple of weeks after AK, antibiotic or antibiotic/steroid drops should be utilized to help reduce the risk of infectious keratitis. A 2-week course of topical antibiotic/steroid drops is typical. If there is any evidence of overcorrection, the antibiotic/steroid drops are discontinued and antibiotic-only drops are begun. Hypertonic saline drops can be helpful if there is any evidence of wound gape and swelling. Also, aqueous suppressants can be helpful in lessening the internal eye pressure that is causing the AK to "bulge" and excessively flatten the previously steep axis. Pharmacological measures can be helpful early on but begin to be less effective after 2 months. Late causes of overcorrected astigmatism include excessive epithelial plug formation (Fig. 14.13A). This can be documented on corneal topography. If the overcorrection is visually significant, the plug can be cleaned out and the AK sutured for better wound edge approximation. When placing a suture in an AK, an intraoperative keratometer can be helpful. The goal is to have a slight overcorrection in the axis of the suture placement, since the suture will relax with time. The author prefers Mersiline suture (11-0) for compression sutures (Fig. 14.13B). It is usually tolerated well over the long term, and if the refractive result is acceptable, the suture can be relied on for long-term, consistent tension (unlike nylon, which will relax and erode more quickly). If multiple sutures are used, selective suture removal can begin about 3 months postoperatively. Topography and refraction serve as important guides in the selective suture removal process.

CONCLUSION

AK is a very powerful tool in reducing congenital or surgically induced astigmatism. It can also be utilized to correct residual astigmatism in patients who have had attempted astigmatism reduction with other modalities (such as the holmium or excimer laser). Attention to the details outlined above will help maximize the chance of a positive surgical outcome. Equally important is to consider the patient's refractive error and how astigmatism-reducing surgery will affect the spherical equivalent. The benefits of AK are maximized in patients with myopic astigmatism. Another option in myopic astigmats is toric ablation with the excimer laser. In these patients, AK will continue to be utilized to enhance the post-toric ablation cylinder. In myopes with large amounts of astigmatism, AK can also be utilized to lessen the astigmatism significantly and a toric ablation performed to complete reduction of the cylinder while also treating the myopia. In hyperopic astigmats the holmium laser may be an option. Hyperopic excimer ablation combined with AK or toric hyperopic excimer ablation (AK can be used to enhance the final result) will also be a consideration for future hyperopic astigmats.

REFERENCES

1. Airy G. On a peculiar defect in the eye, and a mode of correcting it. *Trans Cam Phil Soc.* 1827;2:267–273.

2. Donders FC. *On the Anomalies of Accommodation and Refraction of the Eye.* WD Moore, transl. London: Hatton Press; 1864.

3. Snellen H. Die Richtunge des hauptmeridiane des astigmatishen auges. *Albrecht von Graefes Arch Klin Ophthalmol.* 1869;15:199–207.

4. Bates WH. A suggestion of an operation to correct astigmatism. *Arch Ophthalmol.* 1894;23:9–13.

5. Lans L. Experimentelle untersuchungen uber die entstehung von astigmatismus durch nicht perforirende corneawunden. *Albrecht von graefes Arch Klin Exp Ophthalmol.* 1898;45:117–152.

6. Helmholtz H. *Treatise on Physiological Optics,* vol 1. New York: Dover Press; 1924.

7. Koch DD. Detection and characterization of corneal pathology. In: Sanders DR, Koch DD, eds. *An Atlas of Corneal Topography,* Thorofare, NJ: Slack; 1993.

8. Maguire LJ, Bourne WM. Corneal topography of early keratoconus. *Am J Ophthalmol.* 1989;108:107–112.

9. Thornton SP. Background and theory of corneal relaxing incisions. In: Gills JP, Martin RG, Thornton SP, Sanders DR, eds. *Surgical Treatment of Astigmatism.* Thorofare, NJ: Slack; 1994:1–9.

10. Thompson VM. The surgical correction of myopic and hyperopic astigmatism. *Int Ophthalmol Clin.* 1994;34:87–96.

11. Thornton SP. Astigmatic keratotomy with corneal relaxing incisions. *Int Ophthalmol Clin.* 1994;34: 79–86.

12. Thornton SP. Astigmatic keratotomy with cataract extraction. In: Gills JP, Sanders DR, eds. *Small Incision Cataract Surgery.* Thorofare, NJ: Slack; 1990: 245–258.

13. Nordan LT, Hofbauer JD. Astigmatism: concepts and surgical approach. In: Nordan LT, Maxwell WA, Davison JA, eds. *The Surgical Rehabilitation of Vision.* New York, NY: Gower Medical Publishing; 1991: 23.1–23.30.

14. Lindstrom RL. The surgical correction of astigmatism: a clinician's perspective. *Refract Corneal Surg.* 1990;6:441–454.

15. Agapitos PJ, Lindstrom RL. Astigmatic keratotomy. *Ophthalmol Clin North Am.* 1992;5:709–715.

16. Price FW, Grene RB, Marks RG, et al. Astigmatism reduction clinical trial: a multicenter prospective evaluation of the predictability of arcuate keratotomy; evaluation of nomogram predictability. *Arch Ophthalmol.* 1995;113:277–282; correction 577.

17. Troutman RC, Buzard KA. *Corneal Astigmatism. Etiology, Prevention, and Management.* St Louis, MO: CV Mosby; 1992;180.

18. Fine BS, Yanoff M. *Ocular Histology,* 2nd ed. Hagerstown, MD; Harper & Row, Publishers, Inc; 1979:308–315.

19. Lindquist TD. Complications of corneal refractive surgery. *Int Ophthalmol Clin.* 1992;32:97–114.

20. Rashid ER, Waring GO. Complications of refractive keratotomy. In: Waring GO, ed. *Refractive Keratotomy for Myopia and Astigmatism.* St Louis, MO: CV Mosby, 1992;863–936.

15

Photorefractive Keratectomy for Astigmatism

Rasik B. Vajpayee
Hugh R. Taylor

Astigmatism is a refractive anomaly caused by unequal refraction of the incident light by the refractive elements of the eye. Astigmatism is termed *regular* when the two principal meridians of refraction are oriented at right angles to each other. If the two principle meridians are not at right angles to each other, astigmatism is termed *biblique*. Irregular astigmatism occurs when incident light is brought to focus at different points by various regions of the cornea, leading to asymmetrical refraction. In normal individuals an average difference of 0.5 to 0.75 D is usually seen in the refractive power of the two principal meridians. A difference of 1 D is considered the upper limit of normal.

Most young people have *with-the-rule* astigmatism, in which the axis of least curvature is located in the horizontal plane and the axis of steepest curvature is located in the vertical plane of the anterior corneal surface. Steepening of the horizontal meridian and flattening of the vertical meridian occur with increasing age, changing the configuration of the astigmatism, which is termed *against-the-rule* astigmatism.

The posterior surface of the cornea also shows some astigmatism that varies from 0.25 to 0.5 D. Posterior corneal astigmatism partially neutralizes anterior corneal astigmatism, as its principal meridians are oriented opposite to those of anterior corneal meridians.

Astigmatism causes both blurring and distortion of the visual image. It can be measured by the manifest refraction (*refractive astigmatism*), keratometry, or corneal topography of the anterior corneal surface (*topographical astigmatism*). The disparity between the refractive astigmatism measured at the anterior corneal plane and the topographical astigmatism is called *residual astigmatism*. Thus residual astigmatism represents the sum of astigmatic errors present on the posterior corneal surface, lens surfaces, and the astigmatism caused by varying refractive indices of media and by the decentration of the optical media. Some of these factors are present in optimally ablated eyes that present a spherical cornea on corneal topography and yet still show astigmatism on manifest refraction.

Astigmatism can occur naturally or can result from trauma, infection, or ocular surgery. Some degree of astigmatism is present in more than 90% of eyes, with an average corneal astigmatism of 1.04 D, and residual astigmatism of 0.61 D is present in young adults.[1] The magnitude of the astigmatism also varies greatly; approximately 85% of the population has less than 1.25 D of refractive astigmatism. A large astigmatic error is usually associated with an increased amount of spherical refractive error. The most common form of astigmatism is compound myopia (39%), followed by compound hypermetropia (27%), simple hypermetropia (14%), mixed hypermetropia (11%), and simple myopia (10%).

Available options to correct astigmatic error include spectacles, contact lenses, a variety of conventional keratotomy procedures, toric laser photoablative keratectomy, and the evolving techniques of thermal keratoplasties. The ability to treat the astigmatic component of myopic astigmatism by using an excimer laser is an important advance for the refractive surgeon, as many myopic patients have coexisting astigmatic errors. The first description of the use of the excimer laser to create toric ablations on the cornea was presented by McDonnell and colleagues in 1991.[2] The initial good results of this study encouraged many surgeons around the world to start treating myopic astigmatism with the excimer laser.

PRINCIPLES OF SURGICAL PLANNING

The first step toward correcting astigmatic error with the excimer laser involves the determination of the spherical and cylindrical errors of the individual eye by subjective refraction, mydriatic refraction, and corneal topography. However, creating only a spherical anterior corneal surface may leave a residual astigmatic error from the ocular surfaces. Vector analysis is essential to understand the astigmatic changes induced by surgery.[3] These analyses can be performed by a calculator but are much better performed with either a computer package or by custom programming a computer. The formulas used are available from the literature (e.g., Ref. 3) and commercially (e.g., Assort).

Astigmatic Vector Terminology

Vector analysis is useful in evaluating the results of photorefractive astigmatic keratectomy. The various relationships between the target-induced astigmatism (TIA) and the surgically induced astigmatism (SIA) provide the information about the magnitude of astigmatic correction and the axis alignment.

TIA: The planned astigmatic correction expressed as a vector.

SIA: The achieved astigmatic change expressed as a vector that results after refractive surgery.

Difference vector: The astigmatic correction still required to achieve the initial goal of surgery (TIA-SIA).

Correction index: SIA/TIA.

Percentage of astigmatism corrected: correction index (SIA/TIA] × 100.

Index of success: Difference vector/original TIA.

The most important issue in refractive surgery is the determination of the final refraction that needs to be corrected. This is particularly true for the surgery that will correct astigmatism.

Case Example

The refractive surgeon must synthesize information from a number of sources in determining the final refraction. These sources include subjective refraction, cycloplegic (or at least mydriatic) refraction, keratometry, and corneal topography. Corneal topography provides both a simulated keratometry reading and a schematic of corneal curvature indicating corneal regularity. The information from these sources is often quite different in terms of the amount of astigmatism and its axis, often with some compensatory variation in spherical component. The problem is, what does the surgeon select to treat

A final refraction should be performed that reconciles these different measures and the final subjective refraction should be taken as the final refraction. This final or postmydriatic refraction is determined by taking the cylinder indicated by topography, for example, and then refining both the cylinder and the sphere subjectively. The refractionist then takes the cycloplegic refraction and refines it subjectively to determine which of these gives the best duochrome-balanced, subjective refraction (Table 15.1, Fig. 15.1). This final refraction is used to program the laser.

Once the desired topographic and refractive targets are chosen, the desired astigmatic change or correction (TIA) in the corneal curvature is calculated. TIA may be different from the topographical and refractive astigmatic errors, as the surgeon may decide to leave a calculated amount of residual with the-rule-astigmatism in the manifest refraction. The presence of a small amount of residual astigmatism may be advantageous, as it increases the depth of focus.[4] For the same reason, it is also beneficial in pseudophakic eyes that have lost their accommodative powers.

Table 15.1. Example of Patient in Whom the Refractive and Topographic Astigmatism Differ. The Final Refraction is Used to Program the Laser

Subjective refraction	−3.50	−1.25 × 147
Cycloplegic refraction	−3.75	−1.50 × 148
Topographic astigmatism		−2.20 × 163
Final refraction	−3.75	−1.25 × 150

MECHANISM OF ASTIGMATIC CORRECTION

The current approach to treating astigmatism by the excimer laser involves a cylindrical ablation of the superficial cornea. This requires a nonradially symmetrical ablation of the corneal tissue, with greater ablation in the steep axis and minimal or no ablation in the flat axis.

McDonnell and colleagues[2] were the first to use the excimer laser successfully (VisX 20/20) to create toric ablations designed to correct the cylindrical errors. The laser software and hardware were modified to achieve this. In this technique, the excimer beam was passed through a set of parallel blades (Fig. 15.2). These blades create a slit-shaped or elliptical beam, and their movement is controlled by the computer.[2] The width of the slit depends on the movement of parallel blades and is used to control the amplitude of laser energy delivered for corneal ablation. For example, a slower movement of blades for a constant pulse rate will deliver more laser energy and will lead to a higher astigmatic correction. The slit mechanism works on the same principle of iris diaphragm used for myopic corrections, except that in the case of a slit, the cornea is relatively flattened only in the meridian perpendicular to the long axis of the slit. Ideally, no refractive change is expected to occur along the long axis of the slit, which is also called the *mechanical axis*. The slit of the excimer laser can be rotated, and its mechanical axis can be aligned to any given meridian in the cornea.

Initially, astigmatic corrections were performed using a *sequential* method whereby toric ablations were performed first, followed by a second phase of spherical ablation to correct coexisting myopia.[5] The ends of the ablated cylinder were smoothed to create a transition zone.[6] Although the sequential technique was able to correct astigmatism, it produced steep cuts on the ablated cornea which often induced excessive epithelial thickening and a reduction in the final refractive correction. An *elliptical* algorithm was developed that allowed full astigmatic and myopic corrections to proceed simultaneously.[7]

This elliptical algorithm has been incorporated in the VisX 20/20 excimer laser. The modification combines the expansion of inner parallel blades with a controlled contraction of a round diaphragm. Hyperopic astigmatism and myopic astigmatism that is in excess of the myopic error cannot be treated by this technique alone. This technique is best suited for regular astigmatism rather than bioblique or irregular astigmatism.[8]

The Summit excimer laser uses a shape transfer system in the form of an erodible mask for corneal sculpting to correct myopic and astigmatic refrac-

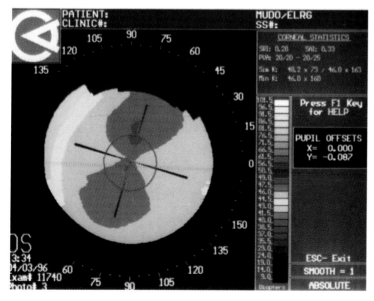

Fig. 15.1. Corneal topography showing corneal astigmatism of −2.2 × 163.

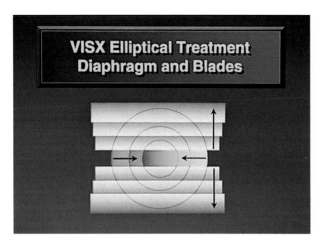

Fig. 15.2. VisX mechanism of astigmatic correction.

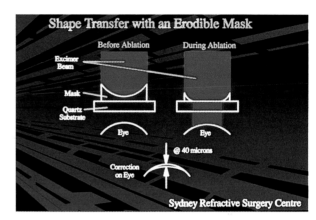

Fig. 15.3. Summit method of astigmatic correction.

tive errors.[9,10] The erodible mask is a thin polymethyl methacrylate (PMMA) button supported by a quartz substrate which is transparent to the excimer laser beam. The mask is placed in a rotatable holder. The ablation rate of the PMMA button is similar to that of the cornea, and its refractive power matches the refractive error to be corrected. The laser beam first ablates the PMMA. After the thinnest part has been ablated, the laser beam is passed to the corneal stroma, which starts to ablate. The process transfers the shape of the mask onto the cornea (Fig. 15.3). This technique may produce a smoother ablation profile than a conventional diaphragm.[11] The initial masks made it difficult to maintain optimal centration of the laser beam, and decentered ablations were encountered.[12,13]

A different mask technique has been developed for use with the Aesculap-Meditec MEL 60 excimer laser.[14] A rotating mask with an hourglass-shaped opening is used (Fig. 15.4) with a scanning slit delivery system. The rotation of the mask is controlled, and when the mask is rotated in equidistant angular steps over 360°, the profile of ablated tissue is symmetrical with the steepest part in the center, thus correcting myopia. However, if the rotation is varied and if the mask is held long in a particular meridian, the depth of the ablation is increased in that meridian. Thus, by selectively allowing more time in a specific meridian, the desired toric ablation can be sculpted on the cornea. Even high astigmatism and astigmatism that is seen after keratoplasty has been successfully treated with this technique, as has hyperopic astigmatism.[14]

In the Schwind excimer laser, the beam profile was initially controlled by means of a series of apertures on a revolving band that passed between the laser and the eye, much like film running through a movie projector. Round apertures were employed to guide their purely myopic ablations, and an oval or slit aperture was aligned at the appropriate axis to treat astigmatic errors.[7] However, a new astigmatism module has been constructed.[15]

A scanning mechanism is used to correct astigmatic errors by the Technolas, Nidek and Lasersight lasers. The scanning beam moves along the axes of astigmatism and differentially ablates the cornea (Fig. 15.5).

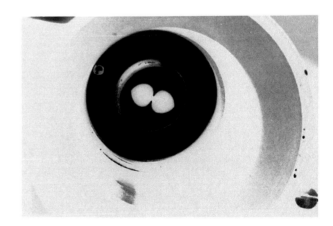

Fig. 15.4. Rotating mask used by the Meditec laser.

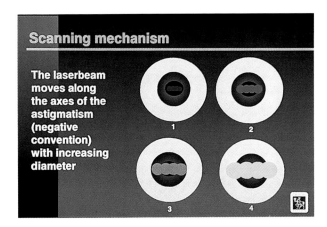

Fig. 15.5. Scanning mechanism of astigmatic correction.

EFFECTIVENESS OF PHOTOREFRACTIVE ASTIGMATIC KERATECTOMY

Myopic Astigmatism

Successful toric sculpting of the cornea with an excimer laser to correct regular corneal astigmatism was first reported by McDonnell and colleagues.[16] An expanding slit was used to flatten the cornea, and in each patient the regular component of the astigmatism was reduced by the surgery. The achieved correction ranged from 63% to 100% of the intended correction (mean, 83% ± 17%). This initial success indicated the potential ability of the excimer laser to treat astigmatic refractive errors, and later many refractive surgeons employed the same principle of toric sculpting of the cornea to correct astigmatism.

Brancato and associates[10] used the erodible mask to control the shape transfer processes. They treated four eyes for the correction of myopia combined with astigmatism. Although the astigmatism was reduced in all eyes, only one eye achieved the attempted correction.

The first major clinical study on excimer laser treatment of myopic astigmatism was published by the Melbourne Excimer Laser Research Group.[17] A VisX 20/20 laser was used, and sequential technique of astigmatic correction was employed to create toric corneal ablations. At 6 months, 85% of their 20 patients treated for myopic astigmatism were within 1 D of plano refraction.

Spigelman and associates also demonstrated the use of the VisX laser to treat myopic astigmatism.[18] Both sequential and elliptical algorithms were used in their study. After 6 months of follow-up, the average cylindrical error decreased from 1.52 D preoperatively to 0.54 D postoperatively.

Carones and associates[11] used a Summit Apex Plus laser incorporating an erodible mask into the laser optical pathway. Compound myopic astigmatism was treated in 67 eyes. Astigmatic attempted correction ranged between −1.00 and −5.00 D (mean, −2.52 ± 1.04 D). The ablation was made sequentially after the myopic correction. At six months the mean cyclinder component was −0.25 ± 0.32 D (range, 0 to −1.00 D). Eighty-nine percent of the best cases had uncorrected visual acuity of 20/25 or better.

The elliptical technique of astigmatic correction was employed by Kim and colleagues,[19] who studied the success of photorefractive astigmatic keratectomy (PARK) in 168 eyes with compound myopic astigmatism. A vector analysis was used to interpret the results. Their 6-month data revealed a wide variation in the range of achieved correction, with both overcorrection and undercorrection detected in some of the cases of the cohort. At 3 months 121 eyes (72%) and at 6 months 58 eyes (65.2%) were within ± 0.50 D of the intended correction. Overall, about 91% of the eyes were within ± 1.0 D of the intended correction.

The results of a 12- to 18-month follow-up of eight eyes that had undergone PARK for naturally occurring compound myopic astigmatism were reported by Pender and group.[20] Although the cylindrical error was reduced in most of the eyes, some residual astigmatism remained.

Dausch and associates[14] used the Aesculap-Meditec laser to treat simple myopic, mixed, or irregular astigmatism successfully. In 30 patients with simple astigmatism, the cylinder was reduced from −3.30 ± 2.40 D (range, −1.00 to −11 D) to −0.19 ± 0.48 (range, 0 to −2.00 D). Three months after treatment, the average cylinder was −0.22 ± 0.59 (range, 0 to −2.75 D). At 12 months, the overall mean cylinder in 19 eyes was −0.30 ± 0.58; 83.3% of the treated eyes were corrected within 0.50 D. In the myopic astigmatism group, the mean preoperative cylinder decreased from −2.10 ± 0.93 D to 0.11 ± 0.41 at 3 months. In these patients 80.6% of the eyes were corrected within 0.50 D.

The Melbourne group has data on 343 eyes for which follow-up has been completed for 1 year or more after PARK. The cohort also includes patients analyzed and reported on earlier.[5,17,21] The results of this study are generally similar to those of the initial studies on the use of the VisX 20/20 excimer laser for correction of myopic astigmatism. While the sequential technique was employed initially, the elliptical algorithm is used now routinely.

The myopic corrections were divided equally into each zone, and the number of zones used depended on the amount of preoperative myopia.[22] When an elliptical astigmatic correction was performed, the cylindrical portion of the treatment, up to 80% of sphere, was included in the largest zone (6 mm). If astigmatic error exceeded 80% of the sphere to be treated in the 6-mm zone, an equal amount of cylinder was entered into the 5- and 6-mm zones. This helped to achieve concentric ellipses and evenly contoured ablation zones. A zone size of 4.5 mm was employed only for the correction of myopia greater than 10.00 D, and no astigmatism was corrected in that zone.

The Alpins method of vector analysis was used to calculate and evaluate the change in cylindrical error in each patient.[3] The initial astigmatic corrections demonstrated an undercorrection of targeted change measured by both refraction and topography. To eliminate this error, a calculated adjustment of 1.2 was factored into the algorithm employed for all the subsequent astigmatic treatments. Prior to adjustment, a geometric mean of 78% correction of astigmatism was achieved, which increased to 90% after the 1.2 adjustment was factored into the corrections. This adjustment has been incorporated into the VisX software and has led to less undercorrection, with SIA moving closer to TIA and a correction index closer to 1.0.

Overall, nearly 60% correction of astigmatism was achieved, and the results were fairly comparable in low, moderate, and high myopes (Figs. 15.6 and 15.7). A difference in undercorrection was noted between the patients treated with sequential and elliptical algorithms. There was less undercorrection, and SIA closer to TIA was achieved by elliptical ablation. However, the sequential technique was still needed for larger cylindrical corrections that exceeded the spherical component. Astigmatic corrections were also less accurate when the intended correction (TIA) was less than 1 D.[22] This may be

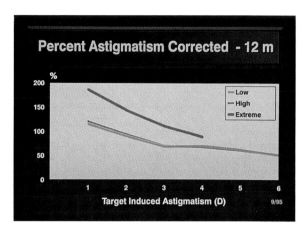

Fig. 15.6. Percentage of astigmatism corrected at 12 months by the VisX excimer laser.

due to irregular epithelial hyperplasia rather than to an effect of the ablation itself.

Problems and Complications

Except for those studies using the VisX 20/20 excimer laser, most of the clinical studies on PARK have not used vector analysis to evaluate the results. Vector analysis is essential for the evaluation of astigmatic correction. Without it, it is not possible to assess the efficacy of a particular laser or technique in treating astigmatism.

The main problem associated with PARK is the apparent undercorrection of the astigmatic component. Axis misalignment of the laser beam may be a

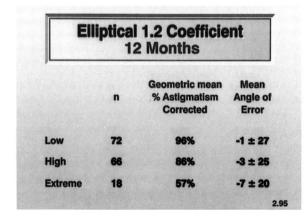

Fig. 15.7. Geometric mean of the percentage of astigmatism corrected by the VisX laser after the 1.2 systemic adjustment in the elliptical algorithm.

potential cause of this problem,[21–25] and with angles of error of 15° there is a 50% reduction in the magnitude of the astigmatism corrected.[7] Also, the effects of meridional healing may contribute to the occurrence of undercorrection.

Recently, the authors used an axis alignment system to try to achieve optimal laser beam alignment before the actual treatment. However, the results did not demonstrate any beneficial effect of this device.[26] The predictability of astigmatic correction is another concern for refractive surgeons. With increasing myopia there is less predictability in the astigmatic correction from the increased inadvertent SIA.[22] The random distribution of axis of such inadvertent SIA may cause overcorrection, undercorrection, or a change in the axis of the intended astigmatic correction. Irregular epithelial healing and epithelial hyperplasia are responsible for irregular corneal surfaces, SIA, and optical aberrations.

Hyperopic Astigmatism

Dausch and colleagues[14] designed a rotating mask for use with the Meditec laser to treat hyperopic astigmatism. Their technique of treating hyperopic astigmatism spares the central cornea, reducing the chances of corneal haze across the visual axis. They treated 23 patients, 13 of whom had hyperopic astigmatism and 10 of whom had mixed astigmatism. Patients with compound hyperopic astigmatism recorded a marked decrease in the mean preoperative SEQ, from +4.00 ± 1.28 D to −0.88 ± 1.73 D. The mean cylinder changed from −2.70 ± 1.23 D preoperatively to 0.40 ± 0.13 D at 3 months. The postlaser axis of astigmatism was within 10° of the prelaser axis in all eyes. At 3 months, more than 60% of patients achieved an uncorrected acuity of 20/40 or better. Overall, the mean uncorrected acuity improved from 20/150 preoperatively to 20/50 at 3 months. For the treatment of mixed astigmatism myopic cylindrical ablation was performed, followed by spherical ablation for hyperopic spherical correction. These eyes had a mean SEQ of +0.47 ± 1.08 D and a mean cylinder of −5.02 ± 0.77 D. At 3 months the mean SEQ was 0.22 ± 0.96 D and the mean cylinder was 0.25 ± 0.60 D. Seventy percent of the patients achieved an uncorrected acuity of 20/40 or better. Of the remaining three eyes, two did not have a 20/40 potential.

Irregular Astigmatism

Gibralter and Trokel[27] described a customized form of ablation to treat irregular astigmatism in two patterns. They used both phototherapeutic keratectomy (PTK) and photorefractive keratectomy (PRK) patterns and based the amount of the tissue to removed on the size and steepness of the irregular corneal surface. Steep areas were identified first by corneal topography, and then PTK was performed over these areas in overlapping, confluent 4.0-mm zones 10 to 20 µm in depth. These superficial ablations smoothed the corneal surface and were followed by a spherical correction in a 6-mm ablation zone. Both patients treated achieved stabilized refraction at 6 months, with uncorrected acuity of 20/50. Postlaser corneal topography demonstrated an improvement in the corneal surface.

The ablatable mask technique has also been used for the correction of irregular astigmatism. Modifying the hardware of the Meditec laser, Dausch and associates[14] treated two patients with irregular astigmatism successfully. The first patient had a preoperative refraction of +2.00/−1.25 × 90. Three months after photoablation, refraction was +0.75/−0.50 × 168. The second patient's refraction changed from +1.25/−7.00 × 130 to +0.50/−1.50 × 180 after 3 months.

Postsurgical Astigmatism

Iatrogenic astigmatism secondary to ocular surgical procedures is usually greater than congenital astigmatism and occurs after cataract and corneal graft surgery. Other surgical procedures—for example, for glaucoma and retinal procedures—can also adversely affect the corneal curvature, causing astigmatism.

Norden and associates[28] treated compound myopic astigmatism after radial keratotomy (RK) and penetrating keratoplasty using a VisX 20/20 excimer laser. They reported that PARK is an effective treatment for correction of postsurgical astigmatism and carries a risk similar to that for eyes having PRK as the initial refractive procedure.

The Melbourne group has 6 month of follow-up data on 51 eyes that had postsurgical astigmatism treated by the excimer laser. Indications for excimer laser correction were astigmatism induced by penetrating keratoplasty (16 eyes), cataract surgery (14 eyes), RK (9 eyes), corneal scars (3 eyes), and glaucoma or retinal procedures (3 eyes). The sequential algorithm was used in 58% of the eyes, and 42% of the eyes were treated by the elliptical method. Despite good numerical results, the visual gain was poor in the postkeratoplasty group. Only two patients achieved an uncorrected visual acuity of 20/40 or better. Most of these patients had irregular astigmatism, which probably could not be effectively treated with the techniques used and was partially responsible for the poor visual gain. Despite the use of postexcimer laser topical steroids, 20% of the eyes went on to have failed grafts due to graft rejection after the excimer laser surgery.

Better results were obtained in the post–cataract surgery group. The regular corneal surface and lower amplitude of errors of both myopia (-2.75 ± 2.27 D) and astigmatism (-3.86 ± 1.22 D) were responsible for the comparatively better results in these patients. At 6 months, about 92% of the patients were within 2 D of SEQ, and the mean postlaser cylinder was -1.56 ± 1.08 DC. The mean postoperative SEQ at 6 months was $+1.36 \pm 1.96$ D. Uncorrected visual acuity of 20/40 or better was achieved in 43% of the patients. The patients with astigmatism after RK also had lower amplitudes of prelaser myopia and astigmatism and achieved good corrections which were similar to those attained with primary PARK. All patients in this group achieved an uncorrected visual acuity of 20/60 or better, with one-third achieving acuity of 20/20 or better at 6 months.

Keratoconus

Keratoconic corneas are usually not suitable for incisional or photoablative surgeries because of the corneal thinning and progressive nature of the disease. However, because of the occurrence of high postoperative astigmatism and the everlasting risk of graft rejection after penetrating keratoplasty, some surgeons have tried excimer laser surgery as an alternative. Mortensen and Ohrstrom[29] treated five keratoconic corneas with the VisX laser and achieved a reduction in astigmatism with an increase in visual acuity in four eyes. No adverse effects or deterioration of keratoconus were observed. Excimer laser surgery may not be an effective long-term treatment for keratoconus, but it may help delay corneal graft surgery and prolong the use of contact lenses. However, the long-term

effects of excimer ablation on keratoconic corneas are yet not known. Until then, the procedure has to be used cautiously for the treatment of keratoconus.

Combination of Excimer Laser and Astigmatic Keratotomy

While the clinical results of PARK have been encouraging, not all excimer lasers are able to correct astigmatism. This has prompted many surgeons to look for alternative techniques. Recently, refractive surgeons have tried to use a combination of excimer laser photoablation and transverse surgical keratotomy to treat astigmatism. To treat compound myopic astigmatism, an incisional astigmatic keratotomy (AK) is performed first, followed by a spherical PRK. Although the predictability of such a combined technique remains questionable, some surgeons have recommended the use of this two-step procedure combining both incisional and laser surgery.[30,31]

Ring and associates[30] performed transverse keratotomy in conjunction with PRK in 40 eyes to correct compound myopic astigmatism. The mean attempted cylindrical correction was -1.73 D. After 6 months, the mean astigmatic error was -0.32 D. The mean SEQ decreased from -5.99 D preoperatively to -0.01 D 6 months postoperatively. Uncorrected visual acuity of 20/40 or better was achieved in 75% of the eyes.

Lipshitz and colleagues[31] treated 11 eyes of nine patients for compound myopic astigmatism. An initial AK was followed 1 month later by excimer laser PRK. The mean cylindrical error decreased from -3.11 ± 1.16 D preoperatively to -0.14 ± 0.9 D postoperatively.

FUTURE OF PARK

Excimer laser surgery to correct astigmatism is still undergoing further modifications and improvements. Improvements are being made to the machine, the algorithms, and the techniques to improve predictability and achieve the desirable astigmatic correction.

However, despite these technological advances, more needs to be known about the biological responses and wound healing. A better understanding of postlaser healing would be of immense help in formulating the ideal algorithms. These algorithms should consider external and internal healing influences on the ablated cornea. These factors will include collateral tissue damage, ablation surface contour, tear-borne and local inflammatory mediators and cytokines, and tear film function, as well as the specific epithelial and stromal wound healing. Pharmacological modulators that can exert a desired influence on the postlaser healing responses may make an impact in the future.

Successful initial clinical results of the treatment of irregular astigmatism have opened the door to the new and exciting possibility for an effective treatment of focal abnormalities of the corneal surface causing irregular astigmatism. Further refinements of the excimer laser algorithms and improvement in corneal topographic analyses may enable effective techniques to optimally change an irregular corneal surface into a predetermined regular, symmetrically curved surface. Patients with idiopathic irregular astigmatism or astigmatism caused by cataract, pterygium, corneal graft surgery, and so forth will benefit from this new technology.

REFERENCES

1. Jackson S. Epidemiology of refractive errors. *JAMA.* 1935;105:1412.
2. McDonnell PJ, Moreira H, Garbus J, et al. Photorefractive keratectomy to create toric ablations for correction of astigmatism. *Arch Ophthalmol.* 1991;109:710–713.
3. Alpins N. A new method of analysing vectors for change in astigmatism. *J Cataract Refract Surg.* 1993;19:524–533.
4. Sawusch MR, Guyton DL. Optimal astigmatism to enhance depth of focus after cataract surgery. *Ophthalmology.* 1991;98:1025–1029.
5. Taylor HR, Kelly P, Alpins N, et al. Excimer laser correction of myopic astigmatism. *J Cataract Refract Surg.* 1994;20:S243–S251.
6. Clapham TN, D'Arcy J, Bechtel L, et al. Analysis of an adjustable slit design for correcting astigmatism. In: Puliafito CA, ed. *Ophthalmic Technologies. Proc SPIE* 1991;1423:2–7.
7. Shimmick JK, Bechtel L. Elliptical ablations for the correction of compound myopic astigmatism by photoablation with apertures. In: Jean Marie Pavel, ed. *Ophthalmic Technologies II. Proc SPIE* 1992;1644:32–39.
8. Seiler T, McDonnell PJ. Excimer laser photorefractive keratectomy. *Surv Ophthalmol.* 1995;40:89–118.
9. Gorden M, Brint SF, Durrie DS, et al. Photorefractive keratectomy (PRK) at 193 nm using an erodible mask. *SPIE Proc* 1992;1644:11–19.
10. Brancato R, Carones F, Trabucchi G, et al. The erodible mask in photorefractive keratectomy for myopia and astigmatism. *J Refract Corneal Surg.* 1993;9:S125–S127.
11. Carones F, Venturi E, Brancato R. Compound myopic astigmatism correction using an erodible mask in-the-rail excimer laser delivery system. *Ophthalmic Surg Lasers.* 1996;27:S530–S531.
12. Seiler T. Photorefractive keratectomy: European experience. In: Thompson FB, McDonnell PJ, eds. *Color Atlas/Text of Excimer Laser Surgery. The Cornea.* New York: Igaku-Shoin Medical Publishers; 1993:53–62.
13. Aron-Rosa DS, Boerner CF, Bath P, et al. Corneal wound healing after excimer laser keratotomy in a human eye. *Am J Ophthalmol.* 1987;103:454–464.
14. Dausch D, Klein R, Landesz M, et al. Photorefractive keratectomy to correct astigmatism with myopia or hyperopia. *J Cataract Refract Surg.* 1994;20:S252–S257.
15. Forster W, Beck R, Borrmann A, et al. Correcting myopic astigmatism with an areal 193 nm excimer laser ablation. *J Cataract Refract Surg.* 1995;21:278–281.
16. McDonnell PJ, Moreira H, Terrance N, et al. Photorefractive keratectomy for astigmatism—initial clinical results. *Arch Ophthalmol.* 1991;109:1370–1373.
17. Taylor HR, Guest CS, Kelly P, et al. Comparison of excimer laser treatment of astigmatism and myopia. *Arch Ophthalmol.* 1993;111:1621–1626.
18. Spigelman AV, Albert WC, Cozean CH, et al. Treatments of myopic astigmatism with the 193 nm excimer laser utilizing aperture elements. *J Cataract Refract Surg.* 1994;20:S258–S261.
19. Kim YJ, Sohn J, Tchah H, et al. Photorefractive astigmatic keratectomy in 168 eyes: six-month results. *J Cataract Refract Surg.* 1994;20:387–391.
20. Pender PM, Excimer Laser Study Group. Photorefractive keratectomy for myopic astigmatism: phase IIA of the Federal Drug Administration study (12 to 18 months' follow-up). *J Cataract Refract Surg.* 1994;20:S262–S264.
21. Snibson GR, Carson CA, Aldred GF, et al. One year evaluation of excimer laser photorefractive keratectomy for myopia and myopic astigmatism. *Arch Ophthalmol.* 1995;113:994–1000.
22. Tabin GC, Alpins N, Aldred GF, et al. Astigmatic

change one year after treatment of myopia and myopic astigmatism with excimer laser. *J Cataract Refract Surg*. In press.

23. Kim JY, Sohn J, Tchah H, et al. Photoastigmatic refractive astigmatic keratectomy in 168 eyes: six-month results. *J Cataract Refract Surg*. 1994;20: 387–391.

24. Chu DF, Gibralter RP, Belmont SC, et al. Excimer laser photorefractive keratectomy for the treatment of astigmatism. *Invest Ophthalmol Vis Sci*. 1993; 34(suppl):799.

25. Krueger RR. The excimer laser: a step-up in complexity and responsibility for the excimer laser surgeon. *J Refract Corneal Surg*. 1994;10:83–86.

26. Vajpayee RB, Aldred G, McCarty C, et al. Evaluation of axis alignment system in photoastigmatic refractive keratectomy. *Ophthalmology*. In press.

27. Gibralter R, Trokel SL. Correction of irregular astig-matism with the excimer laser. *Ophthalmology*. 1994; 101:1310–1315.

28. Norden NT, Binder PS, Kassar BS. Photorefractive keratectomy to treat myopia and astigmatism after radial keratotomy and penetrating keratoplasty. *J Cataract Refract Surg*. 1995;21:268–273.

29. Mortensen J, Ohrstrom A. Excimer laser photo-fractive keratectomy for treatment of keratoconus. *J Refract Corneal Surg*. 1994;10:368–372.

30. Ring PC, Hadden BO, Morris TA. Transverse kera-totomy combined with spherical photorefractive keratectomy for compound myopic astigmatism. *J Refract Corneal Surg*. 1994;10:S217–S221.

31. Lipshitz I, Lowenstein A, Lazar M. Astigmatic kera-tectomy followed by photorefractive keratectomy in the treatment of compound myopic astigmatism. *J Refract Corneal Surg*. 1994;10(suppl):282–284.

16

Keratophakia for Hyperopia

Ricardo Q. Guimaraes
Marcia Reis Guimaraes
Raul D. Castro

INTRODUCTION

Keratophakia (Greek root: *kera*, cornea; *phacos*, lens) was introduced by Barraquer[1-4] in 1949 as a technique based on the same concept as keratomileusis. It involves the intrastromal insertion of a lenticule with refractive power. The lenticule is a piece of corneal stroma tailored by a lathe or microkeratome resection that, once inserted, increases the anterior curvature and consequently the corneal refractive power. Originally, the desired lenticule was obtained by freezing a piece of donor corneal tissue and tailoring it, using a cryolathe.[5,6] A second method was introduced by Krumeich and Swinger.[7] A large disc was obtained with the microkeratome; its thickness was measured; and it was then held, epithelial side down, with suction on a plastic base. The microkeratome was again used to excise the desired lenticule from the disc, according to the needs of the patient and the proposed nomogram. The third method, was developed by Guimarães (oral presentation, International Society of Refractive Keratoplasty Pre-Academy Refractive Surgery Symposium, Anaheim, CA, October 1991). It consisted of using the microkeratome to obtain the lenticule directly from the exposed stroma of a myopic patient undergoing keratomileusis or from a donor eye.

Most of the results of keratophakia that have been published to date concern cases involving the cryolathe technique.

THEORY

The air–cornea interface is responsible for most of the bending of the light entering the eye and directed to the retina. Any attempt to change the refractive power of the cornea should take into consideration the whole structure of the globe.[2,13] It is important for the corneal surgeon to know some basic optical and geometrical principles which affect corneal refractive procedures, although the calculations for these techniques may be done by computer.

The bending of the light at an interface between two media can be calculated by Snell's law (Fig. 16.1). The refractive power of a spherical interface is calculated by the approximation of Littman's formula:

$$D = \frac{(n2 - n1) \times 1000}{R}$$

where D is the refractive power in diopters, $n1$ is the refractive index of medium 1, $n2$ is the refractive index of medium 2, and R is the radius of curvature in millimeters.

If we consider Gullstrand's data for the normal cornea (Table 16.1) and apply Littman's formula to the anterior and posterior surfaces of the cornea, we find the following:

$$\text{Anterior surface} = \frac{1.376 - 1.000}{7.70} \times 1.000$$
$$= 48.83 \text{ D}$$

$$\text{Posterior surface} = \frac{1.336 - 1.376}{6.80} \times 1.000$$
$$= 5.882 \text{ D}$$

If we consider the cornea as a thin lens, we have a total corneal refractive power of 42.95 D (48.83 D − 5.882 D). The anterior surface of the cornea is by far the most important one in terms of refractive power.

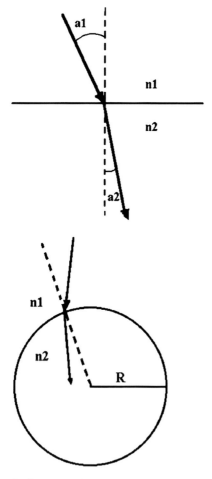

Fig. 16.1. Refraction of light at a plane and at a curved surface.

Table 16.1 Gullstrand's Data for the Normal Eye

Index of refraction of air	1.000
Index of refraction of cornea	1.376
Index of refraction of aqueous	1.336
Radius of anterior corneal surface	7.70 mm
Radius of posterior corneal surface	6.80 mm

A diagram of the postoperative result in keratophakia is shown in Fig. 16.2.

The relevant variables in keratophakia are the diameter of the host disc (Dd), the diameter of the donor lenticule, the thickness of the lenticule (L), the host cap (HC), and the host bed (HB). The usual diameter of frozen lathed lenticules is 6 to 7 mm. In our experience, fresh homoplastic lenticules with an average diameter of 4 mm are most frequently used. The host cap is ideally 8 mm in diameter and 200 μm in thickness. A thicker cap will produce a thinner bed, increasing the risk of posterior ectasia.

What are the theoretical limits of correction with keratophakia? Since steeper radii distort the vision and limit the optical zone, we should consider a maximum preoperative anterior corneal curvature of 9.75 mm and a minimum of 5.8 mm. Using

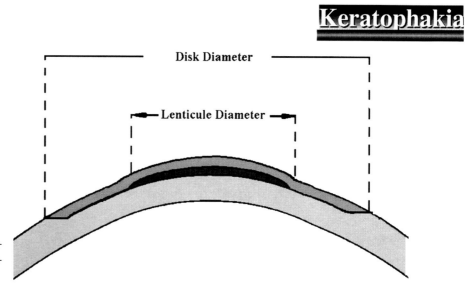

Fig. 16.2. Schematic representation of the cornea after implantation of the lenticule.

Littman's formula and an average index of refraction of 1.331:

$$\text{Flattest cornea} = \frac{1.331 - 1.000}{9.75} \times 1.000$$
$$= 33.95 \text{ D}$$

$$\text{Steepest cornea} = \frac{1.331 - 1.000}{5.8} \times 1.000$$
$$= 57.07 \text{ D}$$

Therefore, the limit of correction obtained with keratophakia depends on the preoperative curvature of the cornea. The highest possible correction is approximately +23 D. In a flat cornea it is possible to achieve a higher correction than in a steep cornea. For example, in an aphakic patient with an initial anterior corneal curvature of 40 D, a maximum correction of 17 D is possible. If the original corneal curvature is 46 D, the maximum correction would be 11 D. When considering a patient for keratophakia, it must be kept in mind that 57 D is the maximum possible curvature.

Precise control of lenticule thickness and diameter is critical for this surgery, as minimal variations may produce significant changes in the final correction.

PATIENT SELECTION

A complete eye examination is mandatory in every case, especially in secondary procedures or traumatic cases. Corneal topography is very important in identifying incipient keratoconus and in follow-up. Cycloplegic and manifest refractions should always be measured, but the surgical plan, as well as the assessment of pre- and postoperative results, are based upon the cycloplegic data. Contact lens use should stop at least 1 week prior to refractive surgery.[14]

The indications for keratophakia include hyperopia, aphakia, and overcorrection after several procedures for myopia (keratomileusis, radial keratotomy, and excimer laser surgery).

With a secondary procedure, there should be an uneventful healing period of at least 6 months, as the transient preoperative rise in intraocular pressure may produce an opening in a cataract incision or split a post–radial keratotomy incision. In terms of patient selection, the best cases involve correction in the range of +2 to +8 D.

As lamellar surgery is not age dependent, it can be used with young patients. In bilateral surgery for congenital hyperopia, we apply the same general rules as in any other refractive surgery.

When preoperative visual acuity is less than 20/100, patients are often disappointed with the postoperative results, even when the proposed objectives for the refractive correction are achieved.

In hyperopic lamellar surgery, corneal thickness is not a critical factor since tissue is added. This is in contrast to the myopic technique, where tissue is removed.

In patients with a decentered visual axis and an abnormal or absent pupil after trauma, centering the lenticule may be difficult.

TECHNIQUE

The technique can be divided in two major steps: preparation of the donor and preparation of the refractive lenticule.

Instrumentation

The key instrument is the microkeratome. Any type of device designed for keratomileusis in situ is suitable for keratophakia. An artificial anterior chamber is necessary for the removal of the lenticule from a donor cornea.

Patient Workup

Patients are given a mild sedative. In patients with a large pupil, diluted myotic drops are used a few minutes before surgery.

Locating the Visual Axis

An important procedure in keratophakia is the centering of the lenticule in the visual axis. The visual axis may be centered or displaced to the temporal or right side and inferior or superior in relation to the pupil.[15] There are several methods of determining the visual axis; the surgeon should use the one he or she is most comfortable with. It should be emphasized that during surgery the disc (host cap) is lifted and no marks should be made in the stroma. We have used a combination of two methods. With one technique, we align the illumination with the optics at the slit lamp, using a small, dim source of light, allowing the patient to look at it comfortably. Either by looking at the reflex or by observing the deviation directly, we can evaluate the position of the visual axis. The second method is used to double-check the first. The location of the visual axis is obtained by keratography, which allows the surgeon to document it through a photograph that can be handled and consulted in the operating room.

Keratectomy

The keratectomy is made with the same technique used for keratomileusis. Because the patient must focus on a reference light (Serdarevic Circle of Light, Mastel, Rapid City, SD) to check for centering, the surgery is done under topical anesthesia using 1 drop of proximetacaine chlorhydrate 0.5% and 3 drops of tetracaine chlorhydrate before surgery. Using a methylene blue ink pen, the host cornea receives an asymmetric mark, which eases the repositioning of the host cap, using at least three lines in different sectors.

The diameter of the host cap should be about 9 mm or larger and never less than 7 mm. Implantation of the lenticule underneath the host cap will raise its central portion, leaving a thin area of exposed stroma in the periphery. The larger the host cap, the smaller the exposed area, reducing the risk of epithelial invasion or any type of discomfort due to the gap formed between the disc and the border of the nonresected area of cornea.

The ideal thickness is about 200 μm. It is strongly advised not to cut too deeply into the cornea to avoid late onset ectasia.

The host cap, should resist manipulation without producing folds. The presence of the intrastromal refractive lenticule decreases the adhesiveness between the host cap and the stroma. Leaving a peduncle at the nasal side is very helpful for repositioning the host cap and stabilization of the refractive lenticule. If a complete resection occurs, more manipulation of the host cap is required, increasing the chance of decentration.

After the keratectomy, the host cap is folded to the nasal side, the stroma is dried with a Merocel sponge, and the lenticule is placed and centered on the visual axis. As the lenticule is very thin, it is sometimes difficult to see it under the strong light of the microscope. It is seen more easily through the refringence of the light at the periphery. In some

cases, a methylene ink mark is placed on the center of the lenticule, enhancing its visualization in the glass plaque or the corneal host cap. Once it is centered, gentle stretching toward the periphery using a semi-wet Merocel sponge is helpful before the disk is repositioned. Care must be taken to avoid any debris or cells in the interface, as it is much more difficult to remove these foreign bodies postoperatively due to the presence of the lenticule. The patient is asked to look at the fixation light of the microscope to allow the surgeon to confirm centration. If the sutureless technique is not used, the ideal suture is the BRA suture described by Guimaraes et al.[16]

Obtaining the Lenticule

All lenticules are obtained using the microkeratome. The desired thickness is determined through microkeratome adjustment. Any type of instrument designed for keratomileusis in situ can be used. Accurate calculation of the refractive power of the lenticule is important for good results. After the initial procedures were performed, in which donor myopic and recipient hyperopic ammetropia were matched, the results were analyzed. A regression formula was developed by the authors to obtain this formula:

$$X = \frac{Y - 2.14}{0.47}$$

where X is the refractive power of the donor lenticule (determined by the myopic keratomileusis nomogram) and Y is the refractive error of the receptor (spherical equivalent at a vertex distance of 12 mm).

From a Myopic Donor

The ideal lenticule for keratophakia is larger than that considered ideal for myopic keratomileusis. Too small lenticules require more critical centration. Refractive power results from the combination of diameter and thickness. The larger the diameter, the smaller the refractive power; in other words, the larger the diameter, the thicker the lenticule must be to provide the same refractive power. A 4.5-mm optical zone (OZ) is the ideal diameter. When a lenticule thinner than 70 μm is used, the tissue is too soft and folds easily. When it is too thick, it tends to produce an abrupt change of curvature in the transition zone. The ideal thickness for easy manipulation is about 100 μm. A lenticule with an OZ of 4.5 mm and a thickness of 100 μm, according to the nomogram, provides a correction of 8.5 D of myopia. When planning the correction of a myopic patient, one must therefore compromise between the ideal diameter and thickness for the myopic donor and for the hyperopic recipient.

From a Donor Cornea

An artificial anterior chamber, as designed by Barraquer, must be used. An initial keratectomy will expose the stroma. The second cut on the stroma will provide the desired lenticule. Donor corneas have different amounts of hydration, depending on the length of storage. It is wise to calculate for overcorrection when working with donor corneas, obtaining a more powerful lenticule than required by the nomogram.

Storing the Lenticule

The lenticule may be obtained fresh from a donor myopic patient or from a donor cornea. In either case, the lenticule can be used immediately after resection or stored in corneal storage medium. Lenticules stored for up to 3 months have been used. Prior to use, the lenticule, regardless of the way it has been obtained, must be placed on a cover glass slide. Its thickness and diameter must be measured, and it must be stored in a Petri plaque to protect it from dust or contamination by microscopic particles present in the air. Before the lenticule is measured, the thickness device tip must be covered with a plastic cover, usually a piece of drape, so that one face of the lenticule lies on the cover glass plaque and the other face is against the plastic. It must be emphasized that very small particles can compromise the optical quality of the lenticule.

After being cut, measured, and stored in the Petri plaque, the lenticule can be used several hours later. Because it dries very quickly while stored in the Petri plaque, the longer the lenticule is kept there, the longer it takes to rehydrate. We have successfully used a dried lenticule 6 hr after its resection. However, we did not succeed when trying to use a lenticule the day after it was resected. It did not rehydrate completely and interfered with corneal metabolism and transparency, requiring replacement.

Storing Lenticules in Corneal Storage Media

Lenticules can be stored in corneal storage medium for months before being used. Lenticules from myopic donors were systematically stored in order to have a wide range of refractive power available. It was noticed, however, that while this tissue was clinically acceptable, there were two problems. Its refractive power decreased in proportion to the time of storage, and it produced much more interface opacities than fresh lenticules.

Placing the Lenticule

The lenticule must be manipulated carefully, as it is very thin and delicate. Any mark produced by forceps manipulation can cause refractive changes. By the time the surgeon takes the lenticule out of the Petri cover plaque, the lenticule will be dehydrated and adherent to the cover glass. It must be rehydrated before any manipulation, which must be always done with a sable brush. A round mark in the center of the lenticule using a methylene blue pen may help center the lenticule in the visual axis. The lenticule should be wet until it is placed and centered. After the desired location is obtained, it should be stretched, avoiding any folds, and dried with a Merocel sponge before the corneal cap is repositioned.

The eye is occluded with a patch and a hard shield until the next day. Antibiotics and anti-inflammatory drops are used three times daily for 1 week.

RESULTS

Hyperopic keratophakia was performed in 85 eyes of 62 patients from 1989 through 1994. Four patients from the original group were excluded due to postoperative visual problems unrelated to the procedure (see Complications). Thirty-three (53.2%) patients were male and 29 (46.7%) were female. The average age was 38 years (range, 6 to 77 years). The average follow-up period was 24 months (range, 1 to 62 months).

The mean preoperative spherical equivalent was +5.56 D (standard deviation, 3.02 D; range, +1.75 to +15.0 D). Fig. 16.3 shows the evolution of refraction (mean spherical equivalent) and mean keratometry during the follow-up period. When the

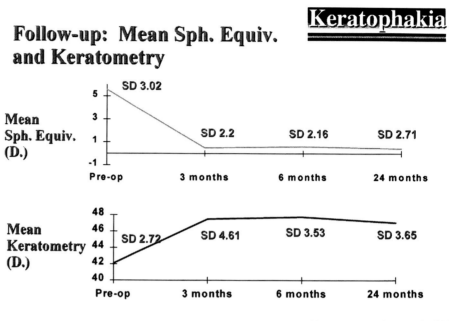

Fig. 16.3. Evolution of the mean spherical equivalent and mean keratometry, with standard deviation.

3-month spherical equivalent median was compared to the 6-month median (Mann-Whitney test), no significant statistical difference between them was found ($p = .5728$) (Table 16.2). This observation is also true for the comparison of the 6-month and 24-month data ($p = 0.5182$) (Table 16.2). These results show that regression is not a problem with keratophakia, as it is with other surgical techniques such as thermal keratoplasty[17–22] and laser thermal keratoplasty.[23–25] Unlike other procedures, in keratophakia, there is an increase in central corneal

Table 16.2. Comparison of the Spherical Equivalent Median Between 3 and 6 Months and Between 6 and 24 Months.

Test	W*	p†
3-month sph. equiv. ✕ 6-month sph. equiv.	470.5	.5728
6-month sph. equiv. ✕ 24-month sph. equiv.	467.0	.5182

*Mann-Whitney measure.
†p value.

curvature due to increased tissue. This added tissue is incorporated by the cornea, as one cannot distinguish the inserted lenticule from the receptor cornea.

The analysis of the uncorrected visual acuity (VASC) of these eyes (Fig. 16.4) showed that only a small percentage of patients (4.61%) could see better than 20/30 before surgery without spectacles or contact lenses. After keratophakia, approximately one-third of the patients had a VASC of 20/30 or better. It is important to note that keratophakia does not correct the astigmatic error, which requires a secondary procedure, such as astigmatic keratotomy, to be refined. Also, it must be emphasized that in this group, only 58.34% of the eyes were able to achieve preoperative vision better than 20/30, as shown by analysis of the best corrected visual acuity (BCVA) (Fig. 16.5). It is well known that amblyopia is a frequent finding in patients with hyperopic anisometropia.

Analysis of the evolution of the BCVA (Fig. 16.5) shows that keratophakia does not interfere significantly with visual acuity. There was a slight decrease in the percentage of eyes which could see 20/30 or better preoperatively. Centration of the lenticule is critical for the final visual result since decentration may cause symptoms such as diplopia, glare, and halos. Some training is necessary to allow the sur-

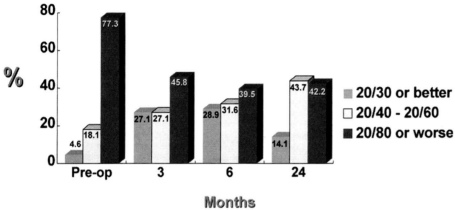

Fig. 16.4. Effect of keratophakia on uncorrected visual acuity.

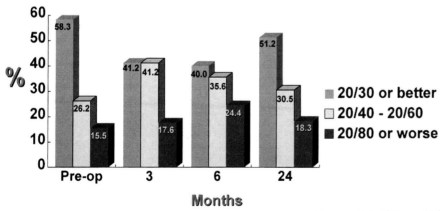

Fig. 16.5. Effect of keratophakia on best corrected visual acuity.

geon to evaluate the positioning of the lenticule, as no reference marks can be done on the stroma, and the patient usually has poor fixation after the superficial corneal disc is resected and put aside.

The table of lines gained and lost (Fig. 16.6) shows that 70.59% of the patients were in the group with +1 to −1 line of visual acuity when the BCVA preoperatively was compared to the 24-month postoperative exam, while 18.82% of the eyes gained 2 or more lines of vision and 10.59% lost 2 or more lines. Irregular astigmatism, due to poor lenticule centration, is the main cause of a loss in visual acuity lines. Contact lens fitting restores preoperative visual acuity in 95% of the patients who lost lines of vision.

Analysis of refractive outcome (Fig. 16.7) shows that, despite being safe, keratophakia does not have high predictability, as with automated lamellar keratoplasty (ALK) that also depends on the microkeratome. In the majority of cases, the lenticules came from myopic eyes that have undergone keratomileusis. Calculation of the refractive power of these lenticules depended on their size and thickness, according to the nomogram for the correction of myopia. Once their refractive power was estimated, a linear regression formula was used (see Technique) to find out how many diopters they would correct on a hyperopic eye. Both the myopic nomogram and the calculation formula played a role in the low predictability of the final result.

COMPLICATIONS

Keratophakia is considered a safe procedure.[12,26–30] Its main advantage is that it is an extraocular procedure. Eventual complications are therefore limited to the surface. Also, it is a completely reversible technique. The implanted lenticule may be removed or exchanged if the refractive power is not appropriate, its transparency is reduced, or it is decentered. Patients will achieve their prior refraction, as the keratectomy itself does not produce any refractive effect. Rigid gas-permeable or soft contact lens fitting presents no special obstacle, when needed in the postoperative period, since an increase in the anterior curvature does not handicap contact lens fitting as much as central flattening does.

In the 85 eyes studied, the complications observed were the following:

- Irregular astigmatism due to:
    Decentered lenticule: 5 cases (5.8%)
    Irregular cut of the superficial disk:
       2 cases (2.3%)
- Interface deposits: 12 cases (14.1%)
- Epithelium in the interface: 5 cases (5.8%)
- Lenticule opacification: 1 case (1.2%)

Irregular Astigmatism

Irregular astigmatism due to a decentered lenticule may be corrected by repositioning or replacing the lenticule. The most frequent complaint related to visual quality. Computerized corneal topography is useful in identifying this problem. If significant irregular astigmatism is caused by a defective cut of the superficial disc, a contact lens is probably the only medical treatment. A lamellar graft or penetrating keratoplasty are the surgical options used to correct it.

In our group, five eyes had the superficial disc lifted and the lenticule repositioned in an attempt to correct irregular astigmatism. In three eyes, the procedure was successful. The other two eyes were fitted with contact lens.

Irregular astigmatism due to defective resection of the superficial disc was noted in two eyes. A rigid gas-permeable contact lens was fitted in these cases, with full recovery of the preoperative visual acuity.

Under- and Overcorrection

As discussed earlier, the predictability of this procedure is somewhat limited. It depends upon the calculation of the dioptric power of the lenticule removed from the myopic patient or donor eye and its correlation with the needs of the hyperopic eye. Significant under- and overcorrection must be treated by lenticule exchange. Radial and astigmatic keratotomy may also be performed after keratophakia in order to correct residual refractive error.

In this study, four eyes had the lenticule exchanged (in one eye the lenticule was exchanged twice) for the correction of significant undercorrection (three eyes) and overcorrection (one eye).

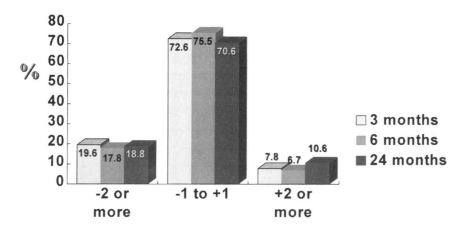

Hospital de Olhos de MG **Fig. 16.6.** Change in BCVA.

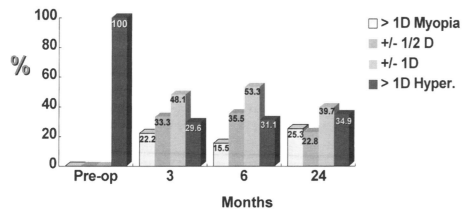

Fig. 16.7. Refractive outcome
Hospital de Olhos de MG (deviation from emmetropia).

Foreign Bodies in the Interface

Interface deposits are a rather common finding in all lamellar procedures. They may consist of metallic particles from the blade, grease from the microkeratome, dust from the air, or mucus from the lachrimal film. Unless the interface is extremely compromised by deposits, complaints or symptoms associated with these deposits are less common and intense than expected. Usually the interface bodies disturb the surgeon more than the patient.

Epithelial cells trapped in the interface may produce significant visual loss and symptoms such as glare. They must be always removed because of the potential risk of island and cyst formation, causing astigmatism and loss of transparency and thus interfering with vision.

Loss of Transparency of the Lenticule

Loss of transparency is rare with fresh-tissue keratophakia. Lenticules kept in corneal preservation medium tend to lose refractive power compared to fresh tissue and have a higher risk of losing transparency.

After its removal from the donor eye and exposure to the environment, the lenticule dehydrates. In our series, lenticules kept dehydrated for a few hours were easily rehydrated after implantation. In one case, a lenticule kept dehydrated for about 24 hr before implantation had to be removed, as it did not recover its normal transparency and interfered with corneal metabolism.

REFERENCES

1. Barraquer JI. Method for cutting lamellar grafts in frozen corneas. New orientations for refractive surgery. *Arch Soc Am Ophthalmol.* 1958;1:237.
2. Barraquer JI. Modification of refraction by means of intracorneal inclusion. *Int Ophthalmol Clin.* 1966; 6:53.
3. Barraquer JI. Keratomileusis and keratophakia. In Rycroft PV, ed. *Corneoplastic Surgery: Proceedings of the Second International Corneo-Plastic Conference.* New York, NY: Pergamon Press; 1969:409.
4. Barraquer JI. *Queratomileusis y Queratofaquia.* Bogotá: Litografia Arco; 1980;409–419.
5. Friedlander MH, Rich LF, Werblin TP, Kaufman HE, Granet N. Keratophakia using preserved lenticules. *Ophthalmology.* 1980;87:687–692.

6. Maguen K, Pinhas S, Verity SM. Keratophakia with lyophilized cornea lathed at room temperature: new techniques and experimental surgical results. *Ophthalmol Surg.* 1983;14:759–762.
7. Krumeich JH, Swinger CA. Nonfreeze epikeratophakia for the correction of myopia. *Am J Ophthalmol.* 1987;103:397–403.
8. Barraquer JI. Keratophakia. *Trans Ophthalmol Soc UK.* 1972;92:499–516.
9. Swinger CA, Barraquer JI. Keratophakia and keratomileusis—clinical results. *Ophthalmology.* 1981; 88:709–715.
10. Friedlander MH, Werblin TP, Kaufman HE, et al. Clinical results of keratophakia and keratomileusis. *Ophthalmology.* 1981;88:716–720.
11. Taylor DM, Stern AL, Romanchuk KG, et al. Keratophakia—clinical evaluation. *Ophthalmology.* 1981; 88:1141–1150.
12. Villasenor RA. Keratophakia—long term results. *Ophthalmology.* 1983;90:673–675.
13. Maguire LJ, Lowry JC. Identifying progression of subclinical keratoconus by serial topography analysis. *Am J Ophthalmol.* 1991;112:41–45.
14. Troutman RC. In Binder P, ed. *Keratophakia in Refractive Corneal Surgery: The Correction of Aphakia, Hyperopia and Myopia*, Vol 23, No 3. Boston, MA: Little, Brown and Co; 1983:11–21.
15. Kaufman HE. The correction of aphakia. *Am J Ophthalmol.* 1980;89:1.
16. Guimarães RQ, Rowsey JJ, Guimarães MFR, et al. Suturing in lamellar surgery: the BRA technique. *Refract Corneal Surg.* 1992;8:84–87.
17. Rowsey JJ. Electrosurgical keratoplasty: update and retraction. *Inv Ophthalmol Vis Sci.* 1987;28(suppl): 224.
18. Newmann AC, Fyodorov S, Sanders DR. Radial thermokeratoplasty for the correction of hyperopia. *Refract Corneal Surg.* 1990;6:404–412.
19. Newmann AC, Sanders DR, Rannan M, Deluca M. Hyperopic thermokeratoplasty; clinical evolution. *J Cataract Refract Surg.* 1991;17:830–838.
20. Feldman ST, Ellis W, Frucht-Pery J, Chayet A, Brown SI. Regression of effect following radial thermokeratoplasty in humans. *Refract Corneal Surg.* 1989;5:288–291.
21. Neumann AC, Sanders D, Raanan M, DeLuca M. Hyperopic thermokeratoplasty: clinical evaluation. *Cataract Refract Surg.* 1991;17:830–838.
22. Durrie DS, Schumer JD, Cavanaugh TB. Holmium: YAG laser thermokeratoplasty for hyperopia. *Refract Corneal Surg.* 1994;10:277–280.
23. McDonnell PJ, Neumann AC. Opinion—radial

thermokeratoplasty for hyperopia. *Refract Corneal Surg.* 1989;5:50–54.

24. Neumann AC, Sanders DR, Salz JJ, Bessinger DJ, Raanan MG, Van Der Karr M. Effect of thermokeratoplasty on corneal curvature. *Cataract Refract Surg.* 1990;16:727–731.

25. Moreira H, Campos M, Sawusch MR, McDonnel JM, Sand B, McDonnel PJ. Holmium laser thermokeratoplasty. *Ophthalmology.* 1993;100:752–761.

26. Troutman RC, Swinger CA, Goldstein M. Keratophakia update. *Ophthalmology (Rochester)* 1981;88:36.

27. Swinger CA. Keratophakia and keratomileusis for hyperopia. In: Saunders DR, Hofmann RF, Salz JJ, eds. *Refractive Corneal Surgery.* Thorofare, NJ: Slack; 1986:495–512.

28. Goldstein M, Troutman RC, Swinger C. Keratophakia: predictability of results. *Cornea.*

29. Troutman RC, Gaster RN, Swinger C. *Refractive Keratoplasty. Transactions of the New Orleans Academy of Ophthalmology.* St Louis, MO: CV Mosby; 1980; 428–449.

30. Troutman RC, Swinger CA, Kelley RJ. Keratophakia—a preliminary evaluation. *Ophthalmology (Rochester)* 1979;86:523.

17

Laser Correction of Hyperopia and Presbyopia

Till Anschütz

The distribution of hyperopic and presbyopic refraction is approximately 70% of all adult refractive errors. Understandably, the surgical treatment of hyperopia and especially presbyopia has aroused a great deal of interest among refractive surgeons worldwide.

One hundred years ago, techniques were described to steepen the central cornea with electrocauterization to shrink peripheral corneal collagen.[1] The results were stable for only a short time. Incisional techniques using peripheral hexagonal keratotomy to decouple the central cornea biomechanically from the periphery[2–4] had limited applicability because of reduced predictability and complications.[5,6] Modifications of nonintersecting spiral hexagonal incisions improved the refractive outcome for the treatment of primary hyperopia, but the need for secondary operations remains high, approximately 30%.[7,8]

Other hyperopic treatments with lamellar techniques such as keratophakia, keratomileusis, and epikeratophakia with donor corneal lenticles were not used extensively because of technical difficulties or side effects.[9–11] Automated lamellar keratoplasty for the correction of hyperopia (H-ALK)[12] simplified the lamellar techniques, but corneal ectasia and iatrogenic irregular astigmatism remained potential problems. Therefore, it was logical to extend the application of photorefractive keratectomy (PRK) and other laser techniques like laser thermokeratoplasty to the correction of hyperopia.

Laser in situ keratomileusis (H-LASIK) as a method of hyperopia treatment has produced encouraging results concerning stability and the preservation of the epithelium and Bowman's layer.

However, there is a long learning curve for surgeons, with inherent technical disadvantages and severe complications.[13–15]

These varied techniques indicate more difficulties with the treatment of hyperopia than with the treatment of myopia. Corneal structure and biomechanics hinder attempts at corneal steepening.

PHOTOREFRACTIVE KERATECTOMY FOR HYPEROPIA

History and Technique

The 7-mm Ablation Approach

The theoretical recontouring of the anterior cornea as a convex lens was first shown by L'Esperance in 1983.[16,17] The principle of hyperopia correction involves steepening of the anterior cornea (Fig. 17.1). This is achieved with an annular-like ablated zone in the corneal periphery. To achieve a sufficient optical zone, a larger ablation zone than in myopic PRK[18–21] is required.

After the first trials of hyperopic PRK on sighted eyes by Dausch and collaborators,[22] Anschütz[23] began performing in 1991 7-mm ablations for hyperopia using a 193-nm excimer laser (MEL 60, Aesculap Meditec, Heroldsberg, Germany), an eye mask holder with a spiral aperture for hyperopic correction, and a suction ring for eye fixation by the surgeon. The scanning-slit technique (Fig. 17.2) of this laser facilitated enlargement of the ablation area. Another advantage was the reduced shock wave impact. The energy of full-sized spot ablations increases to 110 mJ/cm^2 in comparison to 16 mJ/cm^2 in the scanning ablation mode.

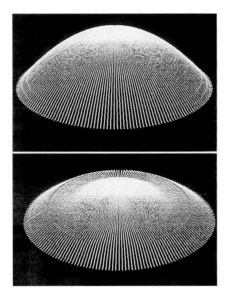

Fig. 17.1. Computer simulation of hyperopic ablation.

Aligned through the rotating spiral mask, the orthogonal scanning laser beam with a slit profile 7 mm in length and 1 mm in width ablated an annular deepening of the peripheral cornea. The energy density of the individual laser beam was 220 mJ/cm^2. The overlap scanning process ensured that the ablation produced smooth surfaces. The aperture rotated at a fixed angle. There was no ablation of the central 1 mm of the cornea. The greatest depth of ablation was at the border of the treated area. The diameter of the zone with full cor-

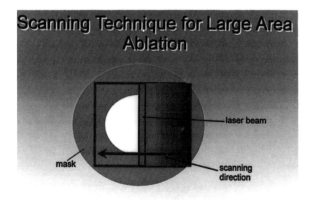

Fig. 17.2. Scanning-slit techniques for ablation of large areas.

rection was 4 mm, and the overall diameter including a transition zone was 7 mm (Fig. 17.3a). There was a 1.5-mm transition zone on all sides, and the repetition rate was 20 Hz. A rectangular field of 7 × 10 mm was scanned with a sweep time of 2 sec. With each sweep, 1 μm of corneal tissue was ablated. The homogeneity and ablation rate were calibrated with a fluence test prior to each procedure.

The 9-mm Ablation Approach

The initial results with the 7-mm ablation zone proved disappointing.[24-27] Suggestions by Serdarevic (presented at the meeting of the American Academy of Ophthalmology, 1989), as well as own observations, enforced our conviction that hyperopic treatments could be improved by widening the optical and ablation zones to 8.5 or 9 mm.[23] This led to a rotating hyperopic template (Fig. 17.4) with a larger optical zone (6 mm) and a larger ablation zone (8.5 mm, later 9 mm) (Fig. 17.3b), which we used for the first time in October 1993. The results were presented at the Society of Cataract and Refractive Surgery Annual Meeting (ASCRS) in 1994.[28]

The scanned rectangular field was enlarged to 9 × 10 mm^2, with a sweep time of 2 sec.

Methods

In all of the author's studies, preoperative testing included cycloplegic and manifest refraction, uncorrected and best corrected visual acuity, slit-lamp examination, fundoscopy, biometry, pachymetry, tonometry, and computerized videokeratography with the Tomey TMS 1 (Cambridge, MA). Informed consent was obtained from each patient after comprehensive verbal and printed explanations and extensive discussions about possible postoperative risks.

Postoperative examinations included the same tests given preoperatively, excluding biometry and pachymetry. Corneal haze was graded from 1 to 4. Since October 1993, preoperative pupil size in scotopic mydriasis was tested with the infrared videoretinoscop (Videorefractor VHP 100, distributed by Tomey AG, Erlangen, Germany). Analysis methods were described previously.[29] Postoperatively, the size of the halo was examined with computerized software, "Glare and Halo" (distributed by Tomey AG). Postoperative examination was carried out on

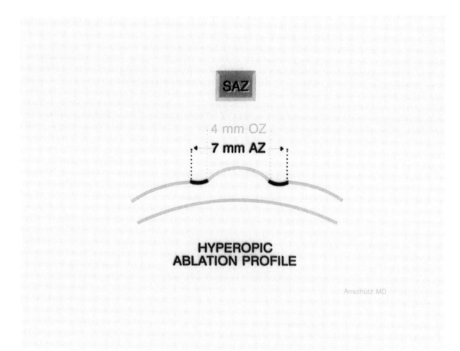

Fig. 17.3(a). Ablation profile of the SAZ: 7-mm ablation zone, 4-mm optical zone.

A

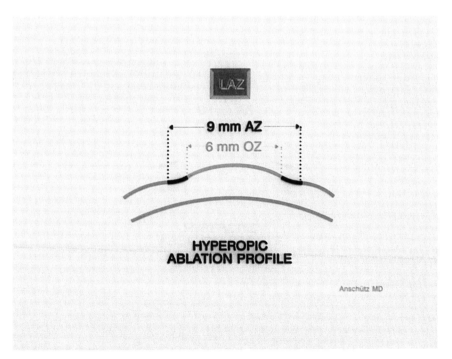

Fig. 17.3(b). Ablation profile of the LAZ: 9-mm ablation zone, 6-mm optical zone.

B

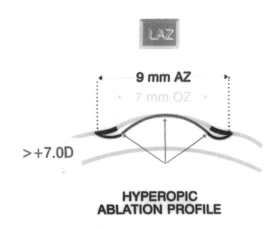

Fig. 17.3(c). LAZ ablation profile of high hyperopic PRK. Increased steepening influences the optical zone through smaller corneal radius.

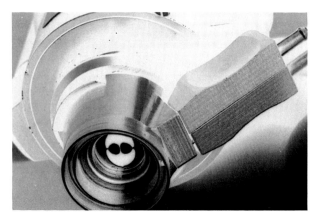

Fig. 17.4. Hand-held eye mask with a rotating hyperopic template providing for a 6-mm optical zone and a 9-mm ablation zone.

days 2 and 3 during months 1, 3, 6, 9, 12, 18, and 24 for the 9-mm large ablation zone (LAZ) group and for the 7-mm small ablation zone (SAZ) group at 30, 36, 42, and 48 months.

The post-PRK regimen in all treated eyes after ablation consisted of viscoelastic agents (Healon, Pharmacia), tobramycin drops (Tobrex, Alcon), protective gels (Actovegin), and disposable soft con-

tact lenses (Acuvue, Newvue) for 2 days. After reepithelialization, the patient started to use fluorometholone drops (FML, Allergan) three times a day for the first 3 months and two times a day for the next 3 months. Tobramicin was administered four times a day until the epithelium was healed. In addition to fluorometholone, patients were treated with heparin drops and protective gels (Actovegin). Topical heparin was used because of studies demonstrating its influence on metabolism in the anterior cornea.[30,31] All refractions, manifest and cycloplegic, were performed with the same chart in the same room.

Surgical Technique

Preoperative surgical management is similar to that in myopic PRK: topical anesthesia with proparacaine, insertion of the eyelid speculum, fixation of the eye in the filament of the operating microscope to find the optical axis, and marking of the optical axis with the 7.5-mm marker for the SAZ groups and with the crosshair 9.5-mm marker for the LAZ groups. After epithelial removal with the hockey knife (Grieshaber), the suction ring was placed after fixation with the hand-held rotating hyperopic mask on the eye (Fig. 17.4). For the SAZ groups the author developed a marker with double concentric rings (2.0 mm and 7.0 mm in diameter). Marking the epithelium facilitates centration of the hand-held masks. For long-term ablation to achieve hyperopic correction, precise fixation of the eye intraoperatively is important. The risk of a "drifting" ablation, with resultant irregular astigmatism and an unpredictable dioptric outcome, is diminished by eye fixation with the suction ring by the surgeon.

Postoperatively, the treated area was immediately rinsed with balanced saline solution. It was then covered with Healon and a therapeutic bandage lens for 12 days.

Results

Aesculap Meditec MEL 60

The author evaluated four groups treated with hyperopic PRK. Groups I and II (SAZ) were treated with the 7-mm ablation diameter. The preoperative refraction ranged from +2.0 D to +4.75 D in group I and from +5 to +8 D in group II. Group I comprised 42 eyes and group II 12 eyes, all treated between April 1991 and October 1992. The ages of the patients ranged from 24 to 70 years (mean, 39 years); the follow-up period was 48 months. Groups III and IV (LAZ) were treated starting in October 1993 with a 9-mm ablation zone. In group III 36 eyes with a baseline refraction ranging from +1.0 D to +6.5 D underwent PRK. In group IV 30 eyes with a baseline refraction ranging from +7.0 D to 10.0 D were treated. The ages of the patients ranged from 22 to 71 years (mean, 36 years). The follow-up period was 2 years.

Small ablation zone–Anschütz During the fol-low-up period of 48 months, both SAZ groups demonstrated increased regression over time. For group I (+2 to +5.75 D) there was a mean regres-sion of 2.1 D and for group II (+6 to +8.0 D) a mean regression of 4.3 D (Fig. 17.5a). The pre-dictability for a range of ± 1.0 D was 62% for group I and a disappointing 1% for group II.[32]

Both groups experienced a very slow return of best corrected visual acuity to preoperative levels. Visual rehabilitation required about 12 months in group I and even longer in group II. The scatter-gram demonstrates relative stability only for low hyperopia (+2.0 to +4.0 D) (Fig. 17.6). In compar-ing the changes in best corrected visual acuity in group I, there was 7% loss of three lines and 24% loss of two lines. The loss of best corrected visual acuity was greater in group II, with 5% loss of four lines and 16% loss of three lines. Postoperative haze ranged between 1.0 and 2.0 and was, on average, lower in group I. The incidence of halo and glare

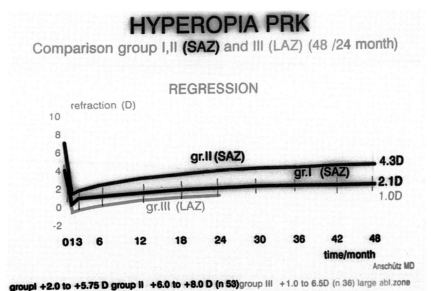

Fig. 17.5(a). Hyperopia PRK regres-sion in SAZ groups I and II (48 months) and in LAZ group III (24 months).

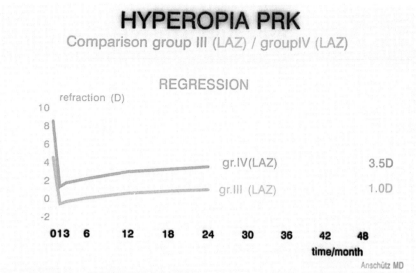

Fig. 17.5(b). Regression in LAZ groups III and IV.

increased with the amount of correction.[29] Results are summarized in Table 17.1.

Large ablation zone–Anschütz There was significantly less regression over a 24-month period after PRK with the large ablation zone than after PRK with the small ablation zone. Group III (+1.0 to 6.5 D) demonstrated a mean regression of +1.0 D and group IV (+7.0 to +10.0 D) a higher regression,

on average, of +3.5 D (Fig. 17.5b). Predictability within ± 1.0 D increased in group III to 84%, and in group IV to 16%.

Best corrected visual acuity returned to preoperative levels much more rapidly in the LAZ groups than in the SAZ groups (Fig. 17.7) because of smooth transition zones and enlarged central zones (Fig. 17.8a–c). There was less loss of best corrected visual acuity in the LAZ groups. In group III there

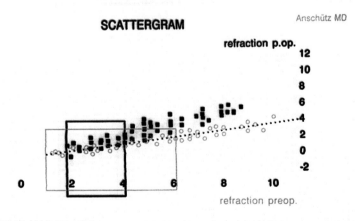

Fig. 17.6. Scattergram of SAZ/LAZ groups I–IV after hyperopic PRK.

was only a 2% loss of two lines and no loss of three or four lines. However, for group IV, the loss of best corrected visual acuity increased to 7% loss of three lines (Fig. 17.9). High hyperopic PRK correction has obviously a limit through reduced optical zone caused to increased cornea steepening (Fig. 17.3c). The incidence of halo and glare decreased with the larger ablation diameter (Fig. 17.10). The reepithelialization time of the LAZ groups was 3.2 days, not significantly higher than that of the SAZ groups. Results are summarized in Table 17.1.

VisX STAR

In 1993 the Food and Drug Administration (FDA)-monitored hyperopic PRK study phase I with the VisX 20/20 laser began with 10 blind patients. This study was done at three sites in the United States. The VisX 20/20 excimer laser projects the laser beam through a spinning spiral shape to masks which spare the central 5 mm of the cornea. Two treatment zones are used, having diameters of 8 mm and 9 mm. The regression using the 8-mm ablation zone was greater than the regression using the 9-mm zone. Because preoperative visual acuity ranged from 20/200 to hand motion, the reliability and validity of the data are limited. All patients achieved hyperopic corrections lasting at least 3 to 6 months. Within the measurement limitations noted earlier, the corrections were quite stable over time.

At the Society of Cataract and Refractive Surgery Annual Meeting in Seattle in June 1996, Jackson[33] presented data on the VisX STAR excimer laser. Twenty-five patients with cycloplegic refractions with SE of +1.0 to +4.0, with +1.0 D or less of astigmatism, best corrected visual acuity of 20/40 or better, and stable refraction for at least a year were enrolled. Ten males and 50 females were treated, with a mean age of 50 years and a mean preoperative SE of +2.50 D (range, +1.0 to 4.0). Epithelial removal of up to 9 mm was accomplished using a Paton spatula either alone or combined with the Amoils rotary epithelium brush. All eyes were patched with an antibiotic steroid ointment, and patients were seen daily until reepithelialization was achieved. FML was used three times daily for 1 week, followed by use of nonpreserved artificial tears. Epithelium healing occurred in 3.56 days (at 1 week, three to seven had a mild myopic refractive shift with marked improvement in uncorrected near

visual acuity). The results are shown in Table 17.1.

Chiron Technolas Keracor 117, Schwind Keratom, Summit Apex Plus

Similar early data have come from Chiron Technolas Keracor 117, which uses a PlanoScan spot beam with an ablation diameter of 8.5 mm and an optical zone of 5 mm to create an annular ablation profile. The first results, from Arbelaez (personal communication), indicate good stability.

The Schwind Keratom laser utilizes a fractal system. The Summit Apex Plus incorporates an optical mask system with an axicon lens.

Novatec Light Blade

Three months of follow-up data from the Novatec solid-state excimer laser were presented by Swinger.[34] PRK was performed on nine eyes that had previous refractive surgery: four myopic PRKs and four failed holmium:YAG thermal keratoplasties. The Novatec Light Blade laser with a small spot (0.3-mm) scanning delivery system and an active eye tracker was used at a fluence of 0.21 μm, a fluence of 100 mJ/cm^2, an optic zone of 6 mm, and a total ablation diameter of 9 mm. Mean preoperative hyperopia of 3.92 D was reduced to −0.11 D at 1 month and to 0.08 D at 3 months. Two eyes lost two lines. At 3 months, six of the nine eyes were within 0.5 D of intended correction and seven eyes were within 1 D.

LASIK FOR HYPEROPIA

In attempting to improve refractive surgery, it was inevitable to extend LASIK to the correction of hyperopia. Ditzen,[13] Knorz,[14] and Condon[15] reported on 12 months data with LASIK. Successful reduction from +8.0 D to plano was achieved in some cases.

Ditzen performed LASIK with the Aesculep Meditec MEL 60 laser and the Chiron Automatic Corneal Shaper in low hyperopes (up to +3.75 D) and high hyperopes (+4 to +9 D). He reported a mean regression of 0.5 D in the low hyperopic group and of 2.5 D in the high hyperopic group at 12 months postoperatively.[13]

Knorz[35] found LASIK to be effective in the correction of hyperopia. The treatment involved using the Chiron Technolas Keracor 116 and the Chiron

Table 17.1. Primary Hyperopia

Study	No. of Eyes	Follow-up (months)	Treatment Zone Ablation Diameter (mm)	Laser Type	Refraction Range (SE) Pre-PRK (D)	Mean Refraction (SE post-PRK (D)
HPRK (I) Anschütz/ Ditzen (1993)	39	12	7	Meditec MEL 60	2.0 to 5.75	1.2
HPRK (II) Anschütz/ Ditzen (1993)	32	12	7	Meditec MEL 60	6.0 to 10.0	3.1
HPRK (I) Anschütz (1996)	42	48	7	Meditec MEL 60	2.0 to 4.75	2.1
HPRK (II) Anschütz (1996)	12	48	7	Meditec MEL 60	5.0 to 8.0	4.3
HPRK (III) Anschütz (1996)	36	24	9	Meditec MEL 60	1.0 to 6.5	1.0
HPRK (IV) Anschütz (1996)	14	24	9	Meditec MEL 60	7.0 to 10.0	3.5
HPRK Jackson (1996)	25	6	9	VisX STAR	1.0 to 4.0	±0.27
H-LASIK (V) Anschütz (1996)	6	9	9	Meditec MEL 60	4.0 to 6.0	0.68
H-LASIK (VI) Anschütz (1996)	5	9	9	Meditec MEL 60	7.0 to 10.0	1.7
H-LTK Anschütz (1996)	12	16	Double ring 6.5/7.5 mm	Sunrise Holmium	1.5 to 2.5	0.8

Predictability (%)				Best Corrected Visual Acuity ≥ 2 Lines Loss	Uncorrected Visual Acuity		
± 0.5	± 1.0	± 2.0	± 3.0		≥ 20/20	≥20/25	≥20/40
10	66	77	90	21%	10%	21%	51%
0	28	31	63	37%	0%	13%	31%
18	62	85	98	31%	10%	33%	64%
0	1	8	64	71%	0%	8%	25%
32	84	96	100	2.7%	55%	83%	94%
0	14	28	71	28%	7%	21%	50%
80	88	100	100	4%	48%	80%	88%
33	83	100	—	16%	17%	50%	67%
0	20	80	100	40%	0%	20%	40%
8	75	100	—	0%	33%	33%	100%

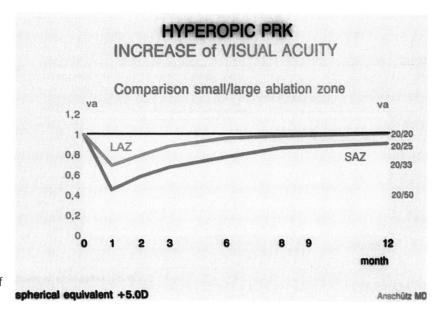

Fig. 17.7. Visual rehabilitation time of SAZ and LAZ groups.

Automatic Corneal Shaper to create a 9- to 9.5-mm flap. The preoperative refraction ranged from +4.0 D to as high as +8.5 D. The eyes, followed up for 12 months, had a mean refraction of +0.7 D (plano to +2 D). Eighteen percent were within +1 D and 100% were within +2 D of the target refraction. Three eyes lost one line of visual acuity but none lost two or more lines.

A prospective hyperopic LASIK study performed with the MEL 60 excimer laser and the Barraquer-Krumeich microkeratome, with 9.0- to 9.5-mm flaps and a follow-up period of 7 months, was conducted by Anschütz and coworkers. In the group treated for hyperopia from +4.0 D to +6.5 D, the mean regression after LASIK was 0.7 D, a result similar to that after PRK with a large ablation zone.

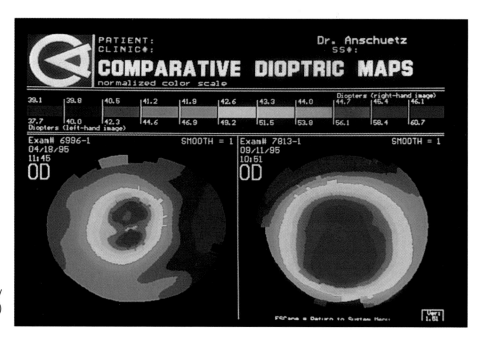

Fig. 17.8(a). Videokeratoscopy of SAZ (left) and LAZ (right) hyperopic PRK.

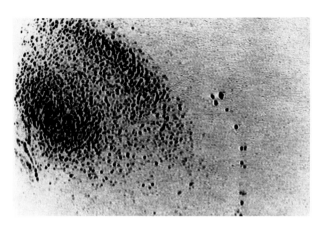

Fig. 17.8(*b*). Peripheral transition zone after LAZ PRK.

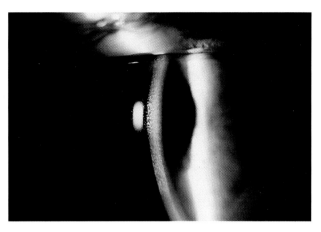

Fig. 17.8(*c*). Enlarged, steepened central zone (slit lamp) after hyperopic PRK.

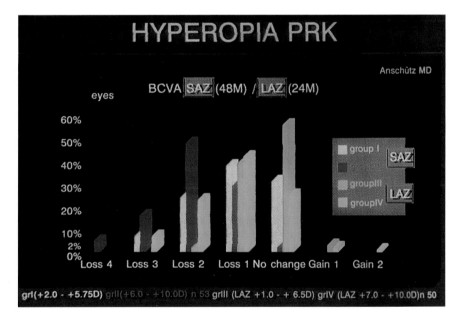

Fig. 17.9. Best corrected visual acuity in groups I–IV.

In the group (VI), treated for hyperopia from +7.0 D to +10 D, there was a mean regression of +2.0 D. In comparison with the non-LASIK group IV (large ablation zone, range from +7.0 D to +10 D), there was less regression after LASIK (Fig. 17.11). In both LASIK groups one eye lost two lines but no eye lost three lines. Complications included one torn flap caused by technical problems (microkeratome, Barraquer-Krumeich), one epithelial ingrowth, and one eye with increasing visual discomfort over time, presumably, due to interface changes.

Hyperopic correction with LASIK requires a 9- to 9.5-mm flap. If the resection is smaller than 9 mm, peripheral ablation can compromise the hinge and reduce additionally the LASIK specific induced smaller optical zone.

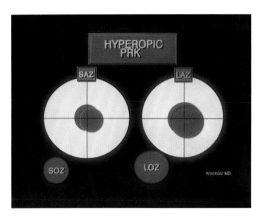

Fig. 17.10. Small optical zones (SOZ) are more susceptible to decentration than large optical zones (LOZ).

PRK FOR SECONDARY HYPEROPIA

The treatment of secondary hyperopia has become a subject of growing interest because of hyperopic shift after RK, myopic PRK overcorrection and hyperopic PRK undercorrection. In several studies starting in 1994, the author compared the effectiveness of PRK and laser thermokeratoplasty (LTK). One study[32] evaluated PRK treatment after previous RK with a mean hyperopic shift of +2.1 D

(range, +1.7 to +2.4 D). The mean subjective manifest refractive change was, on average, −1.9 D after 16 months (Fig. 17.12). Complications included increased haze up to grade 1.5 in two of nine cases. Similar refractive results were obtained after PRK treatment for overcorrected myopic PRK. The initial mean refractive error was +1.86 D; the subjective manifest refractive change after 12 months was −2.0 D (Fig. 17.13). The study of 14 undercorrected hyperopic PRK cases with a mean undercorrection of +1.8 D showed a subjective mean manifest refractive change of −1.6 D after a follow-up period of 16 months (Fig. 17.14). In three cases peripheral haze up to grade 1.5 developed and decreased over time. In all groups, no eye lost more than two lines.[32] Increased haze formation appears to complicate PRK hyperopic treatments in eyes with previus RK or PRK. Results are summarized in Table 17.2.

PRK FOR HYPEROPIC ASTIGMATISM

The author began combined hyperopic astigmatism photoablation in April 1993.[23,27] For the first treatments, the rotating hyperopic template with a 7-mm ablation zone and a 4-mm optical zone was used. This small optical zone produced very poor results, especially with correction of high astigmatism.

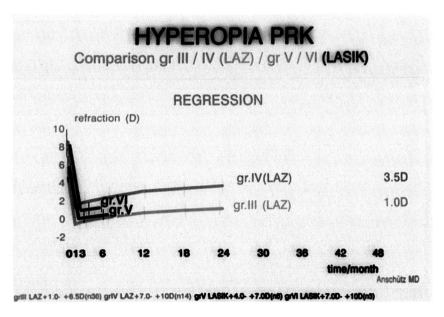

Fig. 17.11. Regression in SAZ/LAZ groups I–IV versus LASIK groups V (+4.0 to +6.5 D) and VI (+7.0 to 10.0 D).

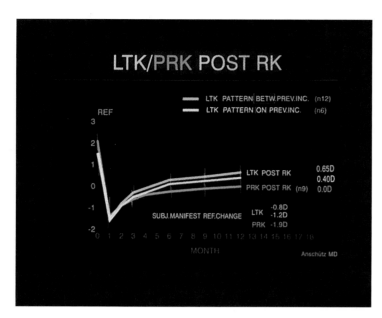

Fig. 17.12. Comparison of regression after PRK and LTK (between and on previous RK incisions) for overcorrected RK.

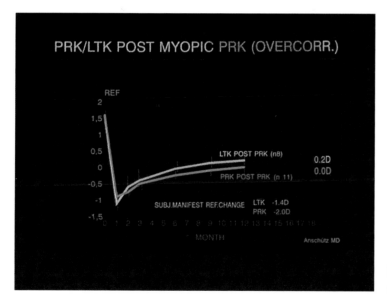

Fig. 17.13. Comparison of regression after PRK and LTK for overcorrected myopic PRK.

Complications were worse than with PRK for hyperopia. To obtain the intended results, it is necessary to perform an oval furrow-like ring zone ablation in the steep meridian. Unequal angle steps and angle distances develop oval ablations because of differences in rotation speed (Fig. 17.15). There are various ablation depths during the rotation in each desired meridian. In myopic PRK the ablation depths are greater in the center and in hyperopic PRK peripherally. These rotating templates are good for correction of cylinders in combination with a spherical component. This elliptical form of the ablation zone further narrowed the central optical zone, with increased visual distortion. Enlarged ablation and optical zones improved the results. In a hyperopic astigmatism PRK study, 12 eyes were treated and followed for a period of 18 months. The preoperative spherical refraction ranged from +1.0 D to +6.5 D, and the cylinder ranged from −1.0 D to −4.0 D. After 24 months the mean

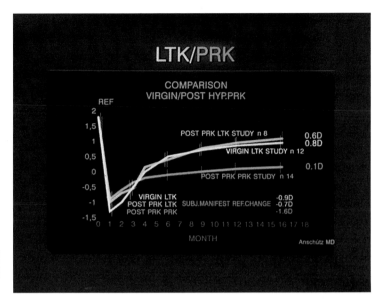

Fig. 17.14. Comparison of regression after PRK and LTK for primary hyperopia and after PRK and LTK for undercorrected hyperopic PRK.

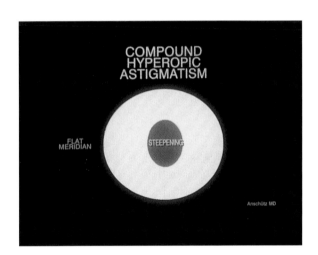

Fig. 17.15(*a*). Circular oval ablation of compound hyperopic astigmatism PRK (both meridians are hyperopic).

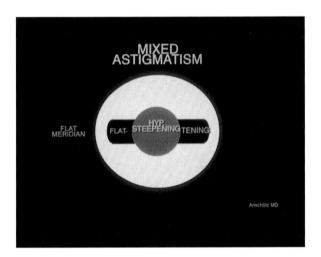

Fig. 17.15(*b*). Circular spherical hyperopia correction (orange color) is combined with rectangular flattening (minus cylinder in the flatter meridian of 0° [blue color]).

spherical refraction was +1.0 D and the mean cylinder was −1.25 D (Fig. 17.16). Higher cylinder corrections were less stable.

Dausch and coworkers[36] reported on the results of combined hyperopic astigmatism PRK in 30 eyes with a follow-up period of 9 months. Six months postoperatively there was good stability, with a mean cylinder of −1.0 D.

The correction of simple and mixed astigmatism, with flattening of only one meridian and no changes in the orthogonal meridian, can be performed with a template (Fig. 17.17) with a slit-shaped opening of 9 × 5 mm. This template allows rectangular band-shaped flattening in the flatter meridian so that the steeper meridian is flattened (Fig. 17.15). The spherical error can be corrected by rotationally

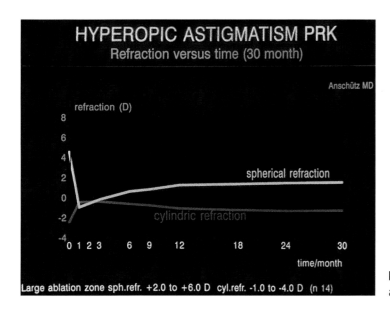

Fig. 17.16. Spherical and cylindrical regression after hyperopic astigmatism PRK.

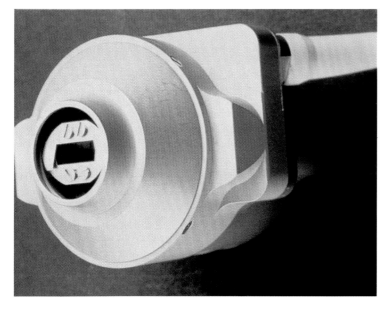

Fig. 17.17. Astigmatism template with slit-shaped opening.

symmetrical *steepening* in cases of mixed *hyperopic* astigmatism or symmetrical *flattening* in cases of mixed *myopic* astigmatism. After 12 months, the mean regression for the spherical refraction was 0.8 D, with a mean cylinder of 0.75 D. The transient 90° change in axis through cylindric overcorrection can produce visual discomfort over a mean period of 2 months, depending on the regression. Longer follow-up is required to evaluate whether cylinderi-

cal corrections of greater than 3 D in mixed astigmatism remain stable.

LTK FOR HYPEROPIA

An alternative laser procedure to correct hyperopia involves thermokeratoplasty using the holmium: YAG Laser. The desired steepening of the central zone is achieved by circumferential coagulation patterns that shrink the stromal collagen in the peripheral cornea.

History and Technique

In his classic cautery experiments in 1898, Lans[1] proved that superficial radial thermal burns change corneal power in rabbits. In 1964 Stringer and Parr[37] reported that the thermal shrinkage temperature of corneal collagen is between 55° to 58°C. This concept was applied to the treatment of keratoconus,[38,39,40] but the refractive effect was only transient[39] and produced corneal scars, pathological changes in the basement membrane with erosions, iritis, melting of the stroma, and even necrosis.[41] The use of radiofrequency probes to perform thermal keratoplasty, which Rowsey and coworkers[42] reported in 1980, was soon abandoned due to lack of predictability and stability.[43]

In 1984 Fyodorov[44] introduced radial thermokeratoplasty for hyperopic correction. The evaluation of Neumann and collaborators.[45] in a retrospective review detected a mean reduction of +3.5 D. Despite increased stability, the disadvantage was the formation of necrotic zones around each coagulation burn.

Lasers were studied for their potential application in thermokeratoplasty.[46–48] Fyodorov[44] studied the use of carbon dioxide and erbium:glass lasers for thermal keratoplasty. Kanoda and Sorokin[49] treated hyperopia over 3 D at a wavelength of 1.54 μm.

In 1990 Seiler and coworkers[48] performed holmium:YAG LTK. They used *contact* devices with a special fiberoptic handpiece and a focusing tip to deliver infrared light (2.1 μm) to the desired locations on the cornea. Treatment consisted of eight spots of irradiation to the circumference of each of two circles centered on the optical axis (Fig. 17.18). Collagen shrinkage of the peripheral cornea has the appearance of a tightened belt (Fig. 17.19).[50] To avoid induced irregular astigmatism, a symmetrical application of radial laser effects is necessary. To achieve symmetrical patterns in the freehand contact method requires experience and precise application.

A modification of *contact* Holmium:YAG thermokeratoplasty was introduced with the Holmium 25 (Technomed, Germany) that uses a special application mask with an optical zone of 8.1 mm.

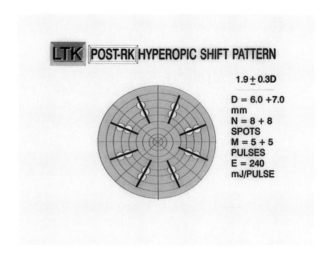

Fig. 17.18. Treatment patterns of LTK. Double ring diameters: *D* = 6.5 + 7.5 mm; spots: *N* = 8 + 8; pulse energy: *E* = 240 mJ/pulse.

The noncontact mode was developed by combining the Holmium:YAG laser with a slit lamp delivery system (Sunrise Technologies, Freemont, CA) (Fig. 17.20).

The principle of LTK is based on empirical studies.[37,51,52] The triple helices of the individual collagen fibrils are heated to the phase transition temperature, also called the *shrinkage temperature*, and the fibers unwind partly from the triple helix configuration into a coiled configuration,[52] depending upon the mechanical properties of the surrounding tissue. The stability of thermokeratoplasty in refractive surgery depends on the long half-life of the thermally processed corneal collagen.[53] Smelser and collaborators[53] reported that collagen turnover in the cornea may occur very slowly, perhaps with a half-life exceeding 10 or more years.

The acute effect of contact LTK has been described based on diferent diameters of spot application.[54] For an inner-zone diameter of 7.5 mm, eight spots result in a 0.64-mm constriction of the inner-zone diameter to 6.36 mm, which leads to steepening of the corneal curvature from a keratometry reading of 40.4 initially to 43.2. Moreira and coworkers[55] evaluated noncontact LTK in 40 human cadaver eyes. They found that the laser treatment produced central corneal steepening with decreased effect as the ring diameter increased. They reported minor endothelial changes at 8 J/cm². Ariyasu and collaborators[56] noted no significant differences in

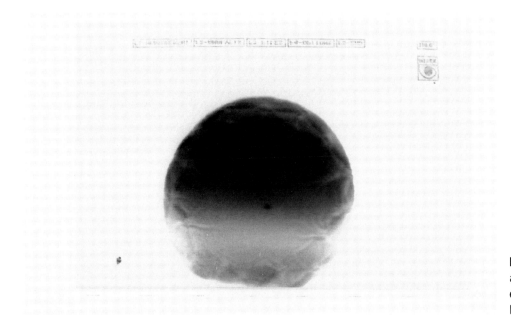

Fig. 17.19. Shrinkage effect after LTK resembling a tightened belt (Schleimpflug slit lamp).

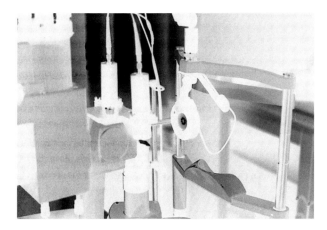

Fig. 17.20. Sunrise slit-lamp delivery system with eight HeNe target lights coincident with the laser spots.

any of the examined endothelial cell indices of poorly sighted human eyes. In vitro experiments with porcine corneas, Koch and coworkers[57] found that at treatment zones of 3.0 and 3.5 mm, central cornea flattening of up to 9 D was produced. A null zone in which no effect was achieved occurred in the 4.0- to 4.5-mm region. At zones of 5 mm or greater, central cornea steepening of over 4 D was achieved. By increasing the number of spots to 16 and by adding 16 additional spots in a second, more peripheral annulus, the effect could be intensified. In compar-

ing the data from Ariyasu, Koch, and Moreira and their associates, it seems apparent that at smaller treatment zones the induced change in central corneal curvature depends greatly upon the number of spots, spot diameter, and pulse energy density.

Surgical Technique

Contact Method

The contact LTK procedure is performed under a surgical microscope with topical anesthesia. An eyelid speculum retracts the eyelid. The patient fixates on an illuminated coaxial ring to allow the surgeon to find the visual axis and to mark the exact location of the coagulation spots with a special optical zone marker. The Holmium:YAG laser from Summit Technology, Inc. (Waltham, MA), is a solid-state laser and operates in 300 μsec at a repetition rate of 15 Hz and a pulse power of approximately 19 mJ with a wavelength of 2.06 μm. The tip of the fiberoptic handpiece, with a cone angle of 120°, is applied orthogonal to the corneal surface, using gentle pressure for delivering up to 60 coagulation spots. The coagulations are shaped as rings with diameters of 6.5 mm and 9 mm.[54,58] Less than 2 sec of exposure is required to treat each spot.

The Holmium 25 YAG laser has a repetition rate of 15 Hz and a pulse power of 20 mJ and 25 pulses.

The coagulation spots are applied with a focusing handpiece on the corneal surface as freehand applications with marked positions or with a metal mask fixed by vacuum with drills for the handpiece (optical zone, 8.1 mm) to enhance the accuracy of the procedure.

Noncontact Method

The Sunrise Holmium:YAG laser operates with a wavelength of 2.12 μm with a pulse power ranging from 100 to 300 mJ and 10 pulses of laser Holmium light at a repetition rate of 5 Hz. The noncontact system simultaneously delivers eight Holmium: YAG laser spots in a symmetrical octagonal array. The laser has a central fixation light (LED) and eight helium neon target lights that are coincident with the eight laser spots. The spot size is 580–630 μm in diameter. The ideal treatment is defined as centration of the eight laser beam spots with respect to the pupillary center.[59] A calibrated green HeNe (wavelength, 543 nm) laser focusing beam is used to focus. The patient fixates on the blinking central target, and the surgeon centers the eight spots around the entrance pupil.

The presence or absence of a tear film can significantly affect laser light delivery into the corneal stroma. Therefore, after inserting the lid speculum, it has been recommended to wait 3 min for dehydration of the cornea (Koch D, personal communication, Houston, 1996). To get a smoother surface, the author uses a moistened cellulose sponge for superficial humidification of the cornea. It is also possible to dry the cornea using an atomizer to blow a gentle air stream on the cornea (Lemagne JM, personal communication, Brussels, 1996).

The postoperative regimen involves the application of topical antibiotics. In addition, a protective gel (Actovegin) is used. No corticosteroids or nonsteroidal anti-inflammatory drugs are given.

Results

Primary Hyperopia: Contact Method

Seiler[58] published 9 months of data on 20 treated partially sighted and 20 sighted eyes (patient ages, 25–70 years) in 1991. The coagulations appeared as cones down to the level of Descemet's membrane. Folds of Descemet's membrane were seen postoperatively and persisted for up to 1 year. After 1 year,

the coagulation cones were replaced by transparent tissue with slightly demarcated borders. No vascularization was noted in the coagulation area. None of the patients lost or gained more than one line in best spectacle-corrected visual acuity postoperatively. One eye showed a plaque resembling a Salzmann nodule at one coagulation site. Endothelial counts were identical and had no tendency to decrease over time.[58]

Regression of the refractive effect occurred during the first postoperative months. The 2-year follow-up results of the Phase IIa U.S. FDA trial detected large 1-month posttreatment mean refractive changes (2.9 to 3.5 D) and modest 2-year posttreatment mean refractive changes of about 1.1 D corresponding to an average regression of 65% of the hyperopic correction over the follow-up period.[60–62]

The treatment of moderate hyperopia[62–64] up to 5 D (Fig. 17.21) showed a poor effect, with high regression (mean refractive outcome at 2 years, +3 D) despite high initial overcorrection (mean initial refractive outcome, −2.0 to −3.0 D).

Contact LTK demonstrated loss of two or more lines of best corrected visual acuity in 24% of patients at the 2-years follow-up,[62] possibly due to irregular induced astigmatism.

Primary Hyperopia: Noncontact Method

The first clinical study with noncontact LTK was conducted by Koch et al.[46] The treatments were performed using a Sunrise Technologies corneal shaping system. One group received the *single* ring treatment (parameters: D = 6-mm center line diameter of treatment spots, N = 8 spots in a symmetrical octagonal array, M = 10 pulses) and the other group received *double* ring treatment (D = 6 + 7 mm, N = 8 + 8 spots in concentric skewed, symmetrical octagonal arrays, M = 10 + 10 pulses. The pulse energy (E) was 208 to 242 mJ, corresponding to Fp = 9 to 10.2 J/cm². In this Phase II FDA U.S. clinical study, 17 patients (age: 55.0 ± 7.0 years mean SD, ranged 45 to 70 years) were treated by LTK unilaterally in their nondominant eye for correction of low hyperopia (up to 3.0 D). Ocular measurements (refraction, visual acuity, keratometry, videokeratography, pachymetry, tonometry, glare contrast sensitivity, and specular microscopy) on both treated and control eyes were obtained before

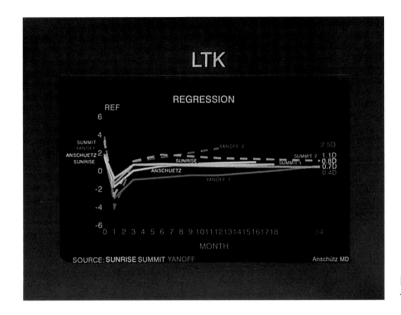

Fig. 17.21. LTK: results of different investigators.

treatment and at follow-up times extending to 18 months posttreatment. In the one-ring group, a mean change in manifest refraction of -0.6 D ($\pm$ 0.3 D) was discovered after 12 months. In the two-ring group, a mean change of -1.6 D ($\pm$ 0.6 D) after 18 months resulted in a mean spherical refractive correction of -0.8 D. The cylindrical component increased from the pretreatment mean of -0.47 D to -1.09 D at 1 day and then regressed/relaxed to a mean reduced astigmatism of 0.08 D at 18 months posttreatment. Cylinder axes were unchanged by LTK treatment for most patients with preexisting astigmatism. None of the patients lost two or more lines of best corrected distance visual acuity.[46]

Anschütz[65] evaluated 12 eyes (5 female 7 male; ages 32 to 56 years; initial refraction 1.5 to 2.25 D mean $\pm$ 1.9 D). In all cases, the treatment parameters were identical double-ring thermokeratoplasty (D = 6.5 + 7.5 mm diameter, N = 8 + 8 spots, M = 5 + 5 pulses, E = 240 mJ/pulse energy, D = 600 μm). The mean manifest refractive change was -1.0 D at 16 months postoperatively (Fig. 17.21). The initial overcorrection in the first 4 weeks was, on average, -1.3 D. Videokeratoscopy demonstrated steepening with rosette-like borders (Fig. 17.22). One patient complained of having much pain for 3 days. The evaluation showed significantly higher regression in patients under 40 years of age. Results are listed in Table 17.1.

Secondary Hyperopia: Noncontact Method

Anschütz assessed the effect of LTK for treatment of iatrogenic hyperopia.[67] The treatment parameters were the same as for LTK for correction of primary hyperopia.

In one study, *RK* eyes that experienced hyperopic shifts of a mean of 1.8 D (n = 6) at 12 months of follow-up were treated with LTK. In three eyes, the laser spot was applied *between* previous incisions, and, in three other eyes, it was applied *on* previous RK incisions. In the latter group, there was a mean refractive change of -1.2 D; in the former group, the mean manifest refractive change was -0.8 D (Fig. 17.12). A study of LTK for *myopic PRK overcorrections* (mean, $+2.3$ D) demonstrated a significant reduction of hyperopia and a mean manifest refractive change of -1.4 D (Fig. 17.13).

Another study (initial refraction mean of $+1.8$ D, n = 12, 16 months of follow-up) to determine the potential of LTK in the treatment of regression-induced undercorrection after hyperopic PRK demonstrated initial good results during the first 4 months. However, over 16 months there was

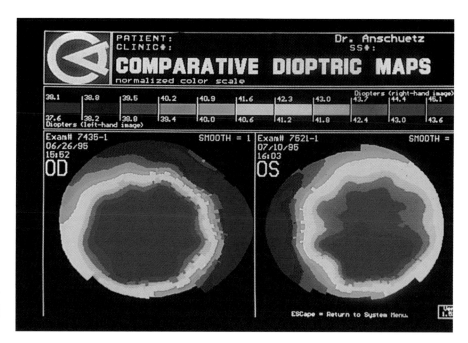

Fig. 17.22. Videokeratoscopy after LTK showing large steepening and typical rosette-like borders.

increased regression. The postoperative refraction after LTK retreatment approached the preoperative value, with a mean subjective manifest refractive change of −0.6 D (Fig. 17.14).

Results are summarized in Table 17.2.

The efficacy of LTK in flat, thin corneas after myopic PRK supports the conclusion that central cornea thickness is an important factor, together with patient age and central keratometer values.

Hyperopic Mixed Astigmatism

LTK patterns for treatment of mixed or hyperopic astigmatism consist of spots along the flat axis. The shrinking effect in the flatter meridian creates an initial marked reduction in astigmatism. However, in most cases, the effects disappear after several weeks and stability is poor.[26] This technique seems to have very limited applicability.

PRK OF PRESBYOPIA

Refractive surgery to correct presbyopia is a universal challenge. Failure to halt the loss of accommodation produces new presbyopic patients each year: in North America, an estimated 4 million; Europe, about 10 million presbyopes.[66] Due to the increasing use of refractive surgery, more must be known about the iatrogenic presbyopic shift after myopic RK or PRK. Surgical approaches to deal with this problem have been developed in addition to treatment with glasses or contact lenses.

History

On the basis of observations of *unintentionally* increased near vision after RK and after early postoperative myopic PRK through increased depth of focus, Anschütz developed a model to conserve residual myopia through bifocal or multifocal photoablation of the cornea. In 1990 the author introduced this model of combined myopia/presbyopia treatment with the excimer laser.[67] After presenting the first data on treated patients in 1991,[68–70] 2 year data was presented in 1993 at the Society of Cataract and Refractive Surgery Annual Meeting.[71]

In 1992 Anschütz presented a model of simple presbyopia PRK.[72,73] The results of a 1992 emmetropia/presbyopia and combined hyperopia/presbyopia study were published in 1994.[23]

Principles and Technique

The principle of the bifocal or multifocal intraocular lens (IOL) or contact lens[74,75] was the basis for *combined myopia-presbyopia PRK*. Considering the possibilities of a *central* near zone with a peripheral distance zone and a *peripheral* concentric near zone with a central distance zone, the author performed physical experiments with a model eye (manufactured by Zeiss) and an infrared laser beam. As a result of these experiments, the author favored a *sector* near zone. This zone represented part of a concentric zone but reached 2 mm within the central zone. The area covered about 2.0 mm^2, which was sufficient for near vision because the energy on the retina is proportional to pupil size.[76] A concentric multifocal zone[77] is not ideal for the human cornea because of the need for smooth transitions zones. Areas smaller than 1.4 mm^2 limit visual acuity to less than 20/20.[78] A small distant central zone 1.5 mm in diameter and an additional transition zone of nearly 0.5 mm implies a pupil diameter of at least 4 mm. The known age-dependent changes that reduce pupil size[79,80] lead to problems due to too small pupils and progressive regression of the small distant zone, with increasing loss of distant acuity and more glare, halo, and scatter effects through the larger border area of the concentric zone. Anschütz abandoned the concentric multifocal concept because of the dependency on large pupil size for optimal performance.[81] The processing of multifocal images is based on the ability of *pseudoaccommodation*.[82–84] Physiological aspects of vision and the interaction of multifocal images have not yet been thoroughly investigated, although some reports seem to confirm the benefit of a bifocal system.[85] Parallel perception is not possible. The author uses the term *polymetropia* to describe the ability of pseudoaccommodation to use a multifocal cornea and to produce distant and near vision. In considering the two types of pseudoaccommodation, *near* dominance and *distant* dominance, two concepts are used: a peripheral-sectorial near zone with pupil size dependence and far visual dominance and a central near zone with less pupil size dependence on visual dominance. The ray model (Fig. 17.23) demonstrates the situation after monofocal myopic PRK and after multifocal myopic/presbyopic PRK. This method should improve the advantages of monofocal myopic PRK with defined, sculptured different corneal power zones. The author started this myopia/presbyopia study in 1991 and to date about 560 patients have been treated.

The technique combining myopic PRK with sectors of under-treated or untreated cornea corresponding to a spherical equivalent of −2.0 to −3.0 D

of residual myopia is called *passive* myopization. Simple presbyopia treatment requires *active* myopization by steepening the cornea to create positive sphericity.

In the early postoperative phases of hyperopic PRK, as with LTK, near vision increases for a short time. The ray model visualizes the near rays pre- and postoperatively for presbyopia treatment (Fig. 17.23b). The physical principles are based on the Gaussian system of cardinal points in the Gullstrand schematic eye,[86] the work of Listing,[87] and the conoid of Sturm (Fig. 17.24). Trials were performed by Anschütz with experimental polymethyl methacrylate (PMMA) contact lenses to simulate presbyopia treatment resulting in partial steepening using a defined sectorial hyperopic ablation with a asymmetric, positive aspheric curvature (Fig. 17.25). After initial treatments with a combination of a hyperopic rotation mask, a nonrotating presbyopic template and an oval aperture, the author developed a special presbyopic rotating template (Fig. 17.26) to treat simple presbyopia. This emmetropia/hyperopia/presbyopia study was started in July 1992 with a study population of 24 cases.[23]

Methods and Surgical Technique

Important treatment factors were patient selection, education, and evaluation of the patient's ability to pseudoaccommodate. Simulations with multifocal contact lenses (Variations Lunelle) were performed but were not always helpful. Preoperative explanation of risks like regression, vision disturbances, and undercorrection or overcorrections was given to each patient. The usual pre- and postoperative measurements were done, as described previously.[23] The investigational nature of the treatment was made clear to all patients, and every patient gave written consent prior to surgery. The postoperative care and regimen were identical to those for hyperopic or myopic PRK. The postoperative examination was carried out over 48 months. The Aesculap-Meditec MEL 60 laser was used for all treatments. Preoperative surgical management was similar to that for hyperopic or myopic PRK.

For the *myopia/presbyopia treatment* a combination of the myopic eye mask holder from myopic PRK and a sectorial or central template based on a cylindrical hand holder—depending on pseudoaccommodation dominance—was used. Through the

Table 17.2. Secondary Hyperopia

Study	No. of Eyes	Follow-up (months)	Treatment Zone Ablation Diameter (mm)	Refraction Range (SE) Pre-PRK (D)	Mean Refraction (SE post-PRK (D)
for overcorr. RK					
H - LTK			double ring 6.5/7.5 mm		
on prev. incision	6	12		1.3 to 2.1	0.4
between prev. inc.	6	12		1.2 to 2.0	0.65
HPRK	14	12	9	1.6 to 2.3	0.1
for overcorr. Myopic PRK					
H - LTK	8	12	Double ring 6.5/7.5 mm	1.5 to 2.4	0.2
H - PRK	11	12	9	1.6 to 2.5	−0.1
for undercorr. H-PRK					
H - LTK	8	12	Double ring 6.5/7.5 mm	1.5 to 2.3	0.6
H - PRK	14	12	9	1.6 to 2.5	0.1

Predictability (%)				Best Corrected Visual Acuity ≥ 2 Lines Loss	Uncorrected Visual Acuity		
± 0.5	± 1.0	± 2.0	± 3.0		≥ 20/20	20/25	20/40
50	100	—	—	0%	50%	67%	100%
20	80	100	—	0%	33%	50%	100%
85	100	—	—	7%	57%	71%	85%
88	100	—	—	0%	88%	100%	64%
91	100	—	—	9%	73%	91%	100%
0	50	100	—	0%	25%	50%	100%
86	100	—	—	14%	50%	64%	78%

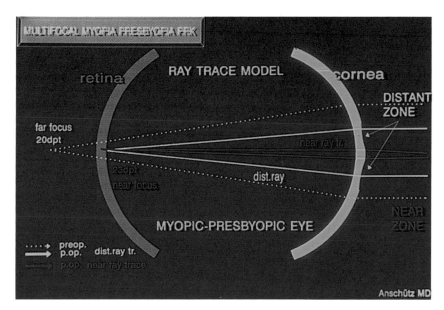

A

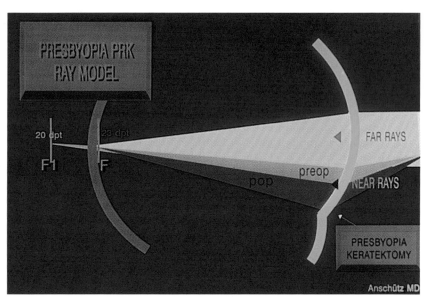

Fig. 17-23. Ray model of multifocal myopic/presbyopic PRK preoperatively and postoperatively.

B

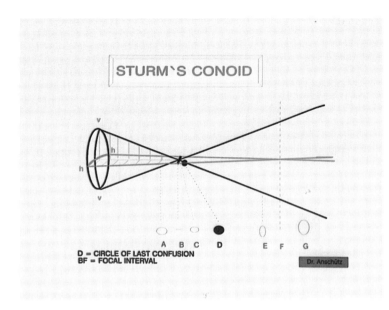

Fig. 17.24. Sturm's conoid: Illustration of the bundle of rays at different points at (*A*). A section of the bundle is in the form of a horizontal oval ellipse. At (*B*) the vertical rays come to a focus while the horizontal rays are still converging (horizontal straight line). Beyond (*B*), the vertical rays diverge while the horizontal are still converging. At first at (*C*), the bundle is a horizontal oval ellipse. At (*D*) the section becomes a circle. The least amount of distortion takes place here. This is called the *circle of least confusion*. Beyond this point divergence of the vertical rays predominates, and an ellipse again is formed (*E*). The horizontal rays up to (*F*) come to a focus; beyond (*G*), both sets of rays always diverge. The section takes the form of a gradually increasing vertical oval.

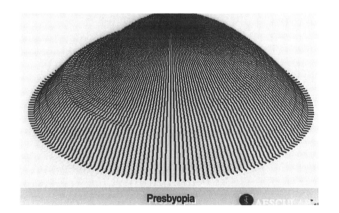

Fig. 17.25. Computerized positive, asymmetric corneal asphericity.

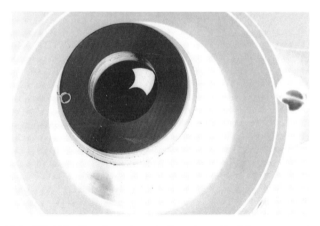

Fig. 17.26. Presbyopic rotating hand-held eye mask with a spear-like aperture.

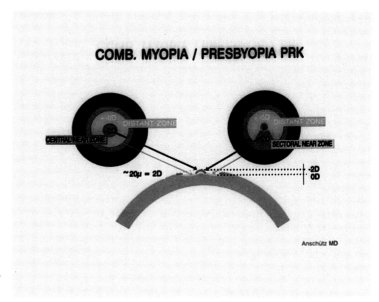

Fig. 17.27(a). Sectoral near zone ablation for combined myopia/presbyopia PRK.

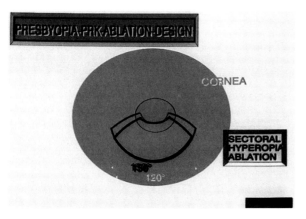

Fig. 17.27(b). Various ablation angles for sculpting semilunar-like corneal steepening.

mask a sectorial or central near zone with an expected residual value of -2.0 -3.0 D and a distant zone with an expected residual value of plano was created (Fig. 17.27a).

For the *emmetropia/presbyopia PRK* and the *hyperopia/presbyopia PRK* initially a combination of hyperopic hand-held rotating mask and a nonrotating presbyopic template with an oval opening was used. Later the rotating presbyopia mask (Fig. 17.26) with a spear-like aperture was designed. Using different rotation speeds, it is possible to create different ablation depths during rotation in the

desired sectorial zone and to achieve a smooth, softer transition to the untreated zones. This system also enables various ablation angles between 80° and 150° to achieve varied, positive, asymmetric asphericity (Fig. 17.27b) in the lower or upper half of the cornea.

Results

Myopia/Presbyopia PRK

The multifocal myopia/presbyopia PRK study, started in April 1991 and followed for 5 years, shows a significant improvement in uncorrected near visual acuity.[23] Group I comprised 31 eyes with a refraction from -2.0 to -6.0 D. Group II comprised eyes with a refraction from -6.5 to -10.0 D. The age range was 45 to 64 years (mean, 54 years) with an intended presbyopic correction from 2.0 to 3.0 D. In group I, after an evaluation of 24 cases, there was a regression similar to that observed after monofocal ablation. The immediate postoperative overcorrection was, on average, $+1.5$ D, and visual acuity regressed over time to a mean of -1.5 D (Fig. 17.28). Average uncorrected near visual acuity after multifocal PRK was J3. A comparative monofocally treated group showed poorer corrected near visual acuity (1.5 lines less). Causes for the decrease in near visual acuity are an additional age-related loss of near visual acuity and

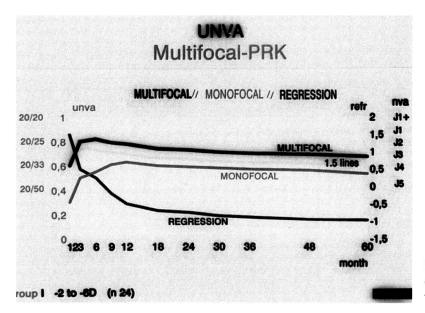

Fig. 17.28. Multifocal myopia/presbyopia. Comparison of monofocal and multifocal treatments and near visual acuity.

epithelialization of the near zone. In the monofocal group after 12 months, there was improved near visual acuity depending on myopic regression. However, over 5 years, there was also a loss of near visual acuity due to age. In the high myopia group II (−6.5 to −10.0 D) similar effecs were seen. However, the higher regression (up to −4.0 D) helped to balance the difference between multifocally and monofocally treated eyes, so the results were not very different. The higher regression in group II led to diminished distant vision without correction and to enhancement of near visual acuity. The comparison of monofocally and multifocally treated eyes with the defocus test (Fig. 17.29) showed significantly better near vision in the multifocally treated eyes. The haze density varied in the different refraction zones. The near zone that had less photoablation developed less scarring. Iron lines were visible in some eyes at the border of the near and distance ablation zones. There was a small loss of contrast sensitivity in the sectorial near zone patients. Retreatment of multifocally treated eyes 2 years later revealed residual sculpting with different surfaces after epithelial removal. Videokeratoscopy (Fig. 17.30) showed the different ablation zones and, over time, the disappearing superficial multifocal effect. Measurement of near visual acuity with full distant correction revealed 1.6 lines better near visual acuity compared to that achieved with mono-

focal treatment. An explanation of this result could be the slower regression rate in the sectorial near zone and different densities of the stroma. With the laser interferometer (Class 1000) it was possible to demonstrate differences in the remaining multifocal refraction zones.

Fifty-four percent of the multifocally treated patients developed more halo and glare effects in the first 6 months, when compared with the monofocally treated patients. After 6 months these adverse effects were reduced in most cases. The decrease in the point spread function measured with the laser interferometer was not marked. After approximately 4 weeks, the brain adapted in most patients to multifocal images. Twenty percent of the patients complained for 3 or 4 months about ghosting and double contours, which later disappeared. In patients with central near zones the complaints about monocular diplopia were significantly more frequent. Patients with small pupils (<2 mm) had poorer distant visual acuity without correction. In four cases the near zone was too large, with residual far visual problems. In three cases the pupil was smaller than 2 mm, with reduced postoperative near visual acuity without correction. Visual recovery in multifocally treated eyes was 2 to 3 weeks longer than that of comparable monofocal myopic treated eyes. In a series of 23 cases, one eye lost two lines through decentration.

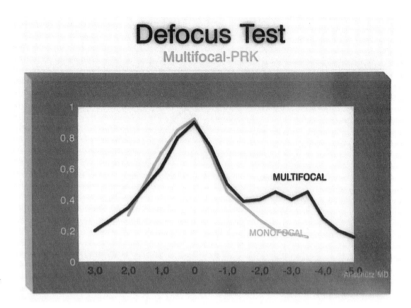

Fig. 17.29. Defocus test. Comparison of monofocal and multifocal ablation.

Simple Presbyopia and Hyperopia/Presbyopia PRK

This presbyopia study started in July 1992 with 20 cases. The age range was 48 to 63 years, and the preoperative baseline refraction varied from plano to +8.0 D. There were three groups: group Ia, plano to +0.5 D; group Ib, +1.0 to +4.75 D; group II, +5.0 to +8.0 D. After a follow-up period of 3 years,

group Ib demonstrated a mean regression of nearly +1.8 D and a mean uncorrected near visual acuity of J4 at a reading distance of 37 cm. Group II developed significantly higher regression of +4.2 D and a significantly lower disappointing near visual acuity of J8. The best results were found in the emmetropic/presbyopic group, with an enhanced

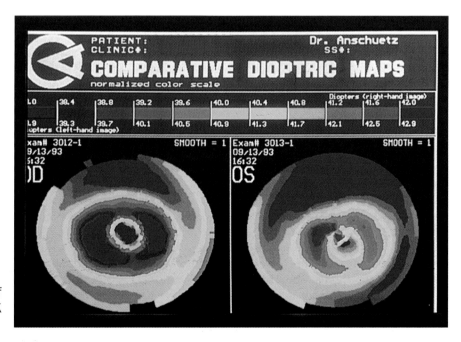

Fig. 17.30(a). Videokeratoscopy of multifocal myopia/presbyopia PRK with a sectorial near zone.

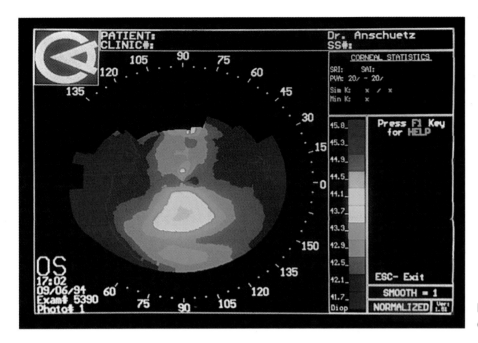

Fig. 17.30(b). Videokeratoscopy of emmetropia/presbyopia PRK.

uncorrected near visual acuity of 2.3 lines over a follow-up period of 36 months (Fig. 17.31). The sectoral steepening of the near zone is visible on postoperative corneal topography (Fig. 17.30b).

Presbyopic PRK affected distance vision during the first 3 months. There was reduced distance vision and improved near vision. After 3 months, distance vision returned to preoperative levels. In this emmetropic simple presbyopic group no eye lost two or more lines. The main problem was that 50% of all treated patients complained about ghost images and double contours, which disappeared by 6 months. In 5% of the treated patients, this effect remained. These phenomena could be caused by the

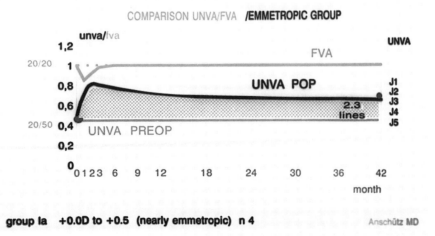

Fig. 17.31. Emmetropia/presbyopia PRK: distance and near vision.

appearance of a bundle of rays at different points, the known adapting phase of pseudoaccommodation, and the slight iatrogenic irregular astigmatism.

An interesting observation concerned the age of treated patients. Less serious problems with ghosting images occurred in patients 45 to 55 years of age. This reinforces the suggestion that the ability to pseudoaccommodate is a complex learning process related to age and intelligence. Most patients over age 60 had problems processing multifocal images. In our study 68% of patients over 70 years complain about ghosting, whereas under 60 years there are only 7%. Recent scientific findings that progressive age diminishes intellectual ability[88] could be an additional explanation.

The first 1-year results of the European multicenter study from Smecka and coworkers (personal communication) demonstrate similar observations. The investigators detected minimal diplopia in the first 2 months. Alteration in distance vision through a small myopic cylindrical shift (−0.5 to −1.0 D spherical, −0.5 to −1.25 D cylindrical) was also seen in the first 2 months. In the group of 35 eyes (initial correction −0.25 to +0.5 D), they reported a very stable correction for near vision within ± 0.25 D of the intended correction. Regression of 0.75 D was observed in only one case. In most cases, semilunar presbyopic PRK was performed in the upper half of the cornea.

After treating more than 560 myopic/presbyopic patients, the author concluded that this method can be used to avoid the disagreeable presbyopic shift after myopic PRK of presbyopic patients and to improve uncorrected near visual acuity. An alternative treatment method to compensate for the presbyopic shift after myopic PRK is unilateral PRK, which conserves myopia at one eye (monovision). The risks are aniseikonia and the anisometropia greater than 1.5 D.[72] After poor outcomes, the author abandoned unilateral PRK in favor of multifocal myopia/presbyopia treatment. However, the dependence on near/far dominance and pupil size, as well as the risks of scatter and halo effects, ghosting, reduced far visual acuity, and regression, must be assessed.

These factors are also important in the symptomatic management of primary or symptomatic presbyopia. This treatment requires careful patient selection. The processing of multifocal images, with the alternate suppression of far and near foci, seems to be a learning process and requires certain intellectual abilities. Treated patients with these abilities are very satisfied with their regained ability to read without glasses.

Tests to exclude patients with the inability to pseudoaccommodate could be helpful to improve the success of treatment. The relation of the treatment to age and intelligence is evident.

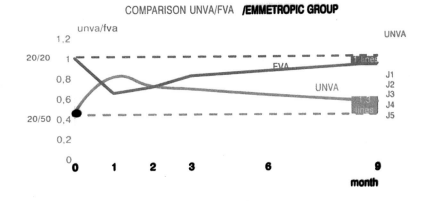

Fig. 17.32. Presbyopic LTK: distance and near vision.

LTK for Presbyopia

There are numerous reports[46,65] of unintentional improvement in near visual acuity after hyperopic LTK treatments. The reason is the increased depth of focus through asphericity and multifocality at the cornea. Unfortunately, these effects are not stable. The author's trials involving eyes with different treated diameters for simple presbyopia without a myopic shift were unsuccessful (Fig. 17.32). Also, sectorial treatments similar to presbyopic PRK models showed only limited applicability. Most of the eyes must be retreated. Few patients are satisfied for a long time.

REFERENCES

1. Lans LJ. Experimentelle Untersuchungen über die Entstehung von Astigmatismus durch nicht-perforierende Corneawunden. *Albrecht Von Graefes Arch Klin Exp Ophthalmol.* 1898;45:117.
2. Yamashita T, Schneider ME, Fuerst DJ, Pearce WJ. Hexagonal keratotomy reduces hyperopia after radial keratotomy in rabbits. *J Refract Surg.* 1986;2:261–264.
3. Gilbert ML, Friedlander M, Aiello JP, Granet N. Hexagonal keratotomy in human cadaver eyes. *J Refract Surg.* 1988;4:12–14.
4. Neumann AC, McCarty GR. Hexagonal keratotomy for correction of low hyperopia: preliminary results of a prospective study. *J Cataract Refract Surg.* 1988; 14:265–269.
5. McDonnell PJ, Lean JS, Schanzlin DJ. Globe rupture from blunt trauma after hexagonal keratotomy. *Am J Ophthalmol.* 1987;103:241–242.
6. Basuk WL, Zisman M, Waring GO III, et al. Complications of hexagonal keratotomy. *Am J Ophthalmol.* 1994;117:37–49.
7. Grandon SC, Sanders DR. Clinical evaluation of hexagonal keratotomy for the treatment of primary hyperopia. *J Cataract Refract Surg.* 1995;21:140–149.
8. Werblin TP. Hexagonal Keratotomy—Should we still be trying? *J Refract Surg.* 1996; 12:613–620.
9. Swinger CA, Barraquer JI. Keratophakia and keratomileusis—clinical results. *Ophthalmology.* 1981; 88:709–715.
10. Barraquer JI. *Keratomileusis. Int Surg.* 1967;48:103–117.
11. Morgan KS, Stephenson GS, McDonald MB, Kaufman HE. Epikeratophakia in children. *Ophthalmology.* 1984;91:780–784.
12. Kezirian GM, Gremillion CM. Automated lamellar keratoplasty for the correction of hyperopia. *J Cataract Surg.* 1995;21:386–392.
13. Ditzen K. Lasik as a secondary operation after normal PRK. Presented at the symposium on "Small Incision Cataract and Refractive Surgery," Rome, 1996.
14. Knorz M. Lasik in the correction of hyperopia, presented at the symposium on "Small Incision Cataract and Refractive Surgery," Rome, 1996.
15. Condon PI. Comparison of ALK and Lasik for the treatment of hyperopia. Presented at the symposium on "Small Incision Cataract and Refractive Surgery," Rome, 1996.
16. L'Esperance FA Jr. *Ophthalmic Lasers*, 2nd ed. St Louis, MO: Mosby-Year Book; 1989:892.
17. L'Esperance FA Jr, Warner JW, Telfair WB, et al. Excimer-laser instrumentation and technique for human corneal surgery. *Arch Ophthalmol.* 1988;107:131–139.
18. Seiler T, Kahle G, Kreigerowski M. Excimer laser (193 nm) myopic keratomileusis in sighted and blind human eyes. *Refract Corneal Surg.* 1990;6:165–173.
19. McDonald M, et al. Excimer laser surface shaping of the primate cornea for the correction of myopia. *Invest Ophthalmol Vis Sci.* 1988;29:310.
20. Dausch D, Klein JR, Schröder E. Photoablative, refractive keratektomy (PRK) for treatment of myopia. A study on 134 myopic eyes with 6-months follow-up time. *Fortschr Ophthalmol.* 1991;88:770–776.
21. Seiler T, Wollensak J. Myopic photorefractive keratectomy with an excimer laser-one year follow-up: *Ophthalmology.* 1991;98:1156–1163.
22. Dausch J, Klein R, Schröder E. Excimer laser photorefractive keratectomy for hyperopia. *Refract Corneal Surg.* 1993;9:20–28.
23. Anschütz T. Laser correction of hyperopia and presbyopia. *Int Ophthalmol. Clin.* 1994;34:105–135.
24. Anschütz T. PRK—results for high hyperopia. *Ophthalmol Times.* 1994;19:7.
25. Anschütz T. Hyperopia-PRK. *Ophthalmol Times.* 1994;8:21.
26. Anschütz T, Ditzen K. Hyperopia PRK results after 1 year. Presented at the ninth European Congress of Cataract and Refractive Surgery (ESCRS), Paris, 1993.
27. Anschütz T. Möglichkeiten und Grenzen der refraktiven Hornhautchirurgie mit dem Excimerlaser. *Augenärztl Fortb.* 1995;18:66–73.

28. Stein HA, Cheskes A, Stein RM. *The Excimer.* Thorofare, NJ: SLACK; 1994:133.

29. Anschütz T. Pupil size, ablation diameter and halo incidence after photorefractive keratectomy. Best papers of session, ASCRS symposium on Cataract, IOL. *Refract Surg.* 1995;1–4.

30. Vannas S. Experimental and clinical investigations into the effect of locally administered heparin on the eye. *Acta Ophthalmol Suppl.* 1952:49.

31. Salomaa S. Experiments with heparin. *Acta Ophthalmol.* 1952;30:33.

32. Anschütz T. Hyperopia PRK: possibilities and limitations presented at the symposium "Small Incision Cataract and Refractive Surgery," Rome, 1996.

33. Jackson WB. Excimer-laser surgery for the correction of low hyperopia of using the VisX Star. Presented at the Society of Cataract and Refractive Surgery Annual Meeting, Seattle, 1996.

34. Swinger C. Surface photorefractive keratectomy for correction of hyperopia using the Novatec laser. Presented at the Society of Cataract and Refractive Surgery Annual Meeting, Seattle, 1996.

35. Knorz M. LASIK found to be effective in the correction of hyperopia. *Ocular Surgery News* 1996;7: 34–35.

36. Dausch D, Klein R, Landesz M, Schröder E. Photorefractive keratectomy to correct astigmatism with myopia or hyperopia. *J Cataract Refract Surg.* 1994; 20(suppl):252–257.

37. Stringer H, Parr J. Shrinkage temperature of eye collagen. *Nature.* 1964;204:1307.

38. Aquavella J. Thermokeratoplasty. *Ophthalmic Surg.* 1976;4:39–48.

39. Gassert AR, Schaw EL, Kaufman HE, et al. Thermokeratoplasty. *Trans Am Acad Ophthalmol.* 1973;77: 441.

40. Kennas R, Dingle J. Thermokeratoplasty for keratoconus. *Ophthalmic Surg.* 1975;6:89–92.

41. Aquavella J, Smith R, Schaw E. Alternations in corneal morphology following thermokeratoplasty. *Arch Ophthalmol.* 1976;94:2082–2085.

42. Rowsey JJ, Gaylor JR, Dahlstrom R, et al. Los Alamos keratoplasty techniques. *Contact Intraocular Lens Med J.* 1980;6:1–12.

43. Rowsey JJ, Doss JD. Preliminary report of Los Alamos keratoplasty techniques. *Ophthalmology.* 1981; 88:755–760.

44. Fyodorov S. Corneal curvature change using energy of laser radiation. Russian patent no. 822407, 1980.

45. Neumann AC, Fyodorov S, Sanders DR. Radial thermokeratoplasty for the correction of hyperopia. *Refract Corneal Surg.* 1990;6:404

46. Koch DD, Berry MJ, Vassiliadis AJ, et al. Non-contact holmium:YAG laser thermal keratoplasty. In: Salz JJ, ed. *Corneal Laser Surgery.* St. Louis, MO: Mosby C.V.; 1995:247–254.

47. Peyman GY, Larson B, Raichand M, et al. Modification of rabbit corneal curvature with use of carbon dioxide laser burns. *Ophthalmic Surg.* 1980;11: 325–329.

48. Seiler T, Matallana M, Bende T. Laser thermokeratoplasty by means of a pulsed holmium:YAG laser for hyperopic correction. *Refract Corneal Surg.* 1990;6: 328–333.

49. Kanoda AN, Sorokin AS. Laser correction of hypermetropic refraction. In Fyodorov SN, ed. *Microsurgery of the Eye: Main Aspects.* Moscow: MIR Publishers; 1987:

50. Schachar RA. Radial thermokeratoplasty. *Refract Surg.* 1990;3:47

51. Allain JC, Bazin S, Lelous M, et al. Isometric tensions developed during the hydrothermal swelling of rat skin. *Connect Tissue Res.* 1980;7:127–133.

52. McCally RL, et al. Stromal damage in rabbit corneas exposed to CO^2 laser radiation. *Exp Eye Res.* 1983; 37:543–55.

53. Smelser GK, Polack FM, Ozanics V. Persistence of donor collagen in corneal transplants. *Exp Eye Res.* 1965;4:349–354.

54. Durrie S, Seiler T, King MC, et al. *SPIE Proc* 1992; 1644

55. Moreira H, Campos H, et al. Homium laser keratoplasty. *Ophthalmology.* 1995;100:752–761.

56. Ariyasu RG, Sand B, Menefee R, et al. Holmium laser thermal keratoplasty of 10 poorly sighted eyes. *J Refract Corneal Surg.* 1995;11:358–365.

57. Koch DD, Abaca A, Menefee RF, et al. Ho:Yag laser thermal keratoplasty: in vitro experiments. *Invest Ophthalmol Vis Sci.* 1993;34(suppl):1246.

58. Seiler T. Ho:YAG laser thermokeratoplasty for hyperopia. *Ophthalmol Clin North Am.* 1993;5: 773–780.

59. Uozato H, Guyton D, Waring GO III. Centering corneal surgical procedures. In: Waring GO III, ed. *Refractive Keratotomy for Myopia and Astigmatism.* St Louis, MO: Mosby-Year Book; 1992:491–505.

60. Thompson VM, Seiler T, Durrie DS, et al. Holmium: YAG laser thermokeratoplasty for hyperopia and astigmatism: an overview. *Refract Corneal Surg.* 1993; 9:S134–S137.

61. Durrie DS, Schumer DJ, Cavanaugh TB. Holmium: YAG laser thermokeratoplasty for hyperopia. *J Refract Corneal Surg.* 1994;10:S277–S280.

62. Thompson VM. Holmium:YAG laser thermokerato-

plasty. Utilizing the Summit system. In: Salz JJ, ed. *Cornea Laser Surgery*. St. Louis, MO: Mosby-Year Book; 1995:254–274.

63. Yanoff M. Holmium laser hyperopia thermokeratoplasty update. *Eur J Implant Ref Surg*. 1995;7:89–91.

64. Thompson VM. Holmium:YAG laser thermokeratoplasty. Paper presented at the American Academy of Ophthalmology meeting, San Francisco, CA, November 3, 1994.

65. Anschütz T. Refractive surgery of hypermetropia. Presented at CISP, Porto, 1996.

66. Pierscionek B, Weale RA. Symposium International de la Presbytie, Opio, France, June 5–9, 1995.

67. Anschütz T. Model of a combined presbyopia correction with the excimer laser and report of treated cases. Presented at the Third International Congress on Laser Technology in Ophthalmology, 1991.

68. Anschütz T. Multifocal excimer PRK: combined myopia-presbyopia treatment. *Germ J Ophthalmol*. 1992;1(3/4):215.

69. Anschütz T. Multifocal excimer PRK, combined myopia-presbyopia treatment. In: Willital GH, Maragatis M, Lehmann RR, eds. *Laser '92*. Aachen, Germany, Shaker; 1992;94.

70. Anschütz T. Multifocal excimer PRK combined myopia-presbyopia treatment. ASCRS 93. *Seattle Abstracts*. 104.

71. Anschütz T. Multifocal PRK-study, experiences and results of 2 years. Society of Cataract and Refractive Surgery, 1993.

72. Anschütz T. Theoretic model of simple presbyopia PRK. Presented at the DELV symposium, 1992.

73. Anschütz T. Presbyopia PRK. *DOG Der Augenspiegel (Kongressbericht)* 1994;40/2:46–48.

74. Holladay JT, Dijk H van, Lang A, et al. Optical performance of multifocal intraocular lenses. *J Cataract Refract Surg*. 1990;16:413–422.

75. Maxwell WA. Introduction to the current status of multifocal intraocular lenses. In: Maxwell WA, Nordan LT, eds. *Current Concepts of Multifocal Intraocular Lenses*. Thorofare, NJ: SLACK; 1991:3–11.

76. Duke-Elder S. The pupil. In: *Textbook of Ophthalmology*. St Louis, MO: CV Mosby; 1954;555.

77. Krüger RR, McDonnell PJ. New directions in excimer-laser surgery. In: Thompson FB, McDonnell PJ, eds. *Excimer Laser Surgery*. Tokyo: Igaku-Shoin Medical Publishers; 1993:143–144.

78. Koch DD, Samuelson SW, Hatt EA, Merin LM. Pupillary responsiveness and its implications for selection of a bifocal intraocular lens. In: Maxwell WA, Nordan LT, eds. *Current Concepts of Multifocal Intraocular Lenses*. Thorofare, NJ: SLACK; 1991: 147–152.

79. Loewenfeld JE. Pupillary changes related to age. In: Thompson HS, Daroff R, Frisen L, Glaser JS, Sanders MD, eds. *Topics in Neuro-ophthalmology*. Baltimore, MD: Williams & Wilkens, 1973:124–150.

80. Loewenfeld JE. *The Pupil*. Detroit, MI: Wayne State University Press; 1993:295–317.

81. Kadlecova V, Peleska M, Vasko A. Dependence on age of the diameter of the pupil in the dark. *Nature*. 1958;182:1520–1521.

82. Knorz MC, Claessens D, Schaefer RC, et al. Evaluation of contrast acuity and defocus curve in bifocal and monofokal IOLs. *J Cataract Refract Surg*. 1993;19:513–523.

83. Knorz MC, Koch DD, Martinez-Franco C, Lorger CV. Effects of pupil size and astigmatism on contrast acuity with monofocal and bifocal intraocular lenses. *J Cataract Refract Surg*. 1994;20:26–33.

84. Chipman RA. Image formation by multifocal lenses. In: Maxwell WA, Nordan LT, eds. *Current Concepts of Multifocal Intraocular Lenses*. Thorofare, NJ: SLACK; 1991;37–52.

85. Roth EH. Sinnesphysiologische Aspekte des Sehens mit bifokalen intraokularen Linsen. *DGII*. 1992: 266–269.

86. Gullstrand. Hb d. physiologischen Optik von H.v.Helmholtz, ed 3. Hamburg, 1 (1909) Einführung in d Methoden d. Dioptrik d. Auges d. Menschen. Leipzig, 1911

87. Listing JB. Zur Dioptrik d. Auges. In: *Wagner's Handwörterbuch der Physiologie*, vol 4. Braunschweig, Germany: 1853:451.

88. Baltes P, Lindenberger U. Im Alter schwindet die Intelligenz. *Welt*. 1996;8

89. Pace PH, Dufier JL. Vergleichende Untersuchung von weichen, diffraktiven Linsen und dem Monovisionssystem. *Conactologia*. 1992;14D:137–140.

90. Nilsson SEG, Söderqvist M. Monovision mit Einmalkontaktlinsen - eine prospektive Studie über 6 Monate. *Contactologia*. 1992;14D:53–62.

18

Correction of Hyperopia and Hyperopic Astigmatism by Laser Thermokeratoplasty

Mahmoud M. Ismail

Juan J. Pérez-Santonja

Jorge L. Alió

INTRODUCTION

Almost 100 years ago, Lans demonstrated that localized heating of the rabbit cornea can change its curvature by inducing thermal shrinkage of the collagen fibers.[1] However, it was many years later when Gasset and Kaufman clinically applied thermal keratoplasty with a heated metal probe as a refractive procedure for flattening keratoconus. After an initial phase of promising results, the refractive outcome proved to be transient, and serious complications occurred such as delayed epithelial healing, corneal scars, recurrent erosions, and corneal neovascularization.[2-4] Electrosurgical keratoplasty, another variation of the same technique, also failed to improve keratoconic corneas due to regression and serious complications.[5,6]

A few years later, Fyodorov popularized radial thermokeratoplasty (RTK) for the management of hyperopia. This technique was refined, standardized by Neumann et al.,[8,9] and used to treat hyperopia in some cases. RTK consists of thermal radial applications in the midperipheral cornea using a fine Nichrome (NiCr) wire probe. This probe penetrates 80–90% of the corneal thickness to apply a resistive temperature of 600°C. RTK proved to be of little clinical value due to regression of the obtained refractive effect, unpredictable outcome, and complications similar to those of thermal keratoplasty, but with endothelial damage, corneal decompensation, and severe corneal necrosis[7-9] in addition.

With recent advances in laser technology, laser thermokeratoplasty (LTK) was studied for the correction of low hyperopia with higher predictability, avoidance of necrosis, and less regression. Erbium, CO_2, and Holmium(Ho):YAG lasers were investigated as potential candidates for this procedure. The CO_2 laser (10.6 μm) LTK was studied by Peyman et al.,[10] who observed a superficial retraction of the corneal collagen and early regression of the refractive effect. By contrast, the cylindrical profile produced by Yr-Erbium-glass laser spots (1.54 μm) led to extensive penetration and tissue necrosis. Also, during the animal studies on this potential approach, iris damage was substantial due to the high penetrative ability of the Yr-Erbium-glass laser[11] (Table 18.1).

In 1990, Seiler and coworkers[12] reported attaining satisfactory effects using the Ho:YAG laser (2.06 μm) for correction of hyperopia up to +5 D. *Contact* LTK involves peripheral treatment with Ho:YAG spots to achieve collagen contraction without substantial stromal necrosis.[12-14] As a new alternative, *Noncontact* LTK with the laser was proposed for the correction of low hyperopia.[15-17] This approach involves the simultaneous application of eight spots using a slit lamp delivery system without probe application. Laser spot penetration ranges from 60% to 80% of the corneal depth. Animal studies of this technique demonstrated mild, limited endothelial damage localized to the site of spot application.[12-17]

Table 18.1. Depth and Profile Correlation for Lasers with Different Wavelengths

	Penetration Depth	Profile	Wavelength
CO_2	Superficial	Cone	10.6 μm
Yr-Erbium	Massive	Cylindrical	1.54 μm
NiCr	Diffuse	Pyramidal	—
Ho-YAG contact LTK	2/3 depth	Pyramidal	2.06 μm
Ho:YAG noncontact LTK	2/3 depth	Cone	2.06 μm

BASIC PRINCIPLES OF LTK

Thermokeratoplasty involves *heat application in order to induce corneal curvature changes*. This effect is based on the ability of the collagen to shrink by 30–45% of its original length at temperatures ranging from 58°C to 60°C. This thermal process produces dissociation of hydrogen bonds, relative unwinding of the triple helix, and significant dehydration of the corneal stroma.[18–20] By this means, the Holmium:YAG laser spots applied on the mid-peripheral cornea produce a "girdle-like" effect, increasing its central curvature. Simultaneously, this process induces a relative flattening of the peripheral cornea outside the new limbus. The girdle can be clearly seen in the slit lamp as a strand passing from one spot to another, especially in the early postoperative period.

Unfortunately, the potential refractive outcome of LTK has two important handicaps; *tissue necrosis leading to a poor refractive result* and *regression of the obtained effect*.

Tissue Necrosis

The collagen shrinkage occurs at temperatures ranging from 58°C to 76°C. This range is directly proportional to age, i.e., there is a higher temperature threshold for induced collagen relaxation because of more stable cross-linked hydrogen bonds. Higher thermal levels, 79°C or more, definitely lead to relaxation of the collagen and complete loss of its elasticity. These temperature profiles induce significant keratocyte proliferation and accelerating collagen turnover, leading to a shorter half-life of its fibers and consequent deposition of new collagen.[19,21]

Regression of the Refractive Effect

This is the major limitation of LTK. Few hypotheses have been developed to explain considerable regression of the obtained effect. Regression is mainly a biophysical mechanism for the following reasons:

1. Regression occurs significantly more often in young adults, in whom stromal tissue and Bowman's membrane are relatively elastic.
2. Anti-inflammatory drugs can accelerate regression of the LTK effect, especially in the early postoperative period. This is achieved by delaying the healing process after LTK by inhibiting fibroblast proliferation.[22]
3. There is a considerable increase in laser spot diameter after regression due to corneal flattening.
4. After regression, the cornea returns to its original preoperative topographic status. Therefore, the corneal topographic "memory" is contained in Bowman's membrane.
5. For the same reason, hyperopia induced after photorefractive keratectomy (PRK) undergoes a large effect when treated by LTK.

TREATMENT PARAMETERS

The LTK treatment parameters, in both the contact and noncontact procedures, are always adjusted in a diopter/energy pattern. The difference between contact and noncontact LTK is illustrated in Table 18.2. Unfortunately, these energy/diopter maps provided by the commercial laser firms ignore the individual parameters of the patient. The authors believe that the parameters for this technique should be

Table 18.2. Comparison Between Contact and Noncontact LTK

	Contact Technique	Noncontact Technique
Application	Contact manual probe	Noncontact slit lamp
Spot size	Variable	Fixed
Spot delivery	Individual	Simultaneous
Endothelium	Localized damage	Mild
Iatrogenic astigmatism	Possible	Unlikely
Patient fixation	Surgeon control	Autofixation
Energy	19 mJ × 25 pulses	25 mJ × 10 pulses
Pulse repetition	15 Hz	5 Hz
Heat irradiance	Strong focus	Weaker focus

adjusted for each patient before treatment (not only according to the patient's refraction).

PATIENT SELECTION

After careful selection of motivated patients, the risk-benefit ratio of LTK should be explained, including the potential regression of the refractive effect. A complete ocular examination is done, with special attention to the following factors:

1. *Age*: The patient should be 18 years of age or older, with stable refraction for at least 1 year. Older patients are expected to have less regression. Presbyopia should be explained to patients over 40 years of age.
2. *Visual assessment*: Both uncorrected visual acuity (UCVA) and best corrected visual acuity (BCVA) are evaluated.
3. *Intraocular pressure (IOP)*: This is tested to exclude hyperopic patients with narrow angle glaucoma. A poor LTK effect is observed in patients with relatively high IOP.
4. *Refraction*: Subjective cycloplegic refraction is extremely valuable in preoperative evaluation and postoperative follow-up.
5. *Videokeratography*: This excludes patients with irregular astigmatism and controls postoperative follow-up of the regression.
6. *Preoperative pachometry*: Thinner corneas usually respond more to LTK than thick ones.

7. *Systemic steroids use or anti-inflammatory treatment*: This should be avoided at least 2 months before surgery and discontinued for 3 months postoperatively.

SURGICAL PROCEDURE

The authors use the Sunrise gLase 210 laser (Sunrise, Fremont, CA). This is a solid-state, pulsed Ho:YAG laser with a wavelength of 2.1 μm. The laser is connected to a noncontact slit-lamp delivery system (Nikon) capable of projecting eight uniform beams in an octagonal array. Each beam has an individual shutter with adjustable optical zone diameters, allowing a variety of geometrical treatment patterns. Alignment-centration and coaxial focusing of the Ho:YAG spots is controlled by two HeNe laser beams (red and green, respectively).

The procedure takes only a few seconds, but considerable patient cooperation is required. Preparation is as follows:

1. Tobramycin eye drops (Tobrex, Alcon, Fort Worth, TX) t.i.d. for 48 hrs before surgery.
2. One hour before LTK, 1 drop of sodium diclofenac (Voltarén, Ciba-Vision, Barcelona) together with a mild analgesic to control postoperative pain and discomfort.
3. One drop of topical anesthetic (tetracaine chlorhydrate 0.1%, Lab. Cusí. Barcelona) every 15 min.

4. For correction of hyperopia, two or three staggered rings of eight spots each at 6, 6 + 7, or 6 + 7 + 8 mm of the corneal diameter are applied. For correction of astigmatism, two rings of four spots, each at the flattest meridian at 6 + 7 mm of the fixation point are applied (Fig. 18.1). The spot size is 600 μm in diameter. The energy varies from 215 mJ to 245 mJ, selected according to the energy/diopter chart of the laser manufacturer.

5. The energy required for treatment is divided into 10 pulses. The authors believe that there is no clinical difference between 10 and 8 pulses. The calibration of the laser should be done before each treatment.

6. The patient is instructed to fixate on the flickering red light as a guide during the laser application. A plastic lid separator is gently applied for 3 min to dry the corneal surface in order to avoid variations that can affect the penetration of the laser beam into the corneal stroma. For convenience, by an ordinary air pulser can be substituted for this maneuver.

7. After the procedure, the eye is rinsed with antibiotic eye drops (Tobrex) and an antibiotic eye ointment is applied (Tobrex). The patient is sent home with an eye patch for 24 hr. A simple analgesic is prescribed (Aydolid Codeina, Fremost, Spain) for patients with eye discomfort. During the first 3 postoperative days, the patient receives the same topical treatment of tobramycin eye drops and ointment.

CLINICAL RESULTS

The authors performed noncontact LTK on more than 800 patients (Fig. 18.2). However, the controlled study with 18 months of followup includes only 386 eyes of 252 hypermetropic patients[23-25] and 38 eyes of 29 patients with simple and compound hyperopic astigmatism.[26] No sight-threatening ocular complications were recorded during the postoperative period even with repeated treatment. Recovery of the preoperative BCVA took 2 to 6 weeks after LTK treatment. Variable amounts of regression of the LTK effect were evident in all cases.

For hyperopia, the preoperative refraction ranged from +1.5 D to +5 D (mean, 3.8 ± 1.2 D), with associated astigmatism of up to +1.5 D. Regression was almost total in 69 patients (17.8%). However, 282 patients (72.7%) achieved their BCVA without correction or with less than +1.5 D of overcorrection in spite of showing some degree of regression. Mean postoperative refraction was +1.82 ± 0.63 D ($p < .005$). In the first few weeks after LTK, a significant increase in the central keratometry readings

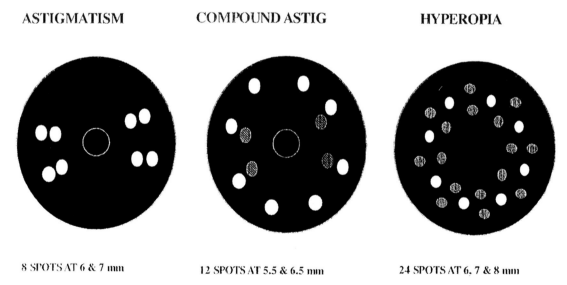

ASTIGMATISM   COMPOUND ASTIG   HYPEROPIA

8 SPOTS AT 6 & 7 mm   12 SPOTS AT 5.5 & 6.5 mm   24 SPOTS AT 6, 7 & 8 mm

Fig. 18.1. Illustration of a spot application pattern.

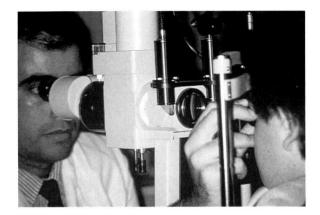

Fig. 18.2. Sunrise Ho:YAG laser model gLase 210.

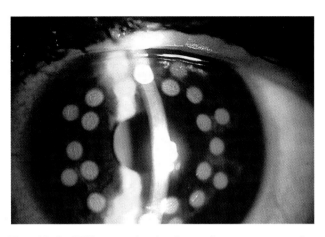

Fig. 18.4. LTK spots in the immediate postoperative period.

was achieved, with subsequent slow regression occurring for up to 1 year postoperatively (Figs. 18.3, 18.4 and 18.5).

Despite regression, videokeratoscopic evidence of corneal multifocality was obtained in many cases, leading to an increase in contrast sensitivity and better near vision. In all eyes, uncorrected visual acuity 18 months postoperatively was significantly better than it was preoperatively. In 41 eyes (10.5%), retreatment was required to achieve a more satisfactory effect between the third and sixth months of the first surgery. The repeat laser treatments were placed between the previous spots.

The residual postoperative cylindrical refraction in simple hyperopic astigmatism cases was +1.67 ± 0.67 D (range, +1.25 to + 3.25 D). For compound

hyperopic astigmatism, the residual spherical refraction was +2.12 ± 1.3 D (range, +0.5 to +3.25 D) (p < .005). The postoperative residual cylinder for compound hyperopic astigmatism was +2.05 D (range, +0.75 to +2.5 D).

The authors have analyzed age, pachymetry, and average keratometry values for the 69 eyes that experienced full or almost full regression (75–100% regression of the effect) and the 82 eyes that regressed ≤25% (Fig. 18.6). Younger patients experienced more refractive regression than older ones (Fig. 18.7). When patients were analyzed according to central pachymetry, thinner corneas were noted to regress less (Fig. 18.8). No statistically significant difference was found when analyzing changes in average central keratometry (Fig. 18.9). The

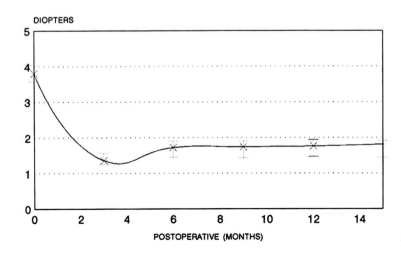

Fig. 18.3. Cycloplegic refraction; follow-up for 18 months.

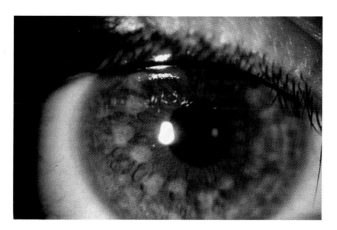

Fig. 18.5. LTK spots 1 year after surgery.

authors developed a formula for preoperative evaluation of the potential amount of postoperative regression:

$$\% \text{ of regression} = \frac{\text{average K}}{15} \times \frac{\text{pachymetry}}{\text{Age}}$$

The authors' results are consistent with those of other investigators[15–17] (Table 18.3). In a 2-year study, Koch et al.[17] induced a mean refractive correction of −1.41 D in 73% of cases. Similar results were achieved by Ariyasu and coauthors[15] in poorly sighted eyes. However, the majority of these results were achieved with only one ring of eight spots.

As for complications, mild photophobia, pain, and a foreign body sensation were reported by many patients. These symptoms resolved within 2 weeks of surgery. However, 5 eyes suffered persistent halos for 3 months due to decentrated applications of the spot. None of the authors' patients lost any lines of preoperative BCVA.

LTK FOR PRK-INDUCED HYPEROPIA

Recently, with the evolving technology of the excimer laser, photorefractive keratectomy (PRK) has offered a new, safe, and precise surgical alternative for the correction of myopia[27–30] and simple myopic astigmatism.[31,32] The results have been highly satisfactory in the treatment of low and moderate myopia of up to −8 D.[31–35] However, some complications occurred, such as dense subepithelial hyperplasia (haze) and decentrated ablation that led to loss of BCVA in some cases. Another significant complication following PRK was induced hyperopia. It is well documented that 2–5% of the patients who undergo PRK may suffer significant and symptomatic overcorrection.[32,33,35] Myopic patients seem to adapt better to residual undercorrection than to overcorrection.[36,37] This could be explained by the sudden demand for extra-accommodative change that occurs when a previously myopic patient

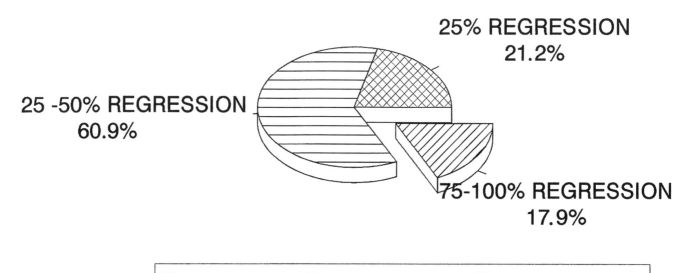

Fig. 18.6. Distribution of the percentage of regression.

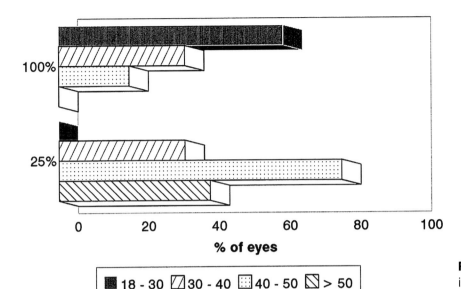

Fig. 18.7. Analysis of the age factor in regression. Significant influence of age on the refractive results.

becomes hyperopic following a refractive procedure.

A total of 14 patients were operated on for PRK-induced hyperopia: 8 females (58.7%) and 6 (41.3%) males. The average age was 32.9 ± 7.9 years (range, 22 to 47 years). Before LTK, the mean spherical refraction of the patients in this series was +4.2 ± 1.8 D (range, +1.75 to +6.25 D) and the mean cylindrical refraction was up to +1.5 D. Mean UCVA was 0.23 ± 0.1 D (range, 0.05 to 0.4 D), and

the BCVA was 0.71 ± 0.12 D (range, 0.2 to 0.9 D). The average keratometry value was 38.98 ± 2.2 D, (range, 36 to 42.25 D).

The Holmium laser spots were always placed outside the previous ablation zone to avoid confluence of haze. No increase in PRK haze was seen in any case.

Improvement in UCVA was achieved in the majority of patients 5 to 7 days after surgery. This improvement reached its maximum in 2 to 6

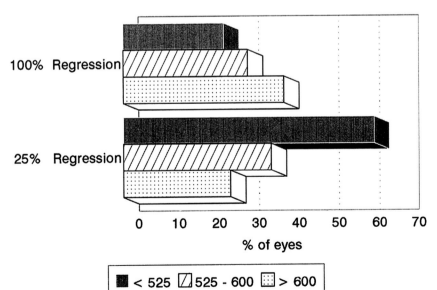

Fig. 18.8. Analysis of the pachymetry factor in regression. Significant influence of thin corneas on the refractive results.

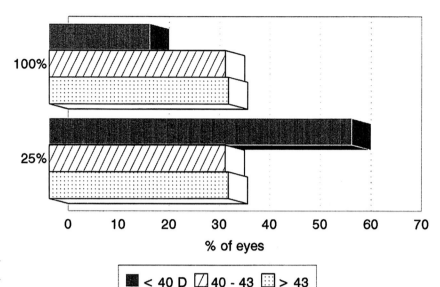

Fig. 18.9. Analysis of the keratometry factor in regression. No significant influence on the refractive results.

■ < 40 D ▨ 40 - 43 ▦ > 43

months. In the immediate postoperative period, a huge myopic shift was recorded (Fig. 18.10). However, 4 to 6 months after surgery, most patients obtained a more stable emmetropic refraction due to partial regression of the effect.

The mean BCVA before LTK was 0.71 ± 0.12 D (range, 0.05 to 0.9 D), and the UCVA after 12 months was 0.65 ± 0.28 D (range, 0.05 to 0.8 D). Twelve patients (85.7%) had a UCVA of 0.6 D or better. The mean cycloplegic refraction before LTK was +4.2 ± 1.8 D (range, +1.75 to +6.25 D), and the mean cycloplegic refraction after LTK was −1.24 ± 0.11 D at 3 months, −0.52 ± 0.17 D at 6 months, 0.23 ± 0.3 D at 9 months, and +0.63 ± 0.16 D at 12 months. At the end of the study, all patients were within ± 1.75 D (range, −1 to + 1.75 D). The mean preoperative keratometric (K) value was 38.98 ± 2.2 (range, 36 to 42.25), and the

mean postoperative K value was 45.94 ± 2.89 at 3 months, 44.02 ± 2.3 at 6 months, 43.96 ± 3.1 at 9 months, and 43.58 ± 1.4 at 15 months. A statistically significant difference was found ($p < .005$) when the preoperative status was compared to the 12-month results. No statistically significant difference was found when we compared the 9- and 15-month results were compared.[27,38]

Overcorrection following myopic PRK can be treated by noncontact LTK. In these cases, a huge effect was obtained with less regression. This was due to the following factors:

1. The lower central pachymetric values, i.e., thin corneas.
2. Absence of Bowman's membrane in these cases helps the cornea respond to the LTK spots.

Table 18.3. Comparative LTK Results of Various Authors

	Seiler[13]	Ariyasu[15]	Koch[17]	Alió[38]
One ring	—	± 1.05 D	± 1.41 D	± 1.8 D
Two or three rings	± 3.7 D	—	± 2.2 D	± 2.4 D
Follow-up	1 year	3 months	2 years	18 months
LTK	Contact	Noncontact	Noncontact	Noncontact

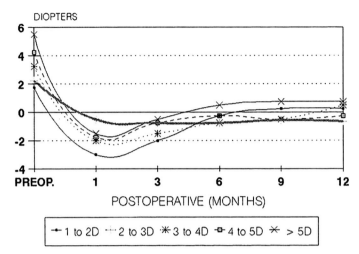

Fig. 18.10. Follow-up of cycloplegic refraction in post-PRK cases. Huge myopic shift in the early postoperative period.

3. Flat post-PRK corneas with low keratometric values demand less curving from LTK than do corneas with normal keratometry readings.

TREATMENT OF RK OVERCORRECTION BY LTK

Overcorrection following astigmatic keratotomy (AK) and radial keratotomy (RK) is a significant complication of these techniques. It is due to the sudden demand for accommodation in myopic patients. In the Prospective Evaluation of Radial Keratotomy (PERK) study, up to 17% of patients became hyperopic.[39,40] The authors treated some of them with corneal Merseline sutures in a controlled study for both RK and AK overcorrections. The suture was adjusted using a placido ring under the operating microscope. All patients were maintained within ± 1 D of emmetropia 6 months after surgery.

However, the refractive result was unpredictable due to suture intolerance. In some cases, the knot of the suture, especially in the purse-string suture, eroded into the epithelium, leading to corneal neovascularization.[41–44]

Noncontact LTK technique was used for the treatment of overcorrections in 38 eyes with post-RK and post-AK hyperopic shifts. Wound gapping occurred in the first three patients treated by LTK and was managed by eye patching for 24 hr. To avoid wound gapping after LTK, the laser spots should be applied on the previous RK incision (Fig. 18.11 and 18.12).

The authors' approach to spot application involves retracting the incision lip to the interior of the cornea, thus preventing wound separation. The obtained correction is less effective but more stable than that in virgen hyperopic cases. More regular corneal topography has been observed in many cases (Fig. 18.13 and 18.14).

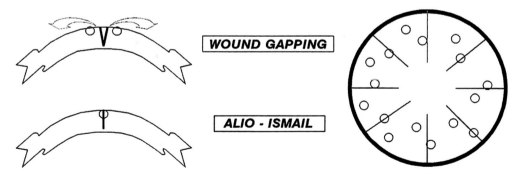

Fig. 18.11. Schematic diagram of spot application in RK patients to avoid wound gapping.

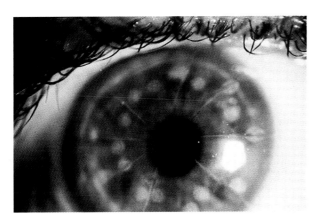

Fig. 18.12. LTK spots 1 year after surgery in a patient with prior RK.

FUTURE REFINEMENT OF NONCONTACT LTK

Results obtained with PRK-induced hyperopia treatment suggest that Bowman's membrane is one important factor in regression of the refractive effect. It holds the topographic memory of the cornea. In an attempt at controlling regression, the authors started a controlled study of young adults with high hyperopia (from +3 to +6 D) that consists of making a lamellar cut with the microkeratotome 2 months before LTK treatment. Initial results are very promising, but 1-year follow-up is mandatory.

INDICATIONS FOR NONCONTACT LTK

Noncontact LTK is a limited alternative for the correction of hyperopia up to +3 D. Algorithms to improve the final results should include an initial calculated hypercorrection adjusted to variables that influence the regression, such as age and corneal thickness. The indications for this technique are as follows:

1. Low hyperopia, especially in patients over 40 years of age.
2. Monovision for low hyperopic-presbyopes.
3. Low hyperopic and mixed astigmatism, especially in patients over 40 years of age.
4. Overcorrections of RK and AK progressive hyperopic shifts.

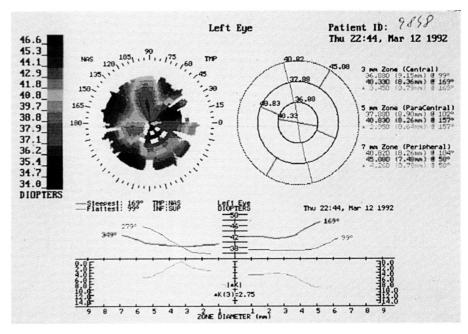

Fig. 18.13. Preoperative video-keratoscopy in an RK patient with irregular astigmatism.

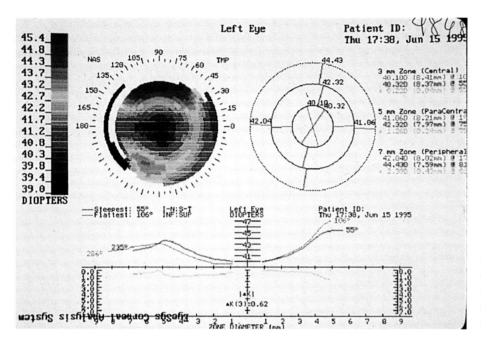

Fig. 18.14. One-year postoperative videokeratoscopy in the same patient. Regular corneal topography with a mild increase in central keratometry.

5. PRK-induced hyperopia and astigmatism.
6. Laser in situ keratomileusis (LASIK)-induced hyperopia and astigmatism.

REFERENCES

1. Lans LJ. Experimentelle Untersuchungen über Entstehung von Astigmatismus durch nicht perforirende Corneawunden. *Graefes Arch Clin Exp Ophthalmol.* 1889, 45:117–152.

2. Gasset AR, Kaufman HE. Thermokeratoplasty in the treatment of keratoconus. *Am J Ophthalmol.* 1975; 79:226–232.

3. Artensen JJ, Laibson PR. Thermokeratoplasty for keratoconus. *Am J Ophthalmol.* 1976;82:447–449.

4. Aquavella JV, Smith RS, Shaw EL. Alteration of corneal morphology following thermokeratoplasty. *Am J Ophthalmol.* 1976;94:2082–2085.

5. Rowesy JJ. Electrosurgical keratoplasty: update and retraction. *Invest Ophthalmol Vis Sci.* 1987; 28: 224–226.

6. McDonnell PJ, Garbus J, Romero N, Rao A, Schanzlin DJ. Electrosurgical keratoplasty clinicopathologic correlation. *Arch Ophthalmol.* 1988; 106: 235–238.

7. Feldman ST, Ellis W, Frucht-Pery J, et al. Regression of the effect following radial thermokeratoplasty in humans. *J Refract Corneal Surg.* 1989;5:288–291.

8. Neumann AC, Fyodorov S, Sanders DR. Radial thermokeratoplasty for the correction of hyperopia. *J Refract Corneal Surg.* 1990;6:404–412.

9. Neumann AC. Thermokeratoplasty for hyperopia. *Ophthalmol Clin North Am.* 1992;5:753–772.

10. Peyman GA, Larson B, Raichand M, Andrews AH. Modification of rabbit corneal curvature with the use of carbon dioxide laser burns. *Ophthalmic Surg.* 1980;11:325–329.

11. Kanoda AN, Sorokin AS. Corneal curvature change using energy of laser radiation. In: Fyodorov SN ed. *Microsurgery of the Eye.* Moscow: Mir Publishers; 1987:147–154.

12. Seiler T, Matallana M, Bende T. Laser thermokeratoplasty by means of a pulsed holmium:YAG laser for hyperopic correction. *Refract Corneal Surg.* 1990; 6:335–339.

13. Seiler T. Ho:YAG laser thermokeratoplasty for hyperopia. *Ophthalmol Clin North Am.* 1992;5: 773–780.

14. Moriera H, Campus M, Sawusch MR, McDonnell JM, Sand B, McDonnell PJ. Holmium laser keratoplasty. *Ophthalmology.* 1993;100:752–761.

15. Ariyasu RG, Sand B, Menefee R, et al. Holmium laser thermakeratoplasty of 10 poorly sighted eyes. *J Refract Surg.* 1995;11:358–365.

16. Kohnen T, Husein SE, Koch DD. Corneal topographic changes after noncontact holmium:YAG laser thermal keratoplasty to correct hyperopia. *J Cataract Refract Surg*. 1996;22:1–9.

17. Koch DD, Abarca A, Villareal R, et al: Hyperopia correction by noncontact holmium:YAG laser thermal keratoplasty. Clinical study with two years follow-up. *Ophthalmology*. 1996;103:731–740.

18. Berry MJ, Fredlin LG, Valderrama GL, et al. Temperature distributions in laser-irradiated corneas. *Invest Ophthalmol Vis Sci*. 1991;32:994–998.

19. Er H, Menefee RF, Valderrama GL, et al. Acute histological changes induced by laser thermal keratoplasty. *Invest Ophthalmol Vis Sci*. 1994;35:2021–2025.

20. Sánchez-Castro P. Efectos histológicos de la termoqueratoplastía con láser de holmio. Estudio experimental. Ph.D. thesis, University of Alicante, Alicante, Spain, 1995.

21. Parel JM, Ren Q, Simon G. Non-contact laser photothermal keratoplasty. I. Biophysical principles and laser beam delivery system. *J Refract Corneal Surg*. 1994;10:511–518.

22. Tervo T, Martaniemi V, Vesaluma M. Inflamaciones en cirugía refractiva. En "Inflamaciones Oculares". Edika Med, Barcelona. *Capítulo*. 1995;9:449–462.

23. Ismail MM, Alió JL. Correction of hyperopia by holmium laser. Presented at the European Congress of Cataract and Refractive Surgery Congress, Lisbon, Portugal, October 2–5, 1994.

24. Ismail MM. Non-contact LTK for the correction of hyperopia. 15 months follow-up. Presented at the ISRS Congress, Minneapolis, July 28–30, 1995.

25. Alió JL, Ismail MM, Sanchez JL. Correction of hyperopia by holmium laser. 15 months follow-up. *J Refract Surg*. In press.

26. Alió JL, Ismail MM. Correction of hyperopic astigmatism Holmium laser thermokeratoplasty (LTK). Presented at One Decade of Excimer Lasers, the International Society for Research on Laser Refractive Surgery, Monaco, March 15–16, 1996.

27. L'Esperance FA, Taylor DM, Del Pero RA, et al. Human excimer laser corneal surgery: preliminary report. *Trans Am Ophthalmol Soc*. 1988;86:208–215.

28. Serdarevic O. Corneal laser surgery. In: L'Esperance FA Jr. *Ophthalmic Lasers*. St. Louis, Mo: The C. V. Mosby Company, 1989.

29. Trokel S. Evolution of excimer laser corneal surgery. *J Cataract Refract Surg*. 1989;15:373–383.

30. Sher NA, Bowers RA, Zabel RW, et al. Clinical use of the 193 nm excimer laser in the treatment of corneal scars. *Arch Ophthalmol*. 1991;109:491–498.

31. McDonell PJ, Moreira H, Clapham TN, D'Arcy J, Munnerlyn CR. Photorefractive keratectomy for astigmatism. Initial clinical results. *Arch Ophthalmol*. 1991;109:1370–1373.

32. McDonnell PJ, Garbus JJ, Hertzog L, Campos M. Photorefractive keratectomy for naturally occurring and post-keratoplasty astigmatism. *Invest Ophthalmol Vis Sci*. 1992;6:334.

33. Seiler T, Kahle G, Kriegerowski M. Excimer laser (193 nm) myopic keratomileusis in sighted and blind human eyes. *Refract Corneal Surg*. 1990;6:165–173.

34. McDonald MB, Lzu JC, Byrd TJ, et al. Central photorefractive keratectomy for myopia. Partially sighted and normally sighted eyes. *Ophthalmology*. 1991;98:1326–1337.

35. McDonnell PJ, Garbus JJ, Salz JJ. Excimer laser myopic photorefractive keratectomy after uncorrected radial keratotomy. *Refract Corneal Surg*. 1991;7:146–150.

36. Maguire LJ, Zabel RW, Paeker P, Lindstrom RL. Topography and raytracing analysis of patients with excellent visual acuity three months after excimer laser photorefractive keratectomy for myopia. *Refract Corneal Surg*. 1991;7:122–128.

37. Lawless MA, Cohen P, Rogers C. Excimer laser photorefractive keratectomy: first Australian series. *Med J Aust*. 1992;156(11):812–815.

38. Alió JL, Ismail MM, Artola A. Correction of PRK induced hyperopia by holmium laser. 15 months follow-up. *J Refract Surg*. In press.

39. Rashid ER, Waring GO. Complications of radial keratotomy and transverse keratotomy. *Surv Ophthalmol*. 1989;34:83–106.

40. Waring GO, Lynn MJ, Gelender H, et al. Results of the Prospective Evaluation of Radial Keratotomy (PERK) study one year after surgery. *Ophthalmology*. 1985;92:177–198.

41. Alió JL, Ismail MM. Management of radial keratotomy overcorrections by corneal sutures. *J Cataract Refract Surg*. 1993;19:195–199.

42. Alió JL, Ismail MM. Management of astigmatic keratotomy overcorrections by corneal suturing. *J Cataract Refract Surg*. 1994;20:13–17.

43. Alió JL, Ismail MM, Artola A. Cirugía de la hipermetropía post-queratotomía radial mediante suturas corneales. *Arch Soc Española Oftalmologia*. 1994;66:211–218.

44. Ismail MM, Alió JL, Artola A. Tratamiento de las hipercorreciones post-queratotomía astigmatica. *Arch Soc Española Oftalmologia* 1994;67:167–172.

19

Prevention and Management of Complications of Laser Thermokeratoplasty

Bernard Mathys

The mechanism of action and results of laser thermokerotoplasty (LTK) have been described in the previous chapters. LTK, however, is not always predictable, and some practical advice can help avoid unsatisfactory results.

CHOOSING THE RIGHT PATIENT: PREOPERATIVE CONSIDERATIONS

The ideal patient is over 40–45 years of age and has less than 3.00 D of hyperopia with less than 1.50 D of with-the-rule astigmatism. Intraocular pressure should be below 15 mm Hg. The keratometry value should be less than 43 D. Central pachymetry should be less than 600–610 μm.

The patient must be aware that he or she will be overcorrected (a very steep cornea immediately after the operation) for at least 4 to 8 weeks. This means that the patient will be able to read without glasses but will have problems with distance vision. Then visual acuity for distance will improve as regression occurs (the cornea flattens) but will diminish for reading. This means that the patient must agree preoperatively that glasses may or will be needed. The patient must also be aware of the fact that the long-term results of the procedure are still unknown.

Patients with high hyperopia (over 4 D) are not very well corrected with LTK. They can achieve a small improvement but will still need glasses after the operation, so it is best to avoid surgery in these cases. Patients with thick corneas also react poorly to LTK. They too should be discouraged from having surgery.

Young patients are happy if their hyperopia is not too high. However, they seem to regress much more than older patients. It is important to be very careful in these cases, as hyperopia can be associated with accommodative strabismus.

Overcorrected patients with radial keratotomy (RK) are not good candidates. The corneal steepening after LTK can open the wounds and create a great deal of astigmatism if the points of application of the laser are between the radial incisions or damage the healing if the laser is focused on the corneal incisions.

By contrast, overcorrected patients with photorefractive keratectomy seem to be very good candidates and show stable refraction with time. This result may indicate that Bowman's membrane plays a role in the regression process. These PRK patients can be treated as having virgin eyes, with the same operative protocol.

In establishing the operative protocol, it seems better to apply one ring for low hyperopia (<2.00 D) and two rings for hyperopia over 2.25 D. The diameter of the inner ring should never be below 6 mm and the outer ring should never be more than 9 mm.

The patient should then sign an informed consent form indicating they understand and agree with the above information.

Antibiotic drops must be given before the operation.

INTRAOPERATIVE COMPLICATIONS

With the noncontact device, it is important that the patient remains quiet and motionless, looking into the fixation light. The cornea must be dry; the eyelids are held with a speculum. The surgeon aims at the center of the pupil; the patient must stay motionless. Then the laser is activated, and eight points are applied simultaneously on the cornea at a prechosen optical zone. If necessary, eight spots in a second optical zone are quickly applied. This should be done radially so that the points are situated on the same axis; this procedure seems to be more stable and to produce a better effect than interpolated optical zones. Antibiotic drops are used after the procedure, and the eye is not patched.

If the patient cannot fixate on the blinking light, it can be very difficult to center the procedure. Preoperative administration of 10 mg of diazepam (valium) can help quiet the patient. The procedure itself takes only 2 sec. If decentration occurs, it is best to stop the treatment and evaluate the cornea over the next few days.

With the contact device, it is mandatory to use markers so that the optical zone(s) can be drawn on the cornea, as for an RK procedure. The use of methylene blue during an operation is very helpful. An eight-incision marker is then applied, intersecting the optical zone(s), showing clearly where to apply the probe during treatment. It is best to use a combined marker; this facilitates the operation.

Then the cornea is dried with a microsponge. The points of application of the probe especially must be dry. A clean probe is then applied on the cornea, and different "burns" are performed. If it is necessary to use two optical zones, the spots are made one after the other in a radial pattern, and the operation is completed. Afterward, antibiotic drops are used and loose epithelial cells are removed with a microsponge. The eye is not patched.

As the procedure takes more time than with the noncontact device, the surgeon has more control during the operation. He or she can stop if the patient moves and ask the patient to look into the light of the microscope.

Centration of the markers is critical to avoid poor results.

If the cornea is not dry, the probe will slip during treatment, inducing astigmatism.

It is also mandatory to apply the probe firmly on the site of application but always with the same pressure; otherwise, astigmatism can be induced. Generally, in with-the-rule astigmatism, the pressure on the cornea can be higher laterally than superiorly and inferiorly. This corrects 1 D of astigmatism.

It is possible to control astigmatism with an intraoperative keratoscope. If this is done, the cornea must be wet; otherwise, there will be a poor light reflex.

POSTOPERATIVE COMPLICATIONS

The main problem following LTK surgery is regression. Very few patients complain after the procedure; the eye may be irritated and sensitive for a few hours. The patient may experience some photophobia.

The slit lamp examination shows some white spots that generally stain with fluorescein, with a "belt" between the different sites of application of the laser. This is responsible for the steepness of the cornea.

After 24 to 48 hr, the achieved steepness can be very high: from 4 D to 10 D following the nomogram, the number of rings, and their diameter. The patient's distance vision is then blurred but generally is very good for reading. Older patients are very happy with this result, but they must be warned that it will diminish over time as regression occurs (Table 19.1).

It is advisable to give antibiotic drops for 5 days after treatment. Cortisone or nonsteroidal anti-inflammatory drugs should not be administered, as they tend to promote regression. On the other hand, it has been found empirically, but not proven, that β-blocker drops can stabilize the effect of the surgery.

Patients must be seen and refracted after 15 days, 1 month, 3 months, 6 months, 1 year, and then every year. A complete eye examination must be carried out, with corneal topography. The topography shows a huge steepening of the cornea postoperatively and sometimes astigmatism. Over time, the cornea flattens and the refraction is modified (Figs. 19.1 and 19.2). Generally, the refraction must be myopic for 1 to 3 months to have a good result afterward.

Patients with low hyperopia, eventually associated with presbyopia, have the best and most stable results. High hyperopes have a lot of regression and achieve only a small gain after the procedure.

Contact LTK initially overcorrects most eyes and requires no retreatments over a followup of 18 months because of the overcorrections lasting 1 to 3 months (Table 19.2). The laser beam penetrates more deeply into the cornea than noncontact LTK.

Table 19.1. Follow-up 18 Months After Contact LTK

	Low Hyperopia 14 Eyes <2 D			Moder. Hyp. 19 Eyes 2.25 <D <3.25			High Hyperopia 32 Eyes >3.5 D		
	Mean Ref	STD	Mean K Value	Mean Ref	STD	Mean K Value	Mean Ref	STD	Mean K Value
Preop value	1.62	0.13	42.6 ± 1.3	2.63	0.42	42.38 ± 1.35	4.03	0.56	42.99 ± 1.35
2 days	−1.37	0.64		−1.32	1.61		−1.57	1.52	
1 month	−1	0.58		−1.03	1.34		−0.75	0.8	
3 months	−0.57	0.41		−0.42	1.02		0.28	1.19	
6 months	−0.12	0.4		0.1	0.35		1.4	0.62	
12 months	0.65	0.57		1.09	0.81		1.77	1.01	
18 months	0.85	0.22	4.35 ± 0.74	1.18	0.37	43.84 ± 2.9	2.23	0.61	44.5 ± 0.47

Table 19.2. Follow-up 18 Months After Noncontact LTK and 8 Months After Contact LTK

	Hyperopia NC <3 D 35 Eyes			Hyperopia NC >3 D 17 Eyes			Hyperopia contact 16 Eyes		
	Mean Ref	STD	Mean K Value	Mean Ref	STD	Mean K Value	Mean Ref	STD	Mean K Value
Preop Value	2.45	0.51	43.11 ± 1.62	4.82	0.72	42.97 ± 1.65	3.40	1.08	43.53 ± 1.67
3 months	0.12	0.1		2.17	1.4		0.25	0.01	
6 months	0.38	0.65		1.79	1.13	67% retreated	0.67	0.53	
12 months	0.38	0.56	16% retreated	1.37	1.23	9% retreated	**8 M 0.71**	0.55	NA
18 months	0.54	0.67	44.54 ± 1.56	1.4	1.51	44.58 ± 1.8			45.7 ± 0.71

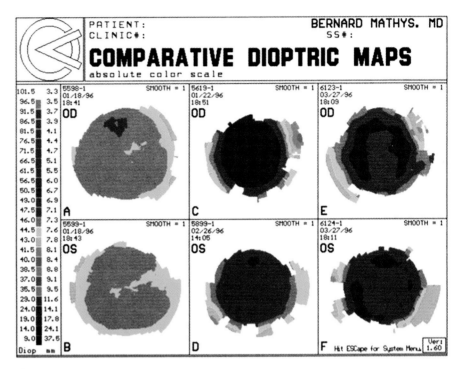

A

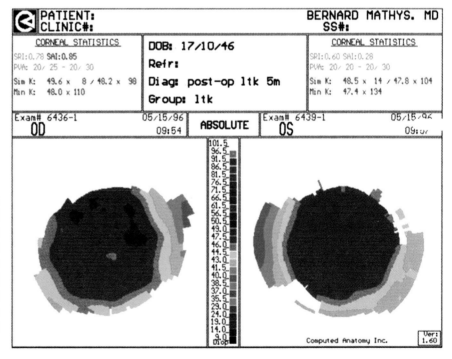

B

Fig. 19.1. Topography maps of a 50-year-old female patient treated with LTK for preoperative hyperopia of +2.00 D in the right eye and +2.75 D in the left eye. Note the large amount of steepening (*A*) immediately after the procedure and stabilization starting 2 months postoperatively. (*B*) Map at 5 months postoperatively.

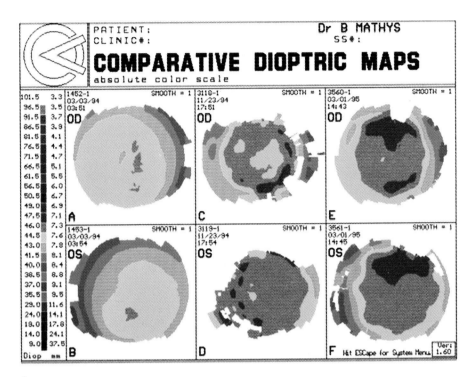

A

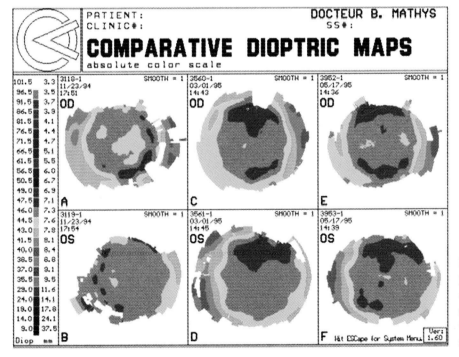

B

Fig. 19.2. Topography maps of a patient treated for 3.50 D of hyperopia in both eyes demonstrating stabilization in the later postoperative period (up to 15 months postoperatively).

Noncontact LTK has less initial effect and requires retreatments by 6 months after LTK.

LTK retreatment gives approximately two-thirds of the correction of the first surgery. In fact, the maximum amount of hyperopia that can be corrected is 2.5 to 3.0 D, because there is a maximum curvature of the cornea that can be obtained and maintained.

In the author's series, no patient lost one line of best corrected visual acuity after treatment, and all patients agree that they had some benefit from the operation, even if the correction was not total. Undercorrected patients treated for hyperopia tend to be more satisfied than undercorrected patients treated for myopia. However, more years of followup will demonstrate whether the technique will remain beneficial. Moreover, it is still unknown how many retreatments can be performed. Long term follow-up of the endothelium after multiple retreatments needs to be evaluated, particularly after deep treatments.

20

Complications of Corneal Refractive Surgery: Emphasis on Corneal Structure

Lee T. Nordan

INTRODUCTION

The past 5 years have presented the anterior segment surgeon with an ever-increasing number of refractive surgery procedures with which to correct ametropia. Many patients will be helped by photorefractive keratectomy (PRK), radial and astigmatic keratotomy (RK, AK), laser in situ keratomileusis (LASIK), intracorneal gel (GIAC), and many other procedures.

Occasionally, however, refractive surgery creates a significant complication, most often overcorrection, irregular astigmatism, and/or a hazy cornea. The increasing popularity of the lamellar refractive procedures, automated lamellar keratoplasty (ALK) and LASIK, demands that these procedures be integrated into a rational plan when combined with PRK and incisional keratotomy. This chapter will explain surgical complications based on the structural abnormality of the cornea and some potentially dangerous and ineffective concepts concerning RK, AK, and lamellar corneal surgery that have been advocated in the past few years, in the author's opinion. In addition, a scheme will be presented whereby the refractive surgeon can easily determine clinically appropriate combinations of refractive surgery and avoid the creation of even greater problems.

Various types of complications may occur following refractive surgery. After incisional keratotomy, complications may include corneal perforation and infection. PRK may create corneal scarring and a decentered optical zone. Lamellar refractive procedures can lead to epithelial inclusion in the stromal interface, a small or decentered optical zone, and even corneal perforation with inadvertent hemi-iridectomy and partial lensectomy. All of these complications have been described in the previous chapters. Yet, the most common complications of refractive surgery relate to the optical ability of the cornea, and less has been written about such problems.

Many mistakes have been made in implementing new refractive surgery techniques that could have been avoided if the development of RK, AK, and keratomileusis had been studied and appreciated. Some surgeons have continued to advocate such concepts as the following:

- RK with less than 3.00 mm optical zone (OZ)
- PRK with less than 6.00 mm OZ
- OZ arcuate incisions greater than 65°
- AK with 5.00 mm OZ
- Hyperopic ALK (H-ALK) to correct overcorrected RK

All of the functional problems arising from the procedures listed above, despite a clear cornea, can be explained by analyzing the structure of the cornea. The principles and experiences related to the problems created by these procedures have been known for more than 10 years. Since the structure of the human cornea and its inherent functional limitations have not changed in hundreds of thousands of years, a paraphrased quotation attributed to President Harry Truman is applicable:

"The only thing not known [about refractive surgery and corneal mechanics] is what has not been learned by studying history."

This chapter attempts to explain the structural limitations of the cornea following corneal refractive surgery and the deleterious effects on function that are associated with extreme corneal change. Hopefully, these concepts can be used by the refractive surgeon to either avoid complications or change a complicated case into a success for both patient and surgeon.

DEFINITION OF A COMPLICATION

A refractive surgery complication may be succinctly defined as any condition created by refractive surgery that is detrimental to intended ocular function. *Undercorrection* is technically a complication, but since it is usually receptive to treatment by performing the original procedure again, it is not as significant as *overcorrection*, which may require a new type of procedure as a remedy. Avoiding a complication is preferable to repairing it.

Since each patient and each cornea is unique, and since refractive surgery is an art as much as a science, complications are a necessary evil that accompany refractive surgery. All refractive surgeons will experience some form of complication if enough operations are performed. It is well within the standard of care for complications to occur, as long as the patient has been prepared with a valid informed consent.

LOSS OF CONTRAST SENSITIVITY AND GLARE

It is astounding that refractive surgery has been performed on a large scale since 1978 with the advent of RK, and yet ophthalmic surgeons continue to judge the results of refractive surgery solely by the Snellen Acuity Test, which is woefully inadequate for the task. The Snellen test is a *high-contrast* test designed to ascertain *visual acuity*.

In general, the Snellen test is an excellent screening test for pathology. Following refractive surgery, however, acuity is often reduced under low-contrast conditions. A contrast sensitivity curve is very difficult to relate to real-world visual performance. A low-contrast acuity test is very valuable in documenting and demonstrating the severity of patients' complaints. For example, a normal preoperative and postoperative refractive surgery patient reading a Snellen-type chart using 6% contrast letters instead of the normal 94% contrast letters will be capable of achieving 20/25 visual acuity instead of 20/20. However, any significant decrease in contrast sensitivity is quickly apparent, which can then be related to the patient's symptoms. Asking a patient with best correction "Which eye sees a black target darker?" is an informal yet very useful contrast sensitivity test.

It will remain very difficult to quantify ocular function following refractive surgery until the testing methods are changed. Much work is needed in this area.

Contrast is the essence of vision, that is, the ability to differentiate light from dark. The greater this ability, the better the ocular function under all lighting conditions. Even though some incoming light may be focused perfectly on the macula, visual function can be reduced significantly by nonfocused light showering the macula. This nonfocused light reduces contrast sensitivity by effectively decreasing the contrast (darkness) of the target. Nonfocused light creates the phenomenon of *glare*. The corneal causes of nonfocused light are central to the complications caused by refractive surgery. Let us examine this issue in greater detail.

A discrete stromal opacity creates very little glare, since light that is blocked out by the opacity has an insignificant effect on visual function. Any light that bounces off the side of the opacity can cause glare. Epithelial irregularity causes significant glare, since a great deal of light scatter is created, amplified by the great disparity between the index of refraction of the tear film and air. Much of the loss of visual function caused by a corneal scar or anterior stromal haze, such as following PRK, is often the result of the associated corneal irregular astigmatism, not the lesion itself. Several situations following corneal refractive surgery which may lead to corneal irregular astigmatism and glare are described in Fig. 20.1.

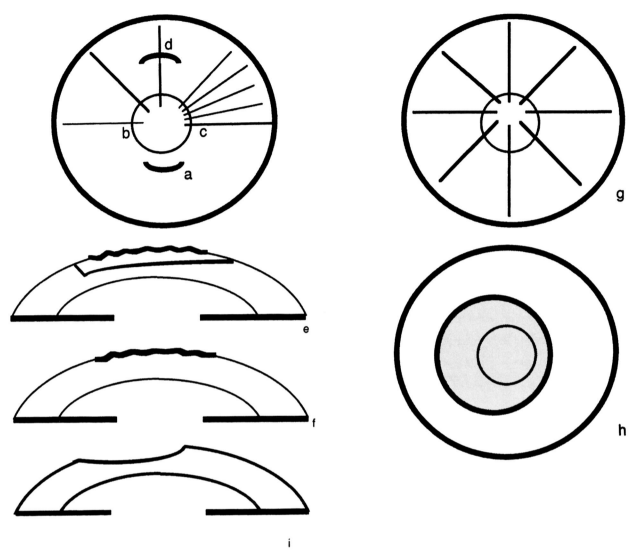

Fig. 20.1. Examples of the various causes of glare in refractive surgery: (*a*) AK with a small OZ; (*b*) RK with a small OZ; (*c*) bridge scarring from RK incisions too close together; (*d*) intersecting corneal incisions close to the visual axis; (*e*) irregular astigmatism following LASIK with a poor keratectomy; (*f*) PRK with significant haze and irregular astigmatism; (*g*) a decentered RK; (*h*) a decentered PRK; and (*i*) a decentered LASIK.

CORNEAL ASPHERICITY

After all forms of corneal refractive surgery, the cornea assumes an aspheric shape; that is, not all areas of the cornea focus light at the same point. This aspheric shape accounts for the poorer night vision often experienced by refractive surgery patients who had about ± 4.00 D or more preopera-

tively), as well as the unexpected improvement in reading for presbyopes as the result of a built-in corneal addition. After refractive surgery, the quality of vision is very sensitive to pupil size (Fig. 20.2).

The aspheric cornea creates compromises in visual function that are important to understand and accept as an integral part of refractive surgery.

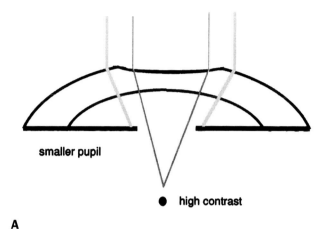

A

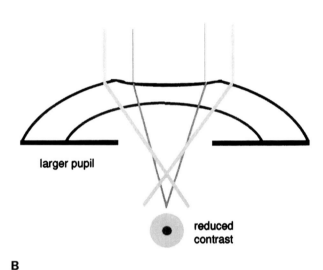

B

Fig. 20.2.(*a,b*) As the result of an aspheric cornea, corneal refractive surgery patients usually have better visual acuity with a smaller pupil.

Corneal asphericity cannot be improved by further surgery and must be differentiated from corneal irregular astigmatism.

CENTRATION OF REFRACTIVE SURGERY: OPTICAL ZONE DIAMETER

As explained above, scattered light which reaches the retina is a significant culprit which causes loss of contrast. The main deterrent for preventing this nonfocused light from reaching the retina is the pupil. Therefore, refractive surgery should be centered about the pupil in order to provide the most

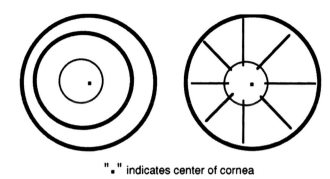

Fig. 20.3. The pupil should be the landmark for centering all corneal refractive surgery procedures, since the symmetry of the relationship between the aspheric cornea and the pupillary margin minimizes glare and loss of contrast. The pupil may be significantly nasal of the geometric center of the cornea, especially in high myopes.

symmetrical and least obtrusive glare pattern (Fig. 20.3). Although the author prefers to use the miotic pupil following the instillation of 0.5% pilocarpine as the guide for surgical centration, other techniques which use the normally constricted pupil are equally acceptable. It is only of academic interest whether the center of these two forms of miotic pupil vary by 0.1 mm, since the pupil changes size in real life and the dioptric value of the cornea overlying the entry pupil varies as a result of asphericity.

The problems caused by a decentered myopic PRK or even a well-centered myopic PRK with a 5.00-mm OZ relate to the "shoulder" of the corneal transition zone, which is in a position within the visual axis to shower nonfocused light upon the retina (Fig. 20.4). For this reason, these patients can function well in bright light with a miotic pupil but do much more poorly when the light is dim enough to cause pupillary dilation. José Barraquer, the father of lamellar refractive surgery, invested a huge amount of time and energy determining that a 6.00-mm OZ was the best compromise between effect and quality of vision for myopic keratomileusis (MKM). It is no coincidence that the same is true for myopic PRK and myopic LASIK, that the bend of the cornea in RK creates about a 6.00-mm OZ, and that the 4.20-mm OZ used in myopic ALK creates serious problems with night vision and should be abandoned in favor of myopic LASIK, with its larger OZ.

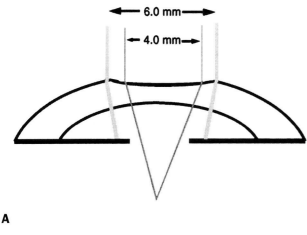

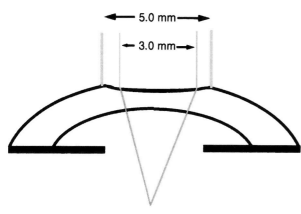

Fig. 20.4. A 6.00-mm OZ in PRK and LASIK provides a functional OZ of about 4.00 mm as a result of the aspheric cornea (*a*). A well-centered 5.00-mm OZ in PRK will provide excellent visual function with a small pupil but an increase in glare when the pupil is relatively dilated (*b*).

CORNEAL IRREGULAR ASTIGMATISM

Corneal irregular astigmatism is undoubtedly the most underrated and overlooked complication following refractive surgery. Irregular astigmatism cannot be seen with the slit lamp, yet it can have a devastating effect on visual function by causing light scatter, with associated loss of contrast and diplopia. Unfortunately, most ocular surgeons document corneal irregular astigmatism only by means of automated topography. These machines are very useful for demonstrating moderate to severe irregu-

lar astigmatism but are not nearly as sensitive as the manual keratometer for discovering subtle irregular astigmatism.

Many talented individuals are currently working to perfect an automated method of documenting subtle levels of corneal irregular astigmatism. Until these methods are available, a high index of suspicion and experience with the manual keratometer are key ingredients for the knowledgeable refractive surgeon. The reader should consult other texts for a more complete treatment of corneal irregular astigmatism.

ADEQUATE CORNEAL STRENGTH

The refractive surgeon should always consider the overall strength of the cornea. The stable, optically smooth cornea acts as a "foundation" upon which the "first floor" of the refractive shape is built. This basic tenet of refractive surgery may be stated as follows:

> If the cornea exhibits irregular astigmatism as a result of structural weakness following refractive surgery, then no subsequent refractive surgery procedure can be successful unless and until the structure of the cornea is repaired.

Let the term *inadequate corneal strength* summarize the situation in which the corneal stroma has been made so thin or weak by a refractive surgery procedure that it cannot sufficiently resist the intraocular pressure, and corneal irregular astigmatism results. In essence, this situation is similar to clinically significant keratoconus.

Not all corneal irregular astigmatism necessarily implies inadequate corneal strength, such as the irregular astigmatism of the front surface of the cornea which may accompany a PRK (often accompanied by corneal haze) or a lamellar corneal procedure (often accompanied by a poor-quality keratectomy). In these two cases, the residual corneal "base" is adequately strong, but it is supporting a defective optical surface (Fig. 20.5).

CLASSIFICATION OF SPECIFIC SURGICAL TECHNIQUES

It is important to classify surgical procedures in terms of whether they weaken, strengthen, or have

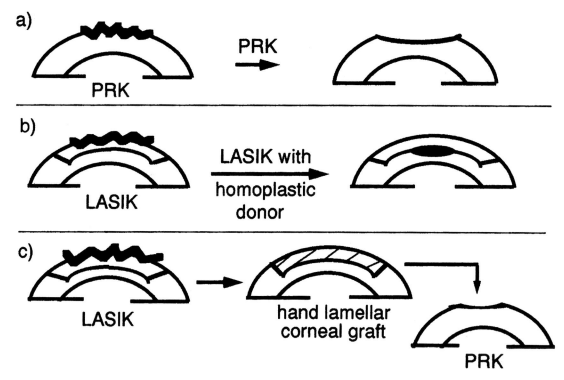

Fig. 20.5. Following PRK or LASIK, the front surface of the cornea may exhibit irregular astigmatism with a normally configured posterior stroma. The irregular astigmatism in this situation may be eradicated by repairing the front half of the cornea by repeat PRK (*a*) or by a repeat lamellar keratectomy (homoplastic donor) with a simultaneous refractive procedure (LASIK) (*b*) or by a subsequent refractive surgery procedure (*c*).

no effect on corneal strength. This is an important step in planning and treating complications.

All refractive procedures which do not add material to the cornea must cause weakening to some extent, since the cornea's basic shape will change. There is no direct clinical correlation between the degree of weakening caused by a valid refractive procedure employed as a primary surgery and its ability to achieve a desired refractive effect. However, it should be emphasized that when various refractive surgery techniques are combined, the potential corneal weakening aspects of the primary and future refractive surgeries may limit certain combinations of such surgeries. In certain instances, a corneal-strengthening surgery may be necessary before the possibility of a second refractive surgery is entertained.

Weakening Procedures

- Incisional keratotomy (RK, AK) is a weakening procedure for the cornea.

- A mechanical lamellar keratectomy (employed with LASIK and ALK) is a weakening procedure for the cornea.

Strengthening Procedures

- A penetrating keratoplasty (PKP) is a strengthening procedure for the cornea.
- A hand lamellar corneal transplant is a relatively strengthening procedure for the cornea.
- (A hand lamellar corneal transplant is a strengthening procedure and an automated lamellar keratectomy is a weakening procedure because the perpendicular scar of the hand lamellar corneal transplant dictates a new central corneal shape (Fig. 20.6). If the preoperative irregular astigmatism is very severe, it is unlikely that a hand lamellar corneal transplant will be capable of correcting all of this irregular astigmatism and a PKP will be necessary. Lamellar corneal procedures do not eradicate the irregular astigmatism of keratoconus.)

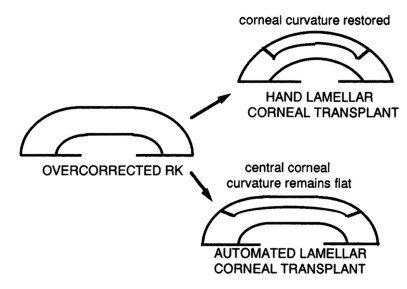

corneal curvature restored

HAND LAMELLAR
CORNEAL TRANSPLANT

OVERCORRECTED RK

central corneal
curvature remains flat

AUTOMATED LAMELLAR
CORNEAL TRANSPLANT

Fig. 20.6. A hand lamellar corneal transplant (*a*) can strengthen the cornea following an overcorrected RK, which an automated lamellar corneal transplant does not (*b*). However, the interface of the hand lamellar corneal transplant may reduce visual acuity by about one Snellen line for 1.5 to 2 years.

- An epikeratophakia donor surgery (hyperopic or plano) is a relatively strengthening procedure for the cornea similar to a hand lamellar corneal transplant (myopic epikeratophakia creates irregular astigmatism and should not be used).

Neutral Procedures

- Myopic photorefractive keratectomy (M-PRK) usually has no effect on corneal strength. If more than 160 μm of central tissue is removed during a PRK or if the thickness of the residual corneal bed following a lamellar refractive procedure is less than 200 μm, then the procedure should be considered a weakening procedure.
- Hyperopic photorefractive keratectomy (H-PRK) has no effect on corneal strength.

Postoperative Result: Weak or Strong Cornea?

In order to treat a cornea that has undergone refractive surgery with an unsatisfactory result, the surgeon must first analyze the situation.

A cornea that has undergone RK and has developed irregular astigmatism now exhibits inadequate corneal strength. A cornea that has undergone RK and is overcorrected without irregular astigmatism also has inadequate corneal strength, since the paracentral cornea is too weak to maintain the desired central corneal curvature.

A cornea that has undergone a lamellar keratectomy at a depth greater than 320 μm or at least 65%

of central corneal thickness is considered to have inadequate corneal strength. This concept fits clinically with the fact that all hyperopic ALK procedures create some degree of irregular astigmatism as the central cornea bows outward (corneal ectasia) to become more steep (and irregular). As a result of this structural defect, hyperopic ALK and hexagonal keratotomy (HEX), which creates similar but even more severe problems, should soon be replaced by H-PRK and H-LASIK, when available.

Successful lamellar refractive surgery (LASIK) must utilize a lamellar keratectomy that is shallow enough so that the residual corneal stroma after laser treatment of the bed will be able to maintain a stable foundation. The minimum thickness of this residual stroma necessary to maintain stability is about 200 μm (Fig. 20.7).

LIMITATIONS OF REFRACTIVE SURGERY

Before planning refractive surgery, it is useful to briefly consider the approximate limitations of current refractive surgery techniques. In some cases, the surgeon may find that combining two different techniques of refractive surgery may provide better results than attempting to extend the range of just one. The surgeon's dilemma in many cases is to achieve an adequate effect that is compatible with good ocular function.

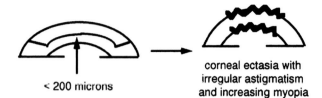

corneal ectasia with
irregular astigmatism
and increasing myopia

< 200 microns

Fig. 20.7. The cornea needs at least 200 μm of residual stroma following a lamellar refractive surgery procedure and 350 μm in overall thickness to ensure corneal stability.

PLANNING COMBINED CORNEAL SURGICAL PROCEDURES

The concepts described above allow the surgeon to develop a rational scheme for legitimate options when dealing with various corneal situations.

The overriding basic concepts are as follows:

- A cornea with adequate strength after a refractive surgery procedure *may* tolerate another refractive surgery procedure.
- A cornea with inadequate strength after a refractive surgery procedure must undergo a restorative (strengthening) procedure before a second refractive surgery procedure is attempted.

Belief in these two basic concepts dictates some very important clinical decisions. Let's explore some of these situations, which have all been borne out clinically (Tables 20.1, 20.2, 20.3). Of course, the situations cited below are the general rule, and specific cases with extreme conditions may warrant alternative individual decisions.

From the perspective of corneal strength:

- An RK which demonstrates overcorrection (hyperopia) with irregular astigmatism is already too weak and cannot be treated by H-ALK or LASIK, which are weakening procedures.
- An RK with irregular astigmatism can be treated by a hand lamellar corneal transplant, PKP, or plano epikeratophakia, which are strengthening (restorative) procedures. After an adequately strong cornea has been achieved and the irregular astigmatism eliminated, refractive surgery may be performed to correct the residual ametropia.

- An overcorrected RK without irregular astigmatism can be treated by an H-PRK, which is neutral relative to corneal strength, or by a PKP, plano epikeratophakia, or a hand lamellar graft, which are strengthening procedures.
- A well-centered but undercorrected PRK may be treated by either another PRK or RK. However, a decentered PRK treated by another PRK will usually result in an area of corneal irregularity still affecting the optical zone (Fig. 20.8). A lamellar corneal graft may be necessary to restore normal corneal architecture to a decentered PRK, followed by another PRK application.
- Treating an undercorrected RK by means of LASIK is risky but may work, depending upon whether the adequate corneal strength is converted to inadequate corneal strength by the keratectomy. In addition, a homoplastic donor *must* be used; otherwise, irregular astigmatism will result from the seriously distorted corneal cap.
- An undercorrected RK may be treated by means of a PRK or another RK.
- An undercorrected AK may be treated by further AK, but an OZ of less than 6.00 mm will cause irregular astigmatism in the visual axis as a result of corneal gape.
- An overcorrected AK may be treated with an AK at 90° to the original if a central "hex" effect is avoided (Fig. 20.9). An overcorrected AK may be sutured for 3–4 months. This will usually reduce the overcorrection by about one-half and improve or eliminate any associated irregular astigmatism by reducing the wound gape.
- An overcorrected H-LASIK may be treated with an RK or M-PRK.
- The myopia of significant keratoconus cannot be treated consistently by RK or lamellar keratectomy, since the weakened cornea is being weakened further.
- Myopia associated with very mild keratoconus (if nonprogressive, which is never certain) may be treated with an M-PRK.
- Irregular astigmatism cannot be treated by an AK, which corrects only regular corneal astigmatism.

Table 20.1. Primary RK

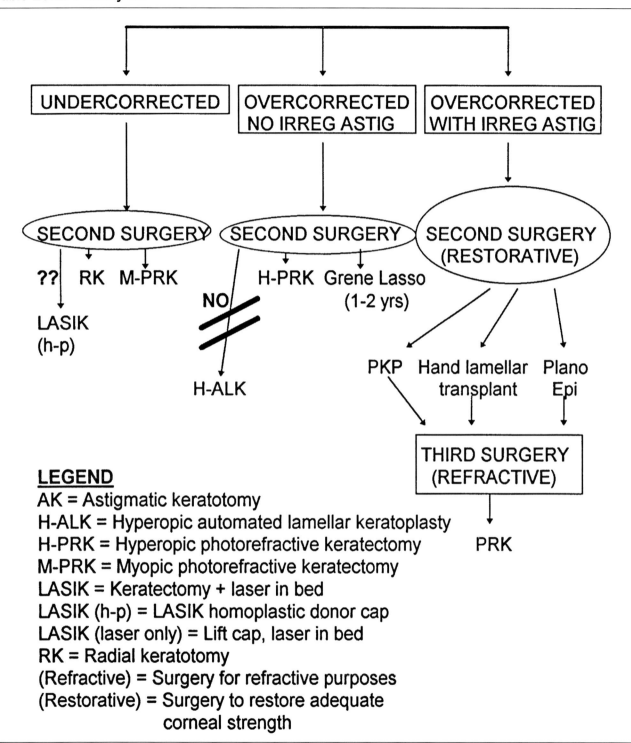

LEGEND
AK = Astigmatic keratotomy
H-ALK = Hyperopic automated lamellar keratoplasty
H-PRK = Hyperopic photorefractive keratectomy
M-PRK = Myopic photorefractive keratectomy
LASIK = Keratectomy + laser in bed
LASIK (h-p) = LASIK homoplastic donor cap
LASIK (laser only) = Lift cap, laser in bed
RK = Radial keratotomy
(Refractive) = Surgery for refractive purposes
(Restorative) = Surgery to restore adequate
                         corneal strength

Table 20.2. Primary PRK

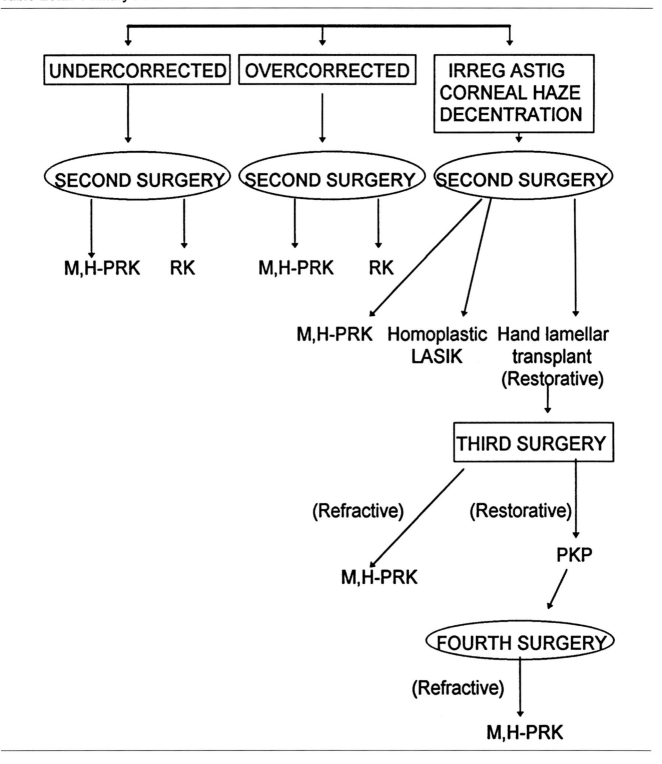

Table 20.3. Primary LASIK

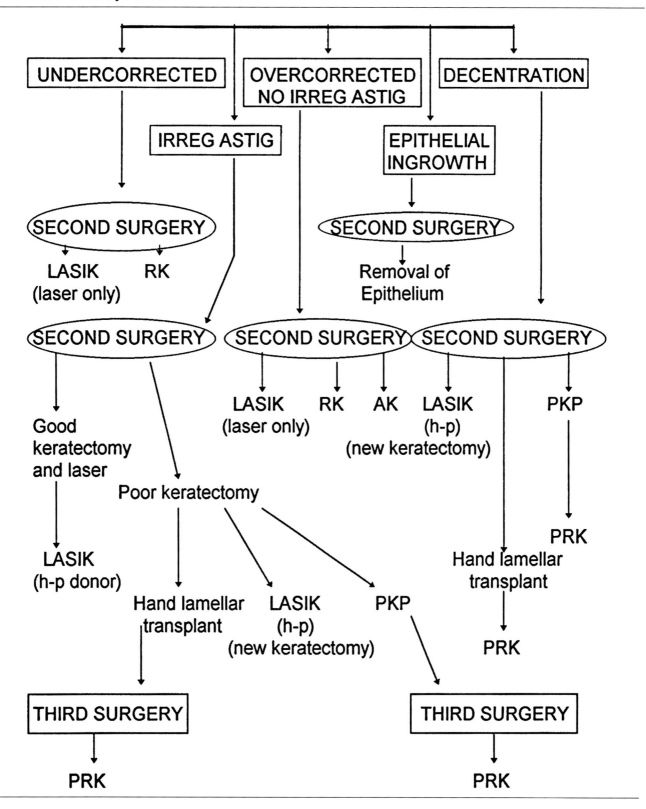

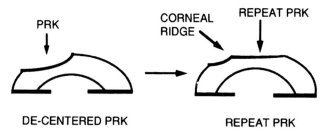

Fig. 20.8. A severely decentered PRK often cannot be fixed completely by a repeat PRK. A lamellar corneal procedure will reconstitute a normal corneal shape, which can then be followed by a refractive surgery procedure.

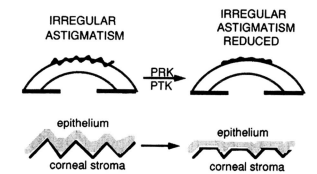

Fig. 20.10. Mild irregular astigmatism may be improved, but not eliminated, by epithelial faceting following PRK.

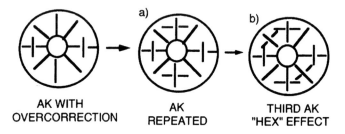

Fig. 20.9. Treatment of residual astigmatism by additional AK incisions may be effective (*a*) as long as a hex effect is avoided (*b*).

SUMMARY

The goal of refractive surgery is to provide the patient with uncorrected, high-quality visual acuity, although certain compromises are always inherent in the process. Although the surgeon wishes to achieve this goal as rapidly as possible, the presence of inadequate corneal strength or poorly conceived refractive surgery can create an optically impure corneal surface which causes light scatter and loss of contrast. Such a corneal condition necessitates restoration of the cornea to a normal structural condition before proceeding with refractive surgery.

Small or moderate amounts of PRK have no clinical effect on corneal strength, but RK, AK, LASIK, and ALK are corneal-weakening procedures to varying degrees. Unfortunately, the corneal-strengthening (restorative) procedures, except for hyperopic epikeratophakia, are not also inherently refractive procedures. This separation of function usually necessitates two surgeries to achieve a satisfactory result once corneal irregular astigmatism has been caused by an initial refractive surgery.

PRK may be the exception to the rule in that the faceting of the epithelium as it spreads over the central cornea may correct ametropia and improve (but never eliminate) mild underlying corneal irregular astigmatism (Fig. 20.10).

The refractive surgeon is urged to consider the principles presented in this chapter when planning refractive surgery and surgical treatment of associated complications. The RK/lamellar keratectomy, keratoconus/refractive surgery, and irregular astigmatism/AK combinations that have been advocated in the recent past should be avoided. Adherence to the basic principles of corneal integrity and structure should allow for improved refractive surgery results in both original cases as well as in those with an initial problem.

21

Refractive Centers: Operations and Management

Stephen F. Brint

Coni Sweeney Fisher

Donald G. Johnson

Jan Ashton

Peter Tseng

W. Bruce Jackson

INTRODUCTION

As ophthalmology practices continue strategic planning for competitive positioning within health care reform, the role of the refractive center is being closely evaluated. A combination of factors have led to renewed interest in refractive surgery. Declining reimbursements for cataract procedures through the impact of RBRVS and expected additional regulations from federal agencies seem to make elective refractive procedures attractive from a revenue standpoint. Two decades of refractive keratotomy (RK) in the United States has demonstrated patient satisfaction. Coupled with this is the surgeons' desire to provide a market-driven elective procedure free of governmental controls. In recent surveys of clinical practices, the number of ophthalmologists performing refractive surgery has continued to increase, as well as the percentage of ophthalmologists identifying their subspecialty area as refractive surgery.

In 1970, a national survey estimated that myopia (nearsightedness) exists in 25% of the U.S. population.[1] Over 20 years of patient demand for contact lenses instead of glasses has fueled the pursuit of new technology and innovative procedures to correct refractive errors. Incisional refractive techniques (RK, astigmatic keratotomy [AK], myopic keratomileusis [MKM], automated lamellar keratoplasty [ALK], and laser in situ keratomileusis [LASIK]) of the past two decades have produced satisfactory results and increasing patient acceptance; today, more than 1 million eyes in the United States have been corrected by refractive surgery. With the recent approval (Summit: October 1995; VisX: March 1996) of excimer laser photorefractive keratectomy (PRK) for the correction of myopia, it is predicted that refractive surgery will become the most frequently performed operative procedure in eye care by the year 2000—with an optimistic estimate of 8 million PRK procedures performed in the first 5 years following the Food and Drug Administration (FDA) approval. In U.S. FDA clinical trials and in more than 300,000 patients in 40 countries worldwide, PRK for the correction of nearsightedness has proven to be a safe, predictable, and effective procedure.

The patients who are candidates for refractive surgery will continue to increase due to several factors:

- Population growth, increasing the number of persons experiencing defective vision (especially myopia).
- Additional protocols and techniques expanding the range of correctable refractive errors with excimer laser technology (PRK and LASIK).

293

- Improved refractive technology and surgical technique, leading to exceptional clinical results and increased patient satisfaction.
- Growing public awareness of and demand for surgical alternatives to glasses and contact lenses.
- Positive public reaction to the FDA regulatory approval of PRK.
- Public perception of the superiority of the laser in medical procedures with nonlaser options.

Continued excellent refractive results have captured the attention of the myopic population. The refractive surgery candidate is a well-informed consumer. Direct marketing to potential patients has been extremely successful. The question to be answered for the future is which refractive procedure will emerge as the procedure of choice for most patients *and* surgeons for the correction of up to 7 D of myopia. In Europe, Canada, and other countries, where PRK has a longer history, it has taken its place with RK in the refractive marketplace or replaced it. Some Canadian surgeons, believing PRK and RK to have equal refractive results, have abandoned RK for the excimer laser procedure for scheduling, marketing, and patient education reasons. In the United States, where RK has reached a high level of predictability and acceptance, RK surgeons will probably be slower to abandon their diamond knives and totally embrace excimer laser technology (PRK/LASIK). The procedures will coexist at least as long as currently trained RK surgeons teach and operate, and the cost of an excimer laser is out of reach for most surgeons. The choice of technique will be influenced by such considerations as patient selection, age, need for astigmatic correction, recovery time, and, last but not least, cost. From a technological perspective, refractive surgery seems positioned similarly to intraocular lenses 15 years ago—exciting technology with both surgeon and patient acceptance.

Just as the 1980s were the decade for advances in cataract surgery, the 1990s are the decade for refractive surgery. With FDA approval of the Summit and VisX excimer lasers in the United States, this reality is now upon us. Within the next 10 years, laser vision correction, whether with an excimer laser or perhaps later with solid-state lasers, will be the refractive surgery of choice.

Therefore, a laser vision correction strategy is essential for the refractive practice. With the extremely high cost of acquiring one of the current generation excimer lasers, as well as its attendant maintenance cost and pillar point fees, determining one's role as a practicing ophthalmologist in this ever-expanding field of refractive surgery can be a source of extreme confusion and frustration. In this age of declining reimbursements, with corresponding increases in practice overhead, one must consider which path is most prudent to follow: individual laser purchase, network participation (open access vs. closed access system), or simply comanaging your refractive surgery patients with an available state-of-the-art laser center and an experienced surgeon. All of these options have advantages and disadvantages; the choice should be the one that provides the greatest advantages to your patients.

IF YOU BUILD IT/BUY IT, WILL THEY COME?

Before seeking refractive surgery as the profit center to replace income loss due to the changes in the health care market for cataract surgery, conduct the necessary internal audits and cost-benefit analysis and assess your particular demographic market. Refractive surgery may or may not be the "field of dreams" for ophthalmology in the future.

In this chapter, the authors share their experience in maintaining levels of refractive surgery as the techniques that we can offer our patients continue to improve. The evolution of the private practice refractive center will be presented based on the experience of the Eye Surgery Center of Louisiana in the United States, the Canadian experience of the London Place Eye Centre in New Westminster, British Columbia, and the Asian experience of the Singapore National Eye Centre in Singapore with PRK. Administrative and clinical issues regarding the incorporation of a refractive center into a private practice will be discussed, in addition to strategy and guidelines for marketing, patient selection and education, staffing, and co-management issues.

Practice Evaluation

Careful internal and external evaluation is important with addition to or enhancement of refractive surgery in the private practice. The review of practice patient demographics with respect to age, diagnosis, insurance coverage, and location can reveal important indicators of refractive surgery potential. Surgical outcomes, revenues, and the current referral base (physicians, screening programs, word of mouth) require concentrated and continual evaluation. The image projected to prospective patients is primarily the perception of the staff and facility; both warrant continual inspection. Externally, population demographics, the competition, and historical considerations are additional areas for research.

Staff Considerations

As the refractive center is "a practice within a practice," careful consideration must be given to staff roles and development. The refractive team includes a coordinator/director, referral liaison, telemarketer(s), educator(s), and technician(s); initially, before volume demands additional staff, multiple roles may be filled by one individual. Figure 21.1 illustrates a typical refractive surgery department.

It is important to note that refractive surgery patients are different from the type of patients that most practices and surgeons are accustomed to or comfortable with. Laser vision correction patients are the ultimate consumers and require quality service plus a lot of "hand holding"; these individuals will be seen quite frequently (an average of seven or eight times the first year). It is imperative that all staff members on the refractive team be very well informed regarding refractive procedures (even those *not* provided) and able to answer most of the frequently asked questions. Most of the prospective patient's questions should be directed to the counselor/educators in the refractive services department; requests or questions of a technical nature may need to be addressed by a senior technician or physician.

The coordinator/director should be responsible for the overall performance of the department. Department functions include all of the contact management, data entry, and mail-outs of the patient information and surveys. With increased volume, the responsibility for data collection and outcome analysis may require a full-time staff member, as well as another full-time employee to maintain the referral and comanagement network. Team

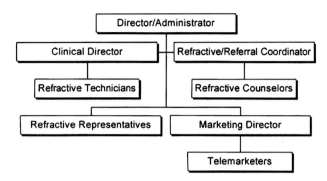

Fig. 21.1. Personnel structure of a refractive surgery department.

responsibilities involve working within the practice (educating the entire staff, identifying current patient candidates, assisting in exams/procedures), working with refractive patients (education/counseling, consultation/testing, support through decision-making processes, monitoring posttreatment satisfaction levels), and working with referral sources (comanagement paperwork, scheduling, communication, educational/promotional materials inventory/distribution).

The training of the laser technician team is critical. These individuals must appreciate sterile technique, and surgical assisting and must pay close attention to detail (particularly important with microkeratome procedures). The technician operating the laser should be somewhat mathematically and mechanically inclined. A three-person refractive surgical team consisting of the surgeon, the laser technician, and a second technician to assist during the procedure is required for PRK, PTK, and LASIK. Additional members of the refractive team include technicians responsible for preoperative preparation and explanation of postoperative instructions.

Candidate Contact

Each member of the refractive team should clearly understand that the purpose of any contact with the potential candidate is to bring the individual to the next level in the decision-making process; the levels of contact or decision making include the initial inquiry (usually by telephone), a seminar or screening (free service), the preoperative exam and testing, and the actual refractive procedure. Scripted communication for patient communications (telephone inquiry, seminar presentation, screening consultation, informed consent, and pre- and postoperative instructions) should be provided for staff training and education. During the specific contact episode, the refractive team member should be trained to determine a category describing the motivational level characterized by the action taken or the appropriate response required. These categories are labeled and ranked as follows:

1. Highly motivated (ready to schedule the procedure).
2. Interested (needs more information).
3. Low interest ("tire kicker").
4. Not a candidate.

If an inquiring person is not a candidate, the reason should be indicated (age/financial/procedure limitations/unreasonable expectations) so that future communication is possible with a situation change. Understanding the reason motivating the patient to seek refractive surgery is also an important issue in counseling the patient regarding realistic expectations and can include any of the following reasons:

- Unhappy depending on glasses or contact lenses.
- Dissatisfied with appearance in glasses.
- Contact lens intolerance.
- Sports/lifestyle considerations.
- Occupational requirements.
- Economic reasons.

At the London Place Eye Centre, the patient flow from initial contact through surgery usually works as follows: When a prospective patient calls requesting information on the procedure, an information package is sent and the dates of the next seminars are given. The information package describes the reasons why people are nearsighted, farsighted, or astigmatic and what can be done to reduce their dependency on glasses or contact lenses. Also included are patient testimonials, results/outcomes, and answers to frequently asked questions regarding the procedure. If this information is sent out first, the patient becomes more educated, reducing telephone time. The return call is usually to schedule a seminar date or consultation appointment or to

have a few additional questions answered regarding the procedure. Refractive team members should be available daily to answer additional questions; the goal should be the arrival of a well-informed individual with reasonable expectations at the consultation screening appointment. Contact management through a computerized patient database is the most effective means of monitoring the patient conversion process. Patient surveys mailed at designated times during this process return important feedback on perceived quality of service.

Refractive Patient Database

Tracking patient inquiry, surgery conversion, outcomes, and satisfaction level are the primary functions of the computer database, whether incorporated into the practice system or kept on a separate personal computer. A manual system is not adequate, but adequate computer software can be generic or custom made. The important issue is to create appropriate data fields for maximum use and advantage. Data fields designed to track patients from inquiry to conversion should include date fields (date of inquiry, date of specific contact levels), contact action fields indicating the action taken in the decision-making progress (appointment scheduled, surgery scheduled, etc.), and response action fields (information mailed, appointment not kept) which indicate some appropriate action from the practice refractive department. The telephone inquiry form should contain information (name, age, home/work phone, mailing address, date of inquiry, inquiry motivation, inquiry source, referral source, current eye doctor, eye history information, level of interest, and potential candidacy for what procedure) which is transferred to the appropriate field. Remember, "garbage in, garbage out" when entering data. An additional but separate database for tracking refractive outcomes (pre- and postoperative refraction, best corrected and uncorrected visual acuity, etc.) will containing many identical patient information fields for easy transfer of an inquiry to a surgical result after conversion. Without a database for tracking, it is impossible to monitor the success of marketing endeavors.

Marketing

Refractive surgery is price sensitive and market driven. Understanding your market is critical, and a commitment to analysis, planning, and an adequate budget (for PRK, plan on $250 per procedure) is essential. The refractive market is somewhat specific for different refractive procedures based on price, clinical aspects (side effects, postoperative management, visual rehabilitation), and patient pool (ametropia, candidacy, and discretionary income). For RK and AK the market niche is defined by the limited amount of correction offered and the inexpensive delivery with an early return to good vision. PRK may appeal to a larger market of candidates due to the high-tech laser image and emphasis on avoiding an incision, but it is more expensive to deliver because of laser purchase, maintenance, and pillar point royalty. More extensive postoperative management and delayed return to best corrected vision and good uncorrected acuity may lead to a short life cycle. LASIK encompasses the largest market niche—all levels of myopia—although the combination of excimer and microkeratome make it the most expensive procedure to deliver. The life cycle of LASIK, characterized by a steep learning curve and significant surgical skill, could be limited by improved outcomes from future technology.

The laser/refractive marketplace for the United States, initially overstated by Wall Street, consultants, and laser center corporations, is represented more realistically by a penetration rate estimated at 1–2% of the target pool, with 0.11% of the general population a good guide for initial predictions (based on the percentage of annual RKs performed in the United States in the total population). Another formula to determine a particular pool of candidates uses the percentage of myopia in the general population and the percentage of qualified candidates by age (35–55 is the typical range) and income (annual income above $35,000) for the specific market. If 44% represents the appropriate age range and 50% can afford the procedure, applying a 1% penetration rate to a population of 1 million predicts 1,100 procedures (550 patients), assuming bilateral application (1.7 eyes per patient is a more realistic prediction).

Intense marketing competition will be driven by advertising, price, and outcomes, as illustrated in the diagram of the refractive surgery market development cycle shown in Fig. 21.2. An increase in the penetration rate can be expected with more advertising dollars in the market, a decrease in procedure

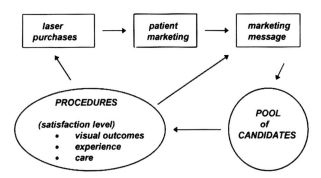

Fig. 21.2. Refractive surgery: market development cycle.

price, outcome success, and an excellent sales support system. Careful attention must be given to calculating the break-even point in order to determine not only a workable volume but a volume that is profitable and financially sound.

Marketing delivers the message to the potential pool of candidates; the particular vehicle that works in one location to inform the myopic population of this exciting new procedure may not be effective in another area. Media placement (print, radio, television) is costly; therefore, professional advice is recommended if experience is lacking. The Eye Surgery Center of Louisiana reports radio to be the most effective media method of reaching candidates, followed by television. In contrast, the London Place Eye Centre reports that radio is unsuccessful and television extremely successful. Both centers highly recommend the 30-min infomercial.

Identifying potential patients captured within the practice is most effective during the patient visit in a routine presentation from the doctor. Direct mail (letters to myopic patients, newsletters) also works well within the comanagement network, and internal marketing provides still another avenue for sending the message via signage, a telephone message-on-hold system, counter posters, brochures, and staff buttons or pins ("Ask me about Laser Vision Correction").

Internal marketing is perhaps the most important and cost-effective method of generating new refractive patients. At the Eye Surgery Center of Louisiana, more than 50% of refractive procedures are generated from patient referrals. A patient whose uncorrected visual expectation has been met is more highly motivated to refer friends and coworkers when those referrals are acknowledged. Patient appreciation techniques—from promotional gift items (T-shirts, refrigerator magnets) to social functions extending special "thank yous"—should be consistently provided, along with surveys to monitor levels of satisfaction.

Patient seminars continue to be an invaluable tool in recruiting refractive patients; their frequency is dictated by the level of education of the prospective patient pool and the maturity of the refractive market. Media announcements (radio and newspaper) commonly provide inquiries. Delivery and location are flexible, depending on the expected attendance and goal. Preregistration is advised to anticipate attendance. Seminars held at the refractive center are effective in introducing the candidate to the quality of the staff and the level of service provided; the free consultation or screening can also be offered toward closure following the presentation. An important purpose of the seminar is to reduce chair time during the consultation and exam, as well as providing information regarding the procedure. An off-site seminar location offers the benefits of reaching beyond the normal geographic limits; this portable seminar can also reinforce referrals when delivered through a comanagement optometric practice. The formal audio/visual presentation should be polished, entertaining, and no longer than 20 min long; this is easily accomplished when the program has been scripted. The goal is to stimulate interest and excitement regarding the procedure, not to present every possible risk, side effect, or complication. As with every patient contact, the goal is to move the inquiry to the next decision-making level. When possible, a former patient should participate by presenting a brief testimonial and answering questions regarding the actual experience; a doctor should be on hand to address clinical/surgical issues, although physician delivery of the presentation is not advised if another practice representative is an accomplished speaker. This individual can describe the experience and quality of the doctor in a less self-aggrandizing manner. The educational seminar should provide the attendee with a warm welcome, an answer to all questions, and written handout exit information for later contemplation. Both American and Canadian markets continue to be successful with educational seminars.

Patient Education and Counseling

There cannot be enough emphasis placed on the importance of informed consent and the role of patient education in refractive eye surgery. Patient marketing communications (ads, brochures, newsletters, videos), as well as clinical communications (informed consent, and pre- and postoperative instructions), must *adequately and accurately present all possible side effects, risks, and potential complications*. The use of videos, patient tests to determine the level of understanding of the procedure, and outcome expectations written by the refractive surgery candidate are excellent tools; however, nothing replaces documentation in the medical record of the discussion of possible risks and complications with the patient by the surgeon. Overlooking any aspect of this crucial patient care information system could lead to severe future problems.

Comanagement

A designated referral coordinator utilized exclusively to maintain the comanagement network is important when a large percentage of refractive patients are comanaged. Two advantages of comanagement are convenience for the patient and freeing up of valuable clinical time for surgery when patients are seen pre- and postoperatively by optometrists. The referral liaison coordinator should have frequent contact with the comanaging doctors to ensure that they are up-to-date on procedures, techniques, drop regimens, etc., and that an open line of communication exists between the comanaging doctor and the surgeon, as well as between the staff of the refractive center and the staff of the comanaging doctor.

Continuing education consisting of both a formal certification course and mini-fellowships increase the consistency and quality of comanaged care. This provides a program allowing comanaging doctors to spend designated times in the refractive center clinic to observe surgery and pre- and postoperative patients, and to determine the quality of the staff and the refractive services program. Most states allow optometrists to receive continuing education credits for the training visits, and the doctors benefit from seeing a wide range of surgical treatments and healing stages of postoperative patients.

Providing a comanagement reference manual, professional newsletters, and updates on surgical technique adds another level of quality to a comanagement program.

Optometrists have not been the predicted referral source expected to fuel laser vision correction. Both the Eye Surgery Center and the London Place Eye Centre initiate more comanagement to optometry than they receive refractive referrals. Patients making initial contact with the refractive center should always be asked for the name of their primary care eye doctor and if they would prefer to be followed by that doctor. This information can then be entered in the inquiry database; therefore, regardless of the date of conversion (it could be 1 year or more), the patient can be returned for comanagement. Individuals from the area of a network optometrist can be given the option of seeing that optometrist for a consultation. When the patient's optometrist is not in the network, an excellent contact opportunity to begin reciprocal referrals is presented.

A patient comanagement agreement should clarify who provides what service and what the respective professional fees cover. The method recommended by the Eye Surgery Center as least apt to trigger an inquiry regarding "incentives to refer" within the U.S. regulatory systems is separate patient payment to each entity (surgeon, facility, and optometrist) providing a service. The London Place Eye Centre uses a fee-for-service basis, paying the comanaging ophthalmologist or optometrist for examinations completed. The information from the exam is transferred to a form which acts both as a billing sheet to trigger payment and as a data form for outcomes, providing the maintenance of a strong outcome database, which is critical in the rapidly advancing field of refractive surgery.

Outcome Analysis

The ability to record and analyze the results of excimer laser surgery is essential in establishing an excimer laser center. The literature regarding the outcome of PRK and PTK is increasing exponentially, and it gives the excimer surgeon a good idea of the results which can be expected with different lasers. However, with continued laser hardware and software changes, these reports do not reflect the current status of PRK. Therefore, it is essential that all surgeons be able to analyze their own results using their laser and be able to present the outcome to patients prior to their surgery. In addition, it is important to be able to review the data if one makes a change in technique, installs a different software version, or makes subtle changes in the level of illumination or level of humidity in the room.

The PRK surgeons at the University of Ottawa Eye Institute, Ottawa General Hospital, recognized this need when they first established their laser center and developed a program running on Microsoft Access not only to record patients' data and produce summary reports, but also to automate the analysis of the results and be in a position to compare their data with other published reports. The following figures show some of the entry screens in the recording database (Fig. 21.3a–e) and the main screen in a separate database established for queries (Fig. 21.4). All information is recorded in the major database. Then the query database is refreshed from one or more of these databases, depending upon the number of centers using this software.

Standard report forms for outcome analysis recording is essential in comparing data from different centers. The surgeon is then able to quickly extract specific information regarding the results of uncorrected visual acuity, best corrected visual acuity, predictability, deviation from intended refraction, haze, and loss of lines of best corrected visual acuity. Graphs showing the spherical equivalent over time, intended versus achieved correction, and haze are instantly displayed and can be imported into Microsoft Power Point for presentations. The software allows various searches to be saved and then rerun with different data.

Outcome analysis is also an effective patient counseling tool. A 45-year-old patient with a -8.00 $+3.00 \times 90°$ prescription could be given the results of all similar patients treated. This information allows the patient to make a more informed decision in electing to pursue refractive surgery.

THREE PERSPECTIVES

The Eye Surgery Center of Louisiana (Stephen F. Brint)

With a busy RK practice for over 10 years and the early experience of having an investigational laser

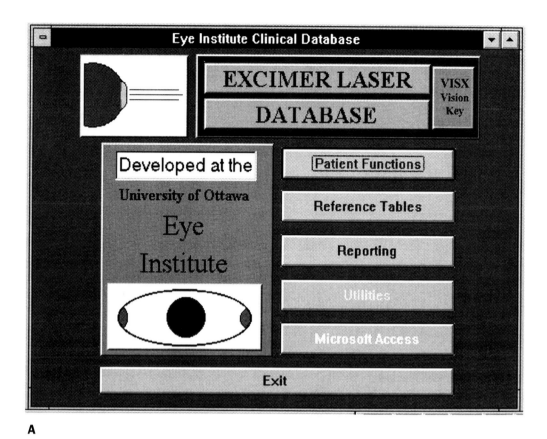

A

Fig. 21.3a–e. Entry screens in the recording data base.

with participation in the FDA PRK clinical trials, understanding that laser vision correction would one day replace RK made choices a little more simple. Experience with both the ability to offer all types of refractive surgery (RK, PRK, ALK, and LASIK) to patients over the last 5 years and the evolution of both staff and patient education regarding exposure to refractive surgery influenced decisions and made them easier than perhaps they are today for someone considering the addition of a refractive center to their practice.

Refractive results at the Eye Surgery Center of Louisiana, for both RK and excimer procedures (PRK and LASIK), have surpassed the expectations dictated by the 10-year Prospective Evaluation of Radial Keratotomy (PERK) and FDA excimer laser clinical trials. Technical advances in instrumentation, corrections in the procedures based on outcomes, and the increased experience of the surgeon have improved performance and predictability.

As a private practitioner in the United States interested in developing refractive surgery in your practice, it is very important to keep an open mind about where we have been and where we are going in refractive surgery. At present, the excimer lasers that are approved for use in the United States are approved only for spherical corrections up to 7 D. This means that for the large group of patients with more than 1.5 D of astigmatism, astigmatic keratotomy performed either before, during, or after the PRK procedure will be necessary, and it is mandatory for the surgeon to be comfortable with and skilled in this technique. Also in selected cases, RK may be the best alternative to refine an undercorrected PRK patient. The place of RK and AK in the future may evolve as an enhancement tool combined with PRK and LASIK.

While it may be relatively easy to become certified in performing PRK techniques, you should expect to either develop incisional surgery expertise or

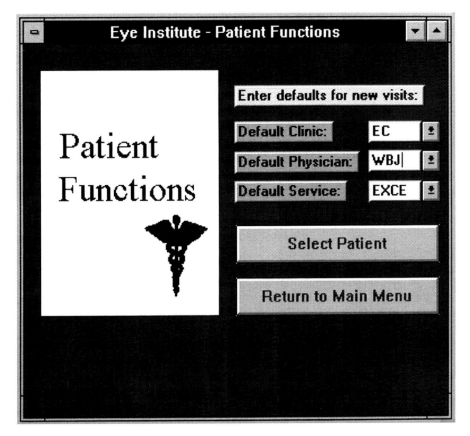

Fig. 21.3b.

Eye Institute - Patient Functions

Enter defaults for new visits:

Default Clinic: EC

Default Physician: WBJ|

Default Service: EXCE

Select Patient

Return to Main Menu

Patient Functions

Excimer Patients Exam Form

Excimer Exam

pts name

01/02/1994

Treatment Eye: Right

Pre-Operative Visit

Display Hints

Excimer Patient Exam Data

Diagnosis:	MYAS		Corneal Clarity (Haze):	0
Uncorrected Visual Acuity:	8	/	400	
Best Corrected Visual Acuity:	20	/	25	
Refraction (Plus Cylinders):				
Manifest:	-10.25	1.00	135	
Auto:	-10.50	0.50	117	
Cycloplegic:	-9.25	0.50	135	

Cancel   Continue

Fig. 21.3c.

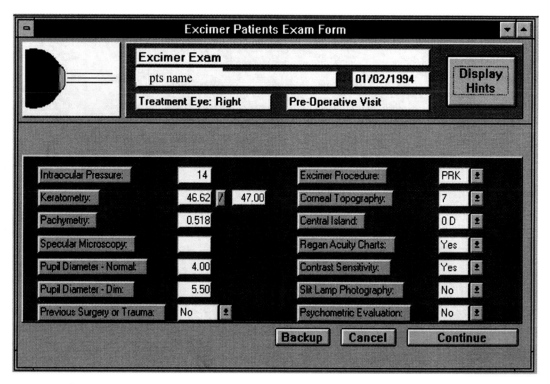

Fig. 21.3d.

Fig. 21.3e.

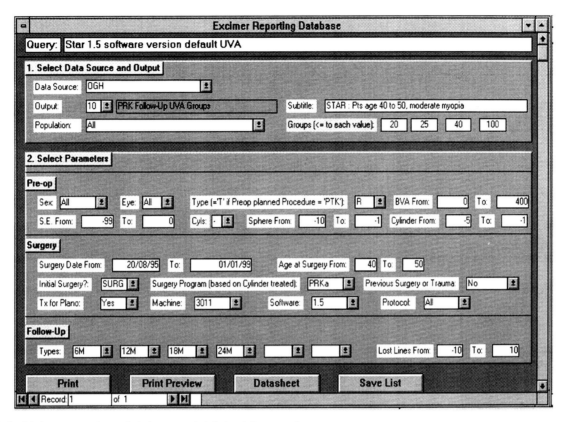

Fig. 21.4. Main screen in a database established for queries.

work with a colleague who is comfortable with incisional surgery in a team effort to offer the best results to your patients. Many physicians believe that LASIK represents the future of refractive surgery because of the quicker rehabilitation of vision it offers compared to PRK, and this is probably true. LASIK, however, requires an even greater commitment to refractive surgery, as both current and future generations of microkeratomes involve a steep learning curve similar to that required for phacoemulsification.

LASIK has been described as 95% microkeratome and 5% PRK, and the use of the microkeratome demands a commitment. This includes not only taking the didactic course and a mini-fellowship, as well as having an experienced microkeratome surgeon with you to oversee your first few cases, but also an ongoing commitment to continuing education and refinement of techniques as this technology continues to evolve, just as phacoemulsification has evolved.

LASIK will perhaps remain, at least for the next 2 to 3 years, in the hands of a relatively small number of surgeons with access to an excimer laser who are highly skilled with the microkeratome, perhaps being involved in one of the ongoing FDA clinical evaluations of this procedure.

With all of this in mind, the joy of refractive surgery, learning new technology and bringing it to your patients to allow them possible freedom from glasses and contact lenses, can be extremely rewarding, both from an emotional and a psychological point of view for your patients, as well as offering new challenges and gratification for you as a physician.

London Place Eye Centre, Inc. (Donald G. Johnson)

The London Place Eye Centre, Inc., began as a medical and surgical eye center in November 1985. During the next few years a variety of private procedures were offered, including cataract surgery, cosmetic lid procedures, and RK. At that time, refractive surgery competition was limited. Only a handful of RKs were being performed on the west coast of Canada, with our closest Canadian competitor being approximately 800 miles east. There was no significant cross-border market during these years.

In November 1990, a VisX Twenty-Twenty (VisX, Inc., Santa Clara, CA) excimer laser was purchased by the London Place Eye Centre. As with any new procedure, Dr Johnson proceeded cautiously with PRK. RK continued to dominate the refractive portion of the practice. However, as PRK proved to be a safe and effective treatment for low myopia, an interesting phenomenon occurred. When RK *and* PRK were offered to patients, there was a decrease in the demand for both procedures. This decrease was attributed to the belief that if the center could not advise what procedure was best for the patient, the patient would opt for neither treatment. No more RKs were performed after May 1992, at which time the center committed to performing only laser refractive surgery.

The competition in the region was negligible during the early years of RK. Patients were generated almost solely by word-of-mouth referrals and the use of press releases and media interviews. No formal advertising or comanagement systems were in place. After 6 years of no refractive competition, the first competitor started performing PRK in Vancouver in June 1991. This may have helped the London Place Eye Centre clinic by increasing awareness of the procedure. There was no drop in the volume of cases.

Throughout the next few years, Canadian regulations allowed the correction of moderate and high myopia using the excimer laser. As results continued to improve even further, the volume of refractive patients increased to the point where the center became a strictly refractive laser surgery clinic. The expanded protocol and experience began to attract patients from the United States who were restricted due to FDA limitations on excimer laser use. This trend has continued today, even after the approval of low myopia treatment in the United States.

Presently, there are four other refractive clinics in the local area and two more within the province of British Columbia. The population of the Greater Vancouver area is approximately 2 million, with a total of 3 million in the province. As the first refractive clinic in the province, with more than 14,000 procedures performed in the clinic, the London Place Eye Centre still has a competitive edge on the market.

Advances in Surgical Technique
This section deals with the evolution of PRK surgical techniques at the London Place Eye Centre, including the advances in total laser epithelial removal, multipass PRK, and multizone PRK.

The Transition from RK to PRK   The decision to commit fully to laser refractive surgery was made by weighing the pros and cons of each procedure. It became clear that the excimer laser represented the future of keratorefractive procedures. The reasons for the switch from RK to PRK are summarized in Table 21.1.

Although the switch from RK to PRK seemed to be a natural progression, the learning curve with PRK was significant. It is a common misconception that excimer laser surgery is a matter of stepping on a pedal and letting the laser do all of the work. The next section describes the advances in surgical technique that have been developed to make this surgery more predictable.

Evolution of PRK Technique   In November 1990, Dr. Johnson began using the VisX excimer laser for low myopia (-1.00 to -6.00 D) with less than 1.00 D of cylinder. The technique used, as per the VisX protocol, included using a suction handpiece that blew nitrogen gas across the corneal surface.[2] This technique was soon abandoned because of a higher incidence of postoperative corneal haze, risk of cyclotorsion of the globe, and patient discomfort with the instrument. Manual epithelial removal was performed using a Beaver blade, followed by irrigation and wiping of the cornea to even hydration. The optical zone sizes used were 5.0 and 5.5 mm. Postoperatively, the eyes were patched and a strong analgesic was prescribed for pain.

In July 1991 astigmatic correction began, and the optical zone size was increased to 6 mm on all eyes. The larger optical zone size decreased the incidence of halos and glare. We also adopted the use of self-fixation instead of holding the eye with a fixation device or forceps. This method was preferred by patients, and decentration was not found to be a

Table 21.1. Comparison of RK with PRK

	RK	PRK
Diurnal fluctuation	Yes	No
Hyperopic shift	Yes	No
Postop pain	Minimal	Controlled with C/L and NSAID
Visual recovery	Rapid	3–7 days
Structural weakening	Yes	No
Retreatment rate	25%	8–10%
Age dependent	Yes	No
Visual aberrations	Halos/starburst	Minimal
Range of myopia	Up to 6 D	Up to 25 D
Surgical skill	High	Moderate
Predictability	Good	Excellent

problem. Postoperative pain and discomfort were lessened by the use of a bandage contact lens and a topical nonsteroidal anti-inflammatory drug[3] every four hours in the immediate postoperative period.

Over the next year, the protocol was expanded to include higher degrees of myopia. Myopic treatments of up to 25 D were performed with reasonable predictability. However, complications such as corneal haze, regression, and central islands still needed to be resolved.

Early in 1993, Dr. Johnson started using laser epithelial removal[4] techniques in selected cases. These procedures were mainly PRK retreatments and RK undercorrections. The rationale was that if a smooth, uniform surface could be created on which to begin the ablation, haze and regression could be reduced. Patients reepithelialized faster and had less discomfort and corneal edema than with the manual method.

By May 1993, all PRKs were being performed using the laser to remove the epithelium. Preliminary results showed less haze and regression; however, predictability was an issue. Dr. Johnson started using a set depth of 50 m on the epithelium, and then moved to 55 and 60 m. Because corneal epithelium did not have a standard thickness, and accurate measurements of it could not be achieved,[5] the method of complete epithelial removal with the laser was developed. This technique, which was described in Chapter 6, allowed the same starting point for the refractive portion of the treatment on all eyes. In May 1994, this method was used routinely in conjunction with a multipass, multizone[6]

ablation pattern. The outcomes have shown this method to be very predictable, with faster healing, less discomfort, and faster return to uncorrected and best corrected visual acuity.

Multiple optical zone sizes were introduced by Piovella for treating moderate and high myopia.[7–10] The objective of this method was, in part, to lessen central depth; however, the benefits of multiple zone sizes extend beyond this reason. The human body is, by nature, not partial to right angles. If we create a sharp "shoulder" on the cornea, it tends to fill in and smooth itself out. This can result in increased keratocyte activity, either generalized or arcuate in nature. By varying the optical zone sizes, a gradual, tapered ablation edge is created, lessening the incidence of haze and regression.

The concept of combining multiple optical zone sizes with multiple passes over the same zone was introduced by Pop. However, using Dr. Pop's method, which he developed for manual removal of the epithelium, resulted in central islands on lower powers when the transepithelial technique was used. This was due to the induced curvature change, as mentioned above. The solution was to start the refractive treatment with smaller optical zone sizes and divide low powers into a minimum of three zones. By delivering more pulses centrally, the incidence of central islands was eliminated.

The next challenge was to improve the final refractions, for the amount of extra correction required to compensate for the transepithelial change in curvature had to be factored in. This method was effective, though the learning curve was quite steep. In January 1996 this procedure was streamlined so that it could be made available to other refractive surgeons. To standardize the treatment, the epithelium was removed as described in Chapter 6, so that it ablated uniformly, without the induced curvature change on Bowman's membrane. The benefits of transepithelial ablations were improved even further, and patients were reepithelialized on average within 48 hr.

To summarize the benefits of this advanced procedure, total laser epithelial removal gives us a definite starting point at which to begin the refractive treatment; creates a smooth surface, with less trauma to the cornea, thereby reducing edema and haze formation; and promotes faster reepithelialization. Multiple zones produce a tapered ablation edge, reducing epithelium and collagen fill; lessen the number of overall pulses and central depth; and deliver more pulses centrally, thereby reducing the incidence of central islands. Multiple passes over a single optical zone smooth the transition between optical zones and create an even smoother surface. This promotes faster healing and quicker return to best corrected and uncorrected vision.

Summary In the last 6 years, refractive surgery has been advancing at a rapid pace. Clinically and administratively, it has been a continual learning experience. Patient education and informed consent are vital to the growth and development of this field. These key elements must be kept in mind when considering marketing strategies and competition.

Department A., Singapore National Eye Centre (Peter Tseng)

Considerations:
There are several factors to consider before setting up a refractive center. These will now be discussed.

- *Sufficient patient pool*: For financial viability, a pool of prospective patients must be available. Highly populated areas are advantageous, as the percentage of myopes will provide a sizable number of potential patients due to the large size of the population. Countries such as China (1.2 billion population) and India (800 million population) are excellent examples. A 10% prevalence rate would equate to about 120 million myopes in China and about 80 million myopes in India. Even a penetration rate of 1% produces very large numbers of patients that would definitely keep many refractive centers very busy and profitable.

- *Patient income*: The affluence of a country is also a very important consideration because potential patients must be able to afford the procedure in order to consider refractive surgery as an alternative solution to the correction of their myopia. Poor and developing countries have difficulty coping with the blindness due to common conditions such as cataracts, trachoma, and vitamin A deficiency; they cannot even consider giving refractive surgery a second thought. There must be a fairly large proportion of affluent myopes who are able to consider refractive surgery as an alternative to spectacle or contact lens wear. In China there is a large number of myopes who have sought refractive surgery because the cost per procedure has been reduced to make it affordable. It is the sheer volume—up to 30 to 50 patients a day being treated—that makes the practice viable.

- *Need*: Ophthalmologists must decide if there is a need to offer refractive surgery. In poor and developing countries, doctors are overburdened by the demand to service the ever-increasing number of cataract patients, so there is little time to concentrate on refractive surgery. The percentage of ophthalmologists in industrialized and developed countries practicing refractive surgery is often less than 10%. This percentage depends strongly on the demand, which is influenced by the above factors.

- *Technical support*: An efficient and effective technical support infrastructure is also very important. The complicated and demanding excimer laser requires constant servicing and maintenance to ensure that it is functioning properly. The demand on the doctor's skill is now much less than the demand on the technician's skill to maintain the equipment and software in perfect working condition.

- *Summary*: Organizing excimer refractive centers requires an in-depth analysis of the above factors, as the initial financial outlay is very high. The number of potential patients and the fee for each procedure must be carefully balanced to allow both affordability and volume to support the center. Many companies that sell these lasers will gladly help the physician to solve these problems, and nonmedical financial backers are willing to invest in the center if funds are not readily available.

Conclusion: Why the Need for Refractive Surgery in Asia?

There is always a place for improving one's perception of life, and there will always be people who want to look and feel better. The need to wear glasses or contact lenses is something which millions of people wish they could do without. As countries become more affluent and society becomes more self-conscious, people will turn to refractive procedures to improve their self-image and eliminate glasses so that they can enjoy the pleasures of life.

As Asia grows increasingly affluent and its people more educated, there is a growing demand for refractive surgery. This is indicated clearly by the huge number of excimer lasers that have been purchased by many countries in this region. Refractive surgery is here to stay. It is only the need to keep up with the latest and newest generation of machines that concerns the refractive surgeon today.

REFERENCES

1. Sperduto RD, Siegal D, Roberts J, Rowland M. Prevalence of myopia in the United States. *Arch Ophthalmol.* 1983;101:405–407.

2. Campos M, Cuevas K, Garbus J, et al. Corneal wound healing after excimer ablation: effects of nitrogen gas blower. *Ophthalmology.* 1992;99:893–897.

3. Ferrari M, Resnati S. Use of topical nonsteroidal anti-inflammatory drugs after photorefractive keratectomy. *J Refract Corneal Surg.* 1994;10(2 suppl): S287—S289.

4. Gimbel HV, DeBroff BM, Beldavs RA, et al. Comparison of laser and manual removal of corneal epithelium for photorefractive keratectomy. *J Refract Surg.* 1995;11(1):36–41.

5. Reinstein DZ, Silverman RH, Rondeau MJ, et al. Epithelial and corneal thickness measurements by high-frequency ultrasound digital signal processing. *Ophthalmology.* 1994;101(1):140–146.

6. Pop M, Aras M. Multizone/multipass photorefractive keratectomy: Six month results. *J Cataract Refract Surg.* 1994;21:633–643.

7. Piovella M. Presented at the American Academy of Ophthalmology Annual Meeting, Chicago, 1991.

8. Kim JH, Hahn TW, Lee YC, et al. Clinical experience of two-step photorefractive keratectomy in 19 eyes with high myopia. *J Refract Corneal Surg.* 1993;9 (suppl):S44–S47.

9. Ch YS, Kim CG, Kim WB, et al. Multistep photorefractive keratectomy for high myopia. *J Refract Corneal Surg.* 1993;9(suppl):S27–S47.

10. Dausch D, Klein R, Schroder E, et al. Excimer laser photorefractive keratectomy with tapered transition zone for high myopia; a preliminary report of six cases. *J Cataract Refract Surg.* 1993;19:590–594.

Comanagement in Refractive Surgery: Delivery Systems for Eye Care

R. Bruce Grene

Comanagement is the cooperative interaction of health care providers to maximize the quality of care and services provided to their mutual patient. At its best, comanagement is one of the highest-quality delivery systems; at its worst, comanagement becomes a kickback scheme. Comanagement exists in all fields of health care. The referral from family practice physician to internal medicine subspecialist to surgeon represents the movement of patients from primary to secondary to tertiary care providers. Similar referral structures are now fully developed for the specialty of refractive surgery. The specific structure, the legal ramifications, and the economic implications vary, depending upon the form of the delivery system involved.

EYE CARE DELIVERY SYSTEMS

Three eye care delivery systems coexist in the United States (Fig. 22.1). The first level of eye care delivery, Level I, is based upon the *independent* relationship of the "three O's": opticianry, optometry, and ophthalmology. In Level I systems each profession keeps to itself, with very little cross-referral. There is little opportunity for comanagement in Level I delivery systems.

It is within Level II and Level III systems that comanagement flourishes. These two systems are quite different from one another, although they may coexist within the same practice. The Level II delivery system is termed *interdependent*. Within the interdependent model, the eye care professions refer back and forth actively to one another. However, despite the referral relationship, there is no formal corporate affiliation among the provider groups. The Level III or *integrated* model reflects the growing integration of eye care professions into unified corporate structures. These structures range from informal networks to full equity-based corporate partnerships. Level III systems may be local, regional, or national, as with companies such as the Physician Resource Group (PRG). In the more formal corporate models of integrated practice, many of the legal and economic problems of referral relationships are diminished.

The interdependent Level II system is based upon the referral of patients from primary to secondary and tertiary care providers. In a patient-centered Level II comanagement system, the patient benefits from the geographic convenience of primary care offices. The trained primary care comanager can support the pre- and postoperative processes and may be more skilled than the surgeon in refraction, contact lens fitting, and other aspects of vision rehabilitation. Continuity of care is another advantage of patient-centered Level II structures.

For high-quality comanagement to exist, the primary care doctor and that doctor's staff must make a strong and ongoing commitment to education. In the rapidly changing world of refractive surgery, a single half-day course is inadequate for the education of the primary care team. Few primary care doctors believe that such a course could prepare them for top-quality contact lens dispensing. In addition, the risk, complexity, and rate of change are much greater in refractive surgery than in contact lens practice.

Even when an excellent comanagement program is offered, the patient sometimes prefers to begin

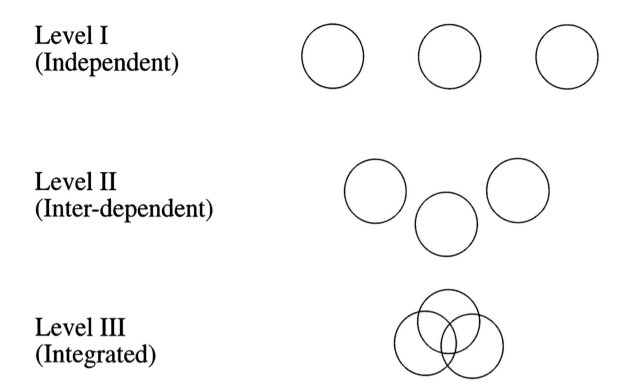

Fig. 22.1. Three delivery systems for eye care. The relationship of the three "O's" takes three forms, and the structure of comanagement varies within each form.

and complete refractive surgery care under the direct supervision of the surgeon. Comanaging primary care doctors must respect the patient's decision. The patient may be informed of the option of comanagement but should not coerced into comanagement by the primary care office.

Because the referral-based Level II comanagement structure is susceptible to abuse, every effort must be made to ensure that the system is truly patient centered. A number of financially centered models have proliferated over the past few years. Some of these are driven by investments in PRK facilities. Other economic incentives include unusually high comanagement fees. These structures are rightfully at risk of prosecution for violation of anti-kickback laws. A small number of PRK companies pander to the political demands of various optometric groups such as support of optometric licensure for surgery. When the focus shifts to economic or political benefit, the comanagement system loses its patient-centered focus.

In the Level II delivery system of eye care, the three professional groups (opticianry, optometry,

and ophthalmology) became vertically and horizontally integrated. This integration can range from loosely structured networks to more formal (MSO) systems. Full integration involves true equity-based partnerships within traditional corporate or limited liability company (LLC) structures. In the more formal integrated systems, comanagement takes on the appearance of traditional group practice. The integrated eye care practice exploits the advantages of partnership to focus completely upon the needs of the patient. In integrated models, both economic and political gain are less likely to contaminate the decision-making process. Compared to Level II referral systems, the Level III integrated model offers fewer legal challenges since there are fewer incentives for abuse for political or financial gain.

Integrated practices can still support referral relationships with independent practices outside the group. When an integrated practice participates in Level II referral relationships, it is best to use a formal referral process so that the patient is identified as part of the comanagement program. This maximizes the likelihood that the patient will be returned to his or her independent primary care source after refractive surgery and not be assimilated into the primary care practices of the integrated group.

THE MECHANICS OF COMANAGEMENT

One of the greatest challenges in developing a comanagement program is the choreography of patient flow. The carefully thought out patient-centered program must balance many factors. Patient flow must address patient education, appropriate provision of services by each participant in the program, geographic convenience, and maximum efficiency for the practices. During 5 years of comanagement, the author has developed a 10-step cycle (Fig. 22.2) to describe the components of comanagement.

Step 1: Awareness

Awareness of the option of refractive surgery has been one of the greatest historical challenges in the refractive surgery practice. With the approval and

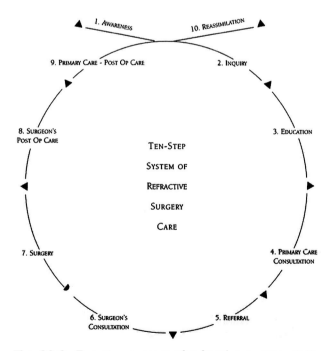

Fig. 22.2. Ten-step system of refractive surgery care.

dissemination of excimer laser technology, there has been a dramatic increase in the general public's awareness of refractive surgery. Nonetheless, the majority of successful, high-quality refractive surgery programs will rely upon advertising to create awareness. Simply waiting for patients to ask about refractive surgery services is unlikely to lead to a sufficient case volume to allow mastery of either the surgical procedure or the component steps of patient pre- and postoperative care.

In both direct contact and advertisements, great care must be taken to balance appropriately the risks and benefits of refractive surgery. The claims made by comanaging practices must be carefully constructed to match the surgeon's marketing program. Each member of the comanagement team is at risk for Federal Trade Commission (FTC) and Food and Drug Administration (FDA) sanctions for the program's advertisements.

Step 2: Inquiry

It is essential that step I (awareness) be carefully linked to step II (inquiry). Many practices have invested both time and money in advertising programs without carefully preparing the entire staff and provider network for the response to the advertising.

The desired effect of a program to increase awareness is to stimulate an inquiry about refractive surgery. Inquiry is the "call to action" of a program designed to build refractive surgery volume.

Step 3: Education

The response to an inquiry should focus upon appropriate and thorough education. The reader is advised to avoid hard-sell techniques which push the patient into a consultation and surgery, bypassing the education process. Within comanagement systems, education can be handled by both the primary care doctor and the surgeon or by the surgeon alone, but the surgeon cannot abdicate his or her responsibility to educate the patient. In some markets, a weekly infomercial provides an excellent starting point for patient education. Print and video materials abound, but the surgeon must choose resources that will fit well into the busy primary care practices of the comanagers. Involve the primary care doctors and their staff in the development of educational resources. The education process should be well underway before the patient is scheduled for a primary care consultation (step IV).

Step 4: Primary Care Consultation

After the patient has had an opportunity to learn the basics of refractive surgery, a primary care consultation should follow. This should occur at a separate appointment, not added to a general eye exam at which the patient makes an inquiry regarding refractive surgery. The primary care consultation is a brief, focused evaluation which allows the primary care doctor to assess the patient's psychological and physical indications and contraindications to surgery. The author has developed a four-step test (Fig. 22.3) which allows the primary care provider

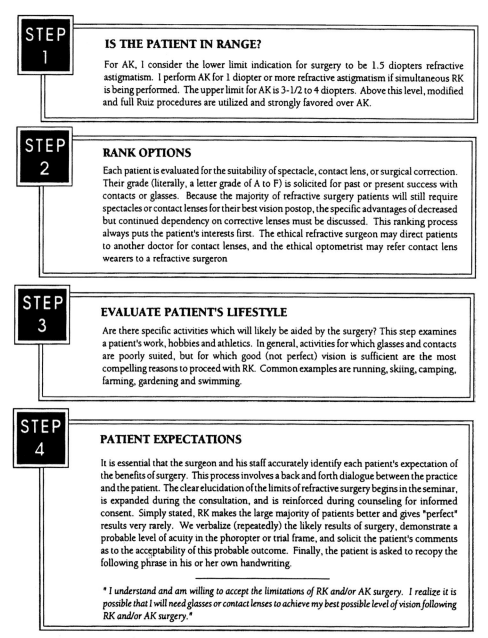

STEP 1

IS THE PATIENT IN RANGE?

For AK, I consider the lower limit indication for surgery to be 1.5 diopters refractive astigmatism. I perform AK for 1 diopter or more refractive astigmatism if simultaneous RK is being performed. The upper limit for AK is 3-1/2 to 4 diopters. Above this level, modified and full Ruiz procedures are utilized and strongly favored over AK.

STEP 2

RANK OPTIONS

Each patient is evaluated for the suitability of spectacle, contact lens, or surgical correction. Their grade (literally, a letter grade of A to F) is solicited for past or present success with contacts or glasses. Because the majority of refractive surgery patients will still require spectacles or contact lenses for their best vision postop, the specific advantages of decreased but continued dependency on corrective lenses must be discussed. This ranking process always puts the patient's interests first. The ethical refractive surgeon may direct patients to another doctor for contact lenses, and the ethical optometrist may refer contact lens wearers to a refractive surgeron

STEP 3

EVALUATE PATIENT'S LIFESTYLE

Are there specific activities which will likely be aided by the surgery? This step examines a patient's work, hobbies and athletics. In general, activities for which glasses and contacts are poorly suited, but for which good (not perfect) vision is sufficient are the most compelling reasons to proceed with RK. Common examples are running, skiing, camping, farming, gardening and swimming.

STEP 4

PATIENT EXPECTATIONS

It is essential that the surgeon and his staff accurately identify each patient's expectation of the benefits of surgery. This process involves a back and forth dialogue between the practice and the patient. The clear elucidation of the limits of refractive surgery begins in the seminar, is expanded during the consultation, and is reinforced during counseling for informed consent. Simply stated, RK makes the large majority of patients better and gives "perfect" results very rarely. We verbalize (repeatedly) the likely results of surgery, demonstrate a probable level of acuity in the phoropter or trial frame, and solicit the patient's comments as to the acceptability of this probable outcome. Finally, the patient is asked to recopy the following phrase in his or her own handwriting.

" I understand and am willing to accept the limitations of RK and/or AK surgery. I realize it is possible that I will need glasses or contact lenses to achieve my best possible level of vision following RK and/or AK surgery."

Fig. 22.3. Four-step test form.

to effectively screen and counsel patients. In order to make comanagement economically viable, it is essential that primary care practices minimize the "chair time" spent with refractive surgery candidates. Reliance upon preconsultation education and an effective surgeon's education program help keep the primary care consultation manageable in length.

Step 5: Referral and Informed Consent

Following the primary care consultation, the comanaging doctor must effectively schedule the candidate with the surgical team. It is also valuable to initiate the informed consent process so that patients have time to review these documents prior to the surgeon's consultation (Fig. 22.4). Primary care offices should be provided with a surgery prep pack to prepare them for the surgeon's consultation and surgery. This education helps make all downstream stages more efficient (Fig. 22.5).

Step 6: Surgeon's Consultation

During the surgeon's consultation, selected testing is repeated to confirm the accuracy of the refraction, manual keratometry, acuities, and intraocular pressure. Special tests such as topography studies or cell count analysis may be performed by the surgeon.

The four-step test is again utilized to determine the suitability of the candidate for refractive surgery. Once it is determined that the patient is a good candidate, then the specific recommended procedure or procedures are discussed. The primary care comanager should avoid telling the patient which procedure will be used. It is the surgeon's responsibility to choose the most appropriate procedure, as the rapidly shifting applications of radial keratotomy (RK), laser in situ keratomileusis (LASIK), photorefractive keratectomy (PRK), and automated lamellar keratoplasty (ALK) make it unwise for comanagers to lock in on a specific procedure. Fee's are explained and collected following the surgeon's consultation (Fig. 22.6).

Step 7: Surgery

The actual surgical procedure is the most important step in the surgery process, but today's refractive surgery armamentarium offers a wide range of brief, painless, and very effective procedures. The selection of a given procedure depends upon many factors. The impact of a comanagement program upon the surgeon's decision includes speed of visual recovery, complexity of postoperative management, rate and complexity of enhancement, ability to do bilateral simultaneous surgery, and complexity of postoperative vision rehabilitation including contact lens fitting.

If one looks at all of the refractive procedures available with regard to ease of comanagement, one finds a spectrum from LASIK to PRK. LASIK is one of the most straightforward procedures for comanagement since it has extremely rapid visual recovery, easy postoperative management, a straightforward strategy for enhancement, the ability for bilateral simultaneous surgery, and straightforward postoperative vision rehabilitation including contact lens fitting. At the other end of the spectrum is PRK, which requires a complex, prolonged interaction of patient, comanager, and surgeon. The PRK patient has much slower visual recovery, a more complex postoperative course including 3 to 4 or more months of steroid use, and a more difficult enhancement strategy. PRK patients are frequently operated on months apart. The visual rehabilitation during this interim is sometimes complex, so PRK requires many more office visits. The immediate postoperative management is more complex due to the initial epithelial defect with exposed stroma. In summary, LASIK is the easiest procedure for a comanagement program, PRK is by far the most difficult, and incisional procedures such as RK and astigmatic keratotomy (AK) are intermediate. Older lamellar procedures such as ALK are also intermediate. Their complexity is due primarily to the very slow visual rehabilitation necessitated by the gradual decrease in irregular astigmatism over many months.

A comanagement program exists primarily to provide geographic convenience for patients. Procedures which require multiple trips to the surgeon certainly diminish the advantages of comanagement. Procedures which are best managed with the full involvement of the surgeon but which are comanaged by optometrists for economic or political reasons place the patient at risk. In the author's opinion, LASIK, followed by incisional techniques, offer the best combination of attributes for comanaged programs.

✔ **I. Pre-Operative Data (See CoManagers Packet)**

___A. Testing:
    1. Complete preop data sheet entirely (please fill in all blanks)
    2. Mail or Fax to Grene Vision Group on the **SAME DAY** you perform your consult.

___B. Estimation of postop uncorrected acuity:
    1. Note "patient demonstrated "20/____ using
        _____ X _____ OD and _____ X _____OS in phoropter.

___C. Discussion documented - use additional pages as needed.
    1. Discussion examples: "Patient understands and accepts that he/she will need thin specs for their best distance vision after refractive surgery. Presbyopia was discussed. Patient (40 years or older) realizes that they will need thin specs for their best near vision."

✔ **II. Fees**

___A. Collect your comanagement fee.
___B. Complete fee agreement sheet, and have patient sign. Retain a copy, give one copy to patient, and mail a copy to Grene Vision Group.

✔ **III. Scheduling Surgeon's Consultation & Surgery**

___A. Call Grene Vision Group at 316-636-2010 to schedule your patient's surgeon's consult and surgery (specify Dr. Grene or Dr. Wellemeyer).
___B. Mail or fax your Preop Data Sheet to Grene Vision Group ASAP. This form must arrive no later than **2 days prior** to the scheduled surgery date. Your patient's surgery maust be postponed if we not receive this data 48-hours prior to surgery.

✔ **IV. Surgery Prep Pack**

___A. Review contents of pack with patient.
    GIVE PATIENT A SURGERY PREP PACK TO TAKE HOME
    SURGERY PREP PACK INCLUDES:

List	Patient Check List
Form A	Patient preop instructions.
Form B	Patient PostOp instructions.
Form C	Patient Consent Form
Form D	Patient homwork and Signature.
	(Instruct Patient: DO NOT SIGN untill surgery consult).
Map	Pharmacy location in your area.
Video	Instruct patient to take home and view in it's entirety. ASAP.
	Video MUST be viewed by patient prior to surgery. It contains important instructions.
Forms	Agreement of Payment
	Surgery Fees
	Surgery Scheduling Sheet

✔ **Instruct patient to bring entire Surgery Prep Pack to surgery day, including video tape. Failure to bring entire Surgery Prep Pack can delay surgery by at least one hour.**

✔ **Remember: Send Preop Data Sheet to Grene Vision Group AT LEAST 2 days before your patient's surgery....or suregry must be postponed.**

Fig. 22.4. Optometric comanagement checklist.

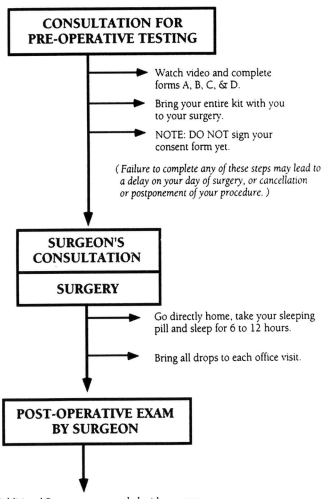

Fig. 22.5. Patient checklist.

	One Eye	Two Eyes
RK/AK	$600	$1100
ALK/LLK	$1000	$2000
PRK/LASIK	$1250	$2500

Fees include surgeon's fee, facility fee, and next day postoperative visit.

■ ■ ■

Follow-up care (any visit after the first postoperative visit) is charged at $45 per visit.

Fig. 22.6. Refractive surgery menu.

Step 8: Surgeon's Postoperative Care

Comanagement programs vary in their allocation of postoperative care responsibilities. The division of fees between surgeon and comanager should reflect the relative contributions of each participant to pre- and postoperative services. Some comanagement systems relegate the surgeon to a technician's role and place most of the responsibility in the hands of the primary care optometrist. Procedures such as RK in the hands of a experienced surgical team may require a surgeon's evaluation only at postoperative day 1. More complex procedures such as PRK may require 3 to 5 days of attention by the surgeon before the patient is released to the care of the comanaging optometrist. Surgeons are well advised to remember that they cannot abdicate their responsibilities for preoperative education, informed consent, patient selection, and postoperative management. Although comanagement exposes the primary care provider to malpractice risk, the surgeon is still held responsible for complications or patient dissatisfaction.

Step 9: Comanager's Postoperative Care

The comanager's postoperative care should entail monitoring of lower-risk aspects of healing, management of visual rehabilitation, and recommendation of enhancement procedures. This means that an entirely new set of clinical skills must be mastered, including but not limited to the diagnosis of regular, macroirregular, and microirregular astigmatism; diagnosis of incision depth and gape with RK; identification of wound-healing stages following PRK; interpretation of multifocal optical systems created by refractive surgery; and clinical judgment regarding the timing and appropriateness of enhancement procedures.

Step 10: Reassimilation

One of the most essential aspects of comanagement is the transfer of patients from the comanagement program back to the regular primary care practice. It is best to plan for step 10 right from the beginning of contact with patients. One must stress clearly, both verbally and in print, the exact duration and extent of comanagement service. Patients will frequently expect a lifetime of eye care at no charge following refractive surgery. Communication

is the key. It is essential that patients understand clearly the services that they are buying in the comanagement package. It is wise to have patients initial this document, which clearly outlines the benefits, duration, and cost of the comanagement program.

SEVEN RULES OF REFRACTIVE SURGERY CO-MANAGEMENT

Although the 10-step model adequately characterizes the structure of comanagement, it does not capture the basic principles which must be understood to have a high-quality, effective, and profitable comanagement program. Based upon 5 years of work with over 100 comanaging optometrists, the author suggests the following seven guidelines for successful comanagement. These guidelines address the basic issues which surgeons should consider with their comanaging colleagues.

1. *Charge a fair comanagement fee.* Refractive surgery is an increasingly competitive arena. The comanager should establish his or her own fee and collect it from the patient. Excessive fees alienate patients and drive them to other providers. Remember that refractive surgery is not a profit center in itself. Retention of refractive surgery patients within the primary care practice is the goal.

2. *Identify and control costs.* Because refractive surgery is a low profit margin service, it is important that every effort be made to monitor costs to the practice. Chair time, staff support, and the cost of printed materials must all be factored in. Some costs can be diminished by participating in a large network of comanaging practices.

3. *Maximize your case volume.* Don't dabble in comanagement. It is difficult to master your clinical skills and the skills of your staff by comanaging only one case every week or two. Approach comanagement as you would your contact lens practice. If you're going to commit, commit fully, since quality and quantity generally keep company.

4. *Offer associated services and products.* Refractive surgery is a marvelous service to patients, but it rarely creates 20/20 emmetropia. This

patient population requires a number of post-operative optical goods and services. Protective sports glasses are essential for shooters and patients involved in sports in which a blow to the eye is possible. Reading glasses are frequently required, as are low-power distance glasses to correct residual emmetropia. Many patients have a loss of contrast and benefit from the variety of high-contrast tints available today. Finally, refractive surgery patients should be seen annually. The average optometric patient is seen approximately every 3 years. Refractive surgery patients required many primary care goods and services.

5. *Retain your patient base.* Failure to participate in refractive surgery comanagement means that your patients will be abandoned at a time when they need your counsel and care. In addition, practices can afford to lose a significant proportion of their existing patient base. Refractive surgery patients, furthermore, are a particularly valuable subset of patients since they frequently come from your most profitable group—today's contact lens wearers. It is possible that more than 50% of your current contact lens population will become refractive surgery patients within the next decade.

6. *Expand your patient base.* The visible, high-quality comanagement program gives a primary care practice a competitive advantage by developing expertise in this field. You will not only retain your existing base but also attract new patients. Few patients are as vocal about their eye care as the refractive surgery population.

7. *Provide first-rate care.* Be sure that your comanagement program is patient centered and not driven by economics or politics. Make a strong commitment for you and your staff to master this complex, rapidly changing field. The golden rule applies: comanage your patients as you would want to be comanaged.

THE FUTURE OF COMANAGEMENT

The future of comanagement will be influenced by the greater forces of change impacting all of medicine and eye care. A decrease in fees coupled with managed care is driving the reorganization of opticianry, optometry, and ophthalmology into horizontally and vertically integrated systems. This is no surprise, since we have witnessed similar consolidation within the rest of medicine. As integration moves forward, there will be a continued shift of Level I and Level II practices into Level III integrated delivery systems. Today's anterior segment surgeon continues to see the world as fee for service and volume driven. This naturally leads to an emphasis upon referral relationships. Tomorrow's integrated practice will live with a greater number of capitated patients and a team-oriented view of care. Refractive surgery comanagement will increasingly involve a well-coordinated team of technicians, optometrists, and refractive surgeons focused on high-quality, efficient, low-cost refractive surgery. Comanagement as a tool to drive referrals will diminish. Comanagement as a tool to enhance quality and efficiency will increase.

23

Medical-Legal Aspects of Refractive Surgery

Alan E. Reider

The challenge of writing a chapter on the medical-legal aspects of refractive surgery for an international text is daunting. While the traditional legal issues of medical liability, such as malpractice and informed consent, have relevance worldwide, today substantial attention is directed to regulatory issues which respond to the constant advances in refractive procedures. Further, to add to the complexity of this area, medical-legal issues must be analyzed in connection with the laws and regulations, as well as case laws which arise from individual jurisdictions. With this introduction, we turn first to regulatory issues which affect refractive surgery, followed by the traditional concerns of malpractice and informed consent. Finally, we summarize the potential impact of the regulatory issues on the traditional liability concerns.

REGULATORY ISSUES

Licensing Concerns

Performing the Procedure

With limited exceptions, the performance of a refractive procedure is not likely to generate significant licensing concerns. State and federal laws generally protect the sanctity of the physician practice and respect the ability of a physician to determine the appropriate care to be rendered to his or patient. Refractive surgery, while now generally accepted by the medical community, had been a subject of controversy in the early 1980s, when conservative ophthalmologists considered the procedure experimental. Nevertheless, states did not interfere with physicians who performed the procedure, as it was within the discretion of the medical

professional. The sanctity of the medical practice also protects from state licensing concerns those ophthalmologists who use custom-made or otherwise adulterated lasers to perform PRK. Perhaps more significantly, because the use of the excimer laser is not a surgical procedure, in some states, notably Idaho and Oklahoma, optometrists may use the excimer laser within the scope of the optometric license.[1] Finally, despite the fact that the Food and Drug Administration's (FDA's) approvals of the excimer lasers do not extend to the laser in situ keratomileusis (LASIK) procedure, and despite the fact that there are currently investigations involving the LASIK procedure, state licensing laws do not prohibit physicians from performing this procedure within the physician's practice.

Comanagement of Refractive Surgery

Chapter 22 of this text is dedicated to comanagement. However, a brief discussion of the regulatory considerations of comanagement and the potential impact on medical-legal issues is appropriate here.

Within the licensing context, the question to be addressed is whether the optometrist comanagement partner is licensed to perform the preoperative and postoperative services. As a general rule, one turns to the State Optometric Practice Act to determine whether specific services fall within the license of an optometrist. Those acts, as interpreted by state boards of optometry, usually support the propriety of an optometrist performing preoperative and postoperative care.

State boards of medicine, however, may take a different approach, and here lies the potential problem. Those boards may take the position that comanagement of any surgical procedure with optometrists is improper, as the postoperative care should be performed only by a licensed ophthalmologist. The basis for this position often is that postoperative care is part of the overall surgical procedure and, therefore, is outside the scope of the optometrist's license.

Several states have struggled with this issue. The attorney general's office in the State of California has issued conflicting opinions in response to requests for guidance; in 1994 it stated that the performance of postoperative care was outside the scope of an optometrist's license, yet, 1 year later, it discussed those situations where optometrists could perform postoperative care without violating that state's anti-kickback law.[2] In 1992 the Iowa Board of Medical Examiners issued a declaratory ruling in response to a petition filed by the Iowa Academy of Ophthalmology concerning the propriety of an optometrist performing preoperative or postoperative care. That ruling and subsequent actions by the Academy have triggered a complaint filed in the federal district court by the Iowa optometric Association against the Academy, alleging anticompetitive activity in violation of Section 1 of the Sherman Act.[3] Litigation involving a dispute between the Board of Optometry and the Board of Medicine concerning comanagement has also taken place in Florida.[4]

FDA REGULATORY ISSUES

Reference is made to Chapter 24. A brief overview of FDA issues is appropriate in the context of medical-legal considerations in refractive surgery.

"Custom Device" Exception

Because of the significant delay in the FDA's approval of the excimer laser for the performance of PRK and the significant technological developments which have taken place but have not yet received approval, many physicians have sought alternative means to provide PRK to their patients. A small number have turned to the "custom device" exception to the food and drug laws, which permits the use of a medical device without obtaining FDA approval. The custom device is defined as a medical device "not generally available in finished form . . . and not offered through labeling or advertising . . . for commercial distribution [which] is intended to

meet the special needs of . . . [a] physician . . . in the course of [his/her] . . . professional practice . . . and . . . is not generally available to or generally used by other physicians."[5]

There is little guidance to allow physicians to determine whether the custom device exception applies to a laser developed by a physician for use in his or her practice. There are no court opinions which define a custom device in this context, and the legislative history is extremely limited. The FDA has defined the term *custom device* narrowly as meaning a device which (1) deviates from devices generally available; (2) is not generally available to or generally used by other physicians; (3) is not generally available in finished form; (4) is not offered for commercial distribution through labeling or advertising; and, most important, (5) is intended for use by an individual patient or "to meet the special needs of the physician."[6] In certain cases, the FDA has issued warning letters to individuals who have developed custom lasers, advising that the FDA believes such practices violate the law.[7]

Performance of LASIK

As noted in the discussion concerning licensing issues, a physician may perform LASIK within his or her own practice without concern about licensing implications. While the analysis of the food and drug laws in connection with the performance of LASIK is not quite so simple, it is generally accepted that the result is the same, at least as long as the physician is using one of the approved excimer lasers.

The performance of LASIK necessarily involves the use of the excimer laser for a purpose other than that for which it was approved. Indeed, the FDA's approvals of the excimer laser were very specific in connection with the indications for use.[8] Furthermore, there are ongoing investigations relating to the LASIK procedure using the excimer laser.

The food and drug laws, however, also recognize the sanctity of a physician's practice and allow a physician to use medical devices which are otherwise approved for any purpose the physician deems appropriate. In other words, even though the FDA approved a device for specific purposes, a physician may use that device in his or her practice for other, nonapproved (i.e., "off-label") uses. The FDA has recently accepted this analysis in the excimer laser area and has now said that a physician's use of "a laser approved only for PRK" for the LASIK procedure is "a practice of medicine issue as long as the physician does not market or promote the laser for LASIK."[9]

With respect to use of a custom device for LASIK, the law is more clouded. In that situation, an unapproved device is used for an unapproved indication. The FDA has said that this use violates the food and drug laws and has threatened to take regulatory action against a physician who uses such a custom device for LASIK. To date, the regulatory action has been limited to warning letters, but the FDA has indicated that it may seek seizures or injunctions in appropriate cases.

MARKETING ISSUES: FEDERAL TRADE COMMISSION OVERSIGHT

Perhaps more than any other ophthalmic procedure, refractive surgery has generated significant attention in the area of marketing. This interest can be attributed largely to the fact that refractive surgery is generally not covered by third-party payers and, therefore, promotion of the procedure is made directly to the public. Further, because of the significant participation by commercial entities in the establishment of laser centers, the traditional business approach to marketing is now being applied to a medical procedure. As a result, the Federal Trade Commission (FTC), which is responsible for policing "unfair or deceptive" practices which affect commerce, has taken a significant interest in the marketing or refractive procedures.[10]

In 1994 the FTC began a nationwide investigation of advertising claims by physicians who perform RK. It appears that the FTC was particularly concerned; among other things, about advertisers' ability to substantiate claims that RK eliminates the need for corrective lenses and provides permanent vision correction.[11] As with other medical procedures that have been the subject of FTC scrutiny, claims regarding the efficacy, safety, and recovery time of the procedure and the degree of pain that it entails may attract the FTC's attention.

It has been widely anticipated that with the approval of the excimer laser there will be new and

perhaps more aggressive advertising of the refractive procedure. If so, the FTC likely will expand its investigation into this area. Undoubtedly, many of the issues raised in the RK investigation must be considered in the context of marketing PRK.

FRAUD AND ABUSE ISSUES

Fraud and abuse concerns involving refractive surgery arise almost entirely from the referral relationship between the optometrist and the ophthalmologist and the establishment of comanagement programs. Generally, this problem can be traced to the erroneous belief that because refractive procedures are paid for almost exclusively by the patient, rather than by the Medicare or Medicaid programs, there are no regulatory issues which apply. In fact, however, many states have antikickback laws which parallel the federal law or have sufficiently broad licensing laws which allow a state board of medicine to interpret a kickback relationship as violating an ethical conduct standard.

Although some may allege that comanagement programs, by their very nature, constitute a kickback, this argument has been effectively rebutted by virtue of the fact that the Medicare program approves of comanagement in the case of cataract surgery by allowing the optometrist to bill for the postoperative care. Further, the Medicare program has specified that the surgical component of cataract surgery is worth 80% of the global fee, while the postoperative component is worth 20%, reflecting the relative value of the two components. It is generally accepted that as long as the referral to the optometrist is not the "price" for the initial referral (i.e., there is no quid pro quo), comanagement of cataract surgery is not an issue.

Applying the parameters of the Medicare program to refractive surgery comanagement should provide a strong defense against the allegation of a kickback. Many practices, however, prefer to bill for refractive procedures globally and pay the optometrist a portion of the fee for performing the postoperative care. Payment to the same optometrist who referred the patient to the ophthalmologist for the procedure, however, may trigger an allegation that the payment, in fact, constitutes a kickback. For this reason, it is generally advised that each professional should bill for the services he or she performs. Similarly, when considering the appropriate proportion of the global fee which should be attributed to the surgery and that which should be attributed to postoperative care, it is important to be able to justify the amounts billed based on the relative intensity and extent of the services performed by each professional. While the 80%/20% split determined by the Medicare program for cataract surgery may not be appropriate in the case of refractive procedures, if the ophthalmologist reduces the surgical fee in order to allow the optometrist to inflate the postoperative fee to an unreasonably high level, both parties could be subject to an allegation that the arrangement constitutes a kickback and violates a state kickback law or constitutes an unethical practice in violation of a state licensing law.

GENERAL LIABILITY ISSUES

Malpractice

Due to the relatively recent evolution of refractive surgery and the length of time it takes for malpractice cases to wind their way through the judicial process, the body of case law in this area is limited. From reported cases and settlements, however, it is possible to identify those claims which are filed most frequently and those which are most likely to result in liability.

In a review of these cases and settlements, four primary claims appear most frequently: (1) negligent performance of the surgical procedure or negligent provision of postoperative care; (2) lack of informed consent; (3) allegations that the patient was an improper candidate for refractive surgery; and (4) nonmedical claims, such as fraudulent advertising, breach of warranty, or breach of promise. While many refractive surgery malpractice cases settle for nominal amounts (less than $100,000) or are dismissed early in the proceedings based on lack of merit, the potential liability exposure can be considerable. For example, there has been one $5.4 million judgment in favor of a plaintiff in California who underwent bilateral RK which "left him functionally blind."[12] And while historically physicians have settled cases because of their nuisance value, today the physician must take into consideration that the settlement will likely trigger a report to the National Health Practitioner Data

Bank. This notice may then result in further inquiry by entities such as a state licensing board, a hospital peer review committee, an insurance company, or a professional society.

Compared to cataract surgery, refractive surgery is associated with greater potential malpractice exposure. This is due to a variety of factors. First, refractive surgery patients are younger, more affluent, and generally more likely to sue. The potential damage awards are significantly greater due to the patient's age and functional visual status before surgery. Moreover, while refractive procedures are generally accepted in the ophthalmic community, it remains relatively easy for a plaintiff's attorney to obtain an expert witness to testify that refractive procedures are not medically indicated or too risky in light of alternative treatment, such as glasses or contact lenses. With this background, we turn to the areas of liability most frequently cited in refractive surgery malpractice cases.

Negligence

Surgery is not an exact science. Unanticipated problems may occur or the care rendered may deviate from the acceptable standard of care. For example, in one judgment in favor of the plaintiff for $175,000, the physician's failure to keep a patient's head steady during the procedure resulted in an extension of the incision into the pupillary zone of the cornea.[13] In another case which resulted in a $214,500 verdict for the plaintiff (and $15,000 for the plaintiff's wife for lack of consortium), the surgeon performed multiple procedures involving a total of 78 incisions on the plaintiff's right eye which caused significant loss of vision and the need for a corneal transplant in the future.[14] While errors which result in harm to the patient occur in certain cases, even in the absence of negligence, patients who obtain a surgical result which is less than they expected are potential plaintiffs.

Based on the malpractice cases reported, the bases for negligence allegations include overcorrection, making too many incisions, making irregular incisions or incorrect placement of incisions, and negligent postoperative care (including failure to monitor properly steroid or antibiotic use and failure to detect and treat complications). From the perspective of a malpractice defense attorney, overcorrection may be a particularly troublesome situation. Obviously, a patient who asserts that he or she is worse after surgery (i.e., needed glasses for only limited purposes, such as driving, before the surgery but now needs glasses to perform all activities at close range) has jury appeal, despite the fact that the patient may have been warned about the possibility of overcorrection, and despite the fact that an overcorrection may occur in the absence of negligence (i.e., the surgery was performed consistent with the standard of care) and the condition may be correctable with subsequent surgery, glasses, or contact lenses. Thus, from a risk management perspective, it appears to be better to err on the side of undercorrection requiring additional surgery than overcorrection.

Lack of Informed Consent

As will be discussed in greater detail later in this chapter, to be legally valid, the consent provided by a patient must be *fully informed* and *voluntary*. That is, a patient must be provided with sufficient information concerning the nature of the procedure, risks, potential complications, benefits, and alternatives in order to form the basis of a reasonable decision on whether or not to proceed with the surgery. For example, a lack of informed consent could be found if the patient contends that he or she would not have undergone surgery had he known that the surgery could result in irreversible loss of vision which was not 100% correctable with glasses, and the physician is unable to document that this information was provided to the patient before the surgery.

Lack of informed consent appears to be a standard allegation in almost all malpractice cases for refractive surgery. Thus, it is critical that the physician develop a comprehensive consent procedure which addresses all legal requirements. Often this procedure includes watching a videotape, completing a questionnaire, talking with the surgeon, and completing a written consent form. Physicians are cautioned that some states have specific statutory requirements which must be followed to ensure informed consent. Thus, when using a commercially produced videotape or form, the surgeon must make sure that all of the state requirements on informed consent are met.

The elements of informed consent involving refractive surgery are discussed later in this chapter. There are, however, certain issues which raise particular concerns in the context of a malpractice claim. For example, the surgeon should not make any guarantees regarding the success or outcome of the procedure or provide a description of an "ideal candidate." In addition, early malpractice cases make it clear that refractive surgery patients must be informed of the potential for subsequent surgery. Finally, the issues addressed in the consent procedure must be discussed using specific examples that the patient understands. It is not enough merely to inform the patient that he or she may have visual problems.

Even if the patient received all of the necessary information upon which to base a consent, a lack of informed consent claim will prevail if the patient can show that the decision to proceed with the surgery was not voluntary; that is, the patient may contend that he or she did not have enough time to comprehend the information that was given and that he or she was unduly encouraged to undergo the procedure without an adequate opportunity to consider the issue fully. This may arise when the informed consent procedure is performed too close to the time of surgery. To address this issue, many surgeons provide all the consent information at the time the patient schedules the surgery, which is often 1 to several weeks before the surgery.

Improper Candidate for Refractive Surgery

A number of malpractice cases contain allegations that the patient was an improper candidate for refractive surgery (e.g., too myopic) or that the patient experienced a poor result of surgery on the first eye. This claim has contributed to decisions in favor of the plaintiff, including the $5.4 million verdict in the *Nicholson v. Simon* case.[12] Unfortunately, there is little definitive guidance for physicians in this area. The cases involving this allegation are too few in number to provide any real instruction. In addition, the standard of care for refractive surgery is evolving, and at this time there do not appear to be any universally recognized criteria to determine an appropriate candidate. Thus, the surgeon must perform an individual assessment of each patient and document the appropriateness of surgery. A consultation with another physician may also be helpful in certain situations.

Nonmedical Claims

In addition to traditional medical oriented claims, a significant number of refractive surgery malpractice cases include nonmedical claims including breach of warranty, breach of promise, false advertising, negligent or fraudulent misrepresentation, and violation of the state's Consumer Protection Act. In these cases, the plaintiffs asserted that the physician promised a result which did not happen, misrepresented the extent of potential complications, or overstated the safety of the procedure. For example, the *Nicholson v. Simon* verdict in favor of the plaintiff included claims that the physician provided fraudulent assurances regarding the safety of RK in his advertising and in his discussions with the patient. In another case, the plaintiff in *Brannon v. Boyd*.[14] who underwent several procedures on his right eye (with a total of 78 incisions) and was awarded $214,500 in damages, alleged breach of promise, negligence, and lack of informed consent; further, the judge awarded an additional $10,000 for violating the state's Consumer Protection Act. Thus, providing inadequate or incorrect information may not only form the basis for a claim of lack of informed consent but also may serve as the basis for an independent claim of a violation of an expressed or implied representation or promise made by the surgeon.

Informed Consent

As discussed earlier in this chapter, to be legally valid, the consent to treatment provided by a patient (or the patient's representative) must be fully informed and voluntary. In order to meet this standard, the patient must be provided with sufficient information concerning the following:

1. The diagnosis of his or her condition.
2. The nature of the proposed course of treatment.
3. The benefits of the proposed treatment.
4. The risks associated with the recommended treatment.
5. The potential complications of the treatment.
6. The alternatives to the recommended treatment.

In performing any refractive procedure, it is important for the ophthalmologist to engage in a dialogue with the patient in which the physician describes, in terms understood by the patient, the nature of the patient's condition; the purpose of the refractive procedure; a complete description of the

procedure, including the equipment to be used; the use of any anesthesia or sedative; the effect of the surgical incisions on the eye, if applicable; and possible postoperative complications. Only after receiving complete information regarding all of these factors can a patient be expected to grant the type of consent which the law requires.

With refractive procedures, it is imperative that the ophthalmologist discuss with the patient the various alternatives to refractive surgery, particularly nonsurgical corrections (such as the use of glasses or contact lenses). Juries can be extremely sympathetic to claims by patients that they would not have permitted the physician to perform surgery had they been advised that their condition could have been treated with noninvasive corrections. In hindsight, glasses or contact lenses appear to be a preferable alternative to a bad surgical result. Thus, it is necessary that the ophthalmologist carefully explain the nonsurgical alternatives to the patient and that the patient acknowledge that those alternatives were discussed with him or her prior to granting consent to surgery.

While it is impossible within the scope of this chapter to address every potential risk associated with refractive procedures, the following list illustrates the issues which should be discussed with the patient:

- Any operative or postoperative pain or discomfort, with instructions on how to recognize it and deal with it.
- Possibility of over- or undercorrection and the necessity for further procedures.
- Commonly experienced visual conditions following the procedure, even if temporary (such as blurred vision or the starburst effect), along with instructions on what to do if such conditions occur.
- The possibility that such temporary visual conditions might become permanent; and, if so, the recommended course of treatment, including potential additional procedures.
- Description of potential serious complications (even if an infrequent occurrence) such as corneal vascularization, corneal ulcer, perforation of the cornea, irregular astigmatism, cataract, retinal detachment, partial or total loss of vision, and complications requiring additional treatment and/or surgery.

- The chance that glasses or contact lenses may still be required after the procedure.
- The possibility of hyperopic shift.
- The potential for monovision.
- The likelihood that additional procedures (enhancements) may be necessary.

If the physician uses a customized or adulterated laser (see the earlier discussion), it is wise to disclose this fact to the patient and explain that the laser has not been approved by the FDA. Further, if the ophthalmologist has received a warning letter from the FDA regarding the use of the customized laser, it is advisable to disclose this fact as well to the patient. In addition, the physician should discuss with the patient the potential limitations of using a laser for conditions for which the device has not been approved, such as a limitation on how much vision correction can be achieved in one procedure or treatment and the fact that follow-up procedures may be needed.

As stated earlier in this chapter, LASIK involves the use of the excimer laser for a purpose beyond the scope of the FDA approval for that device. This fact should be disclosed to the patient and discussed in detail. Even though the law recognizes the right of a physician to utilize an approved medical device for an off-label use, within his or her professional judgment, it is best to err on the side of disclosure when communicating with patients.

If the ophthalmologist is using a treatment protocol or procedure which is the subject of clinical investigation or trial, it is imperative that this fact be disclosed to the patient. Furthermore, the patient should be informed about how his or her participation in the clinical trial procedure will be treated or reported. The patient must grant approval for the use of data derived from the procedure and the dissemination of that information (even when the patient is not identified).

It is interesting to note that states have developed different approaches to determine the standard for the adequacy of the informed consent. Some jurisdictions apply the *medical community standard* of disclosure. This test is based on what ophthalmologists practicing in that medical community customarily disclose to patients with the same medical condition. Other state courts apply the *patient need standard* of care. This view requires the ophthalmologist to disclose to the patient that information

which a reasonable person in the patient's position would consider to be material in arriving at an informed decision to grant consent to the treatment or procedure. Regardless of the jurisdiction, however, the elements of informed consent apply in all cases, and the physician who fails to meet those standards risks an allegation of inadequate informed consent.

IMPACT OF REGULATORY ISSUES ON GENERAL LIABILITY

As is evident from the discussion above, medical and technological developments involving refractive surgery are evolving, just as the rules which regulate refractive surgery are evolving. And while the traditional theories of liability apply to refractive procedures, the development of the rules which apply to refractive procedures may have an impact on the effect or extent of liability.

Licensing Issues

In connection with licensing considerations, the risk of liability may be increased when an optometrist performs the postoperative care and a state board of medicine has taken the position that such care constitutes the practice of medicine. Aside from the regulatory and enforcement risks, if a complication arises during the postoperative period, both the ophthalmologist and the optometrist will almost certainly face the allegation that the ophthalmologist was negligent by allowing the patient to be treated by an individual who is not qualified to provide postoperative care or by failing to provide adequate information about the need for the ophthalmologist to provide postoperative care as part of the informed consent.

Food and Drug Law Issues

Food and drug law issues create particular risks for increased exposure. A malpractice suit involving a patient who was treated by a physician using a custom laser will almost certainly include an allegation that the laser was not approved by the FDA, and that despite the extent of information provided in the informed consent documents, the physician had a higher duty to ensure that the patient was not subjected to an unapproved device. Certainly, a physician who has received a warning letter from the FDA in connection with the custom laser faces a still higher risk of exposure in such cases.

Food and drug law concerns also may arise in connection with the off-label use of the excimer laser, either for patients whose visual acuity is beyond the range approved by the FDA or in connection with the LASIK procedure. While both procedures fall within the scope of the physician's license and may be exempt from regulation by the FDA, a liability claim will almost certainly focus on the fact that the excimer laser was not approved for the particular procedure.

A physician's off-label use of a medical device, however, does not automatically result in negligence liability. Courts have recognized that the manner in which a physician chooses to use a federally approved drug or medical device is within the scope of the physician's medical judgment. Thus, in order for a physician to be liable for medical negligence, a jury must determine that the physician's treatment did not meet the standard of care of the medical community and that the physician's breach of the standard of care caused the patient's injuries. In most jurisdictions, whether or not the physician's use was federally approved is only one of several factors that the jury considers in making this determination.[15] Other factors include information in the medical literature and the actual practices of other physicians in the community.

Off-label use of a medical device also raises issues of informed consent. Patients have based claims of lack of informed consent upon the failure of a physician to disclose that a proposed treatment involved a device or procedure which was not FDA approved.[16] At this time, however, there does not appear to be any reported decision that has found that failure to disclose the off-label use of a medical device or drug is presumptively a violation of the doctrine of informed consent. In fact, a number of courts have held that the physician is not required to disclose the FDA labeling status because this regulatory description is not a "risk" of the treatment.[17] Furthermore, courts have specifically noted that FDA-approved indications "were not intended to limit or interfere with a physician's practice of medicine."[18]

FTC Concerns

Publicity concerning the FTC's investigation of RK marketing may also increase exposure under liability theories, particularly relating to informed consent. The FTC's scrutiny of marketing refractive procedures has sensitized lawyers to the theory that failure to provide balanced information in advertising to the public may jeopardize the adequacy of the physician's informed consent process. To the extent that the advertising is not consistent with the informed consent information, the patient may claim that he or she relied on the information in the advertising, rather than in the informed consent, and, therefore, the informed consent process was inadequate.

Fraud and Abuse Issues

Finally, fraud and abuse concerns may have an impact on liability theories. Allegations of negligent referral to optometrists may arise in connection with postoperative complications that are not detected or treated adequately by the optometrist. This theory may be further supported if it can be shown that the referral to the ophthalmologist was conditioned on the referral back to the optometrist.

CONCLUSION

As technological advances in refractive procedures continue, liability issues will become still more complex. The regulation of these developments further complicates the liability issues associated with refractive procedures. Physicians should be aware of all of the ramifications and take appropriate steps to protect themselves to the extent possible.

REFERENCES

1. Idaho Code § 54-1501(3); Written Interpretation of Law, State Board of Optometry, Bureau of Occupational Licenses, State of Idaho (Oct. 6, 1995); Okla. Stat. Ann. tit. 59, §§ 581–583.
2. *See* Letter to Physicians from the California Department of Consumer Affairs, February 22, 1994; Letter to the Executive Director of the Medical

Board of California from the Staff Counsel of the California Department of Consumer Affairs, March 15, 1995.

3. *Iowa Optometric Association et al. v. Iowa Academy of Ophthalmology et al.*, Civil Action No. 4-94-CV-10123, United States District Court for the Southern District of Iowa, Central Division. As of this writing, both parties have filed motions for summary judgment, and on November 21, 1995, the court granted summary judgment for the Iowa Academy of Ophthalmology with respect to its members' actions in petitioning the Board of Medical Examiners. However, the court denied the Academy's request for summary judgment in connection with alleged concerted threats or otherwise anticompetitive activity outside of the board's declaratory ruling. Those issues must now be resolved at trial.

4. *Florida Bd. of Optometry v. Florida Bd. of Medicine*, 616 S.2d 581 (Fla. App. 1993).

5. 21 U.S.C. § 360j(b)(1) and (2).

6. 21 C.F.R. § 812.3(b).

7. Warning letters constitute notices to individuals and have no legal significance other than an expression of the agency's view of the law. Often, the individual and the FDA are able to reach a mutual resolution without the need for adjudication of whether the FDA's position is correct.

8. "This laser is not indicated for use in a new procedure for correcting nearsightedness called LASIK, which is a refractive surgical procedure in which a flap of cornea is created with an automated lamellar keratome and then a laser is used to remove underlying corneal tissue."

9. Memorandum from Sara Thornton, Center for Devices and Radiological Health, FDA, to Marie Rosenthal dated January 26, 1996.

10. 15 U.S.C. § 41.

11. These FTC concerns evidently grew out of reports of a continuing, gradual hyperopic shift in RK patients, as well as many patients' eventual need for reading glasses, regardless of the effect of refractive surgery on their nearsightedness. Recently, the investigation was concluded with the understanding that professional societies would develop appropriate marketing guidelines.

12. *Nicholson v. Simon*, No. 279, 359(Super. Ct., Contra Costa County (CA) 1992).

13. *McCauley v. Simons*, No. 86-CV-11000, (Denver Dist. Ct. (CO) 1988).

14. *Brannon v. Boyd*, No. 87-2-07562-1 (King County Super. Ct. (WA 1990).

15. One limited line of case law recognizes a prima facie case of medical negligence if the FDA-approved package insert contains clear and explicit warnings against the use that allegedly caused the patient's injury. For a general discussion of the cases, *see Ramon v. Farr*, 770 P.2d 131, 134 (Utah 1989).

16. *See, e.g., Retkwa v. Orertreich*, 584 N.Y.S. 2d 710 (1992).

17. *See, e.g., In re Orthopedic Bone Screw Prods. Liab. Litig.*, 1996 U.S. Dist. LEXIS 2825 (E.D. Pa. Mar. 8, 1996).

18. *Weaver v. Reagen*, 886 F.2d 194, 198 (8th Cir. 1989).

24

Regulatory Aspects of Refractive Surgery: Refractive Devices and the FDA

Mark D. Stern

INTRODUCTION

Recent developments in refractive surgery have sparked an interest within the ophthalmic community about the regulatory process involved in introducing new refractive devices into the commercial market in the United States. The information void concerning the regulatory process has contributed to some frustration within the ophthalmic community. To remedy this situation, a chapter on the regulatory process has been included in this book. This chapter will focus on the congressional mandate given to the Food and Drug Administration (FDA) and the mechanics of the process to regulate medical devices so that they are safe and effective as labeled for their intended use. The choice of a particular regulatory vehicle used for the evaluation of a medical device reflects the level of concern about safety and effectiveness. Finally, current regulatory issues facing refractive devices will illustrate the regulatory process in action.

GLOBAL ISSUES AND THE FDA

The eyes of the world have recently focused on the FDA. Our regulatory system serves as a prototype for many countries. However, the system that has evolved in America may not be feasible or even desirable in another country. The search for the best method of serving patients and protecting public health balances many issues for which no one answer is universally suitable. The regulatory process selected for a given country reflects more on the individual political, economic, and sociologic realities of that culture than on the delivery of medical care.

In this era of global communication, the world community would benefit from agreeing upon certain standards and accepting common methodologies. The goal is to be able to share information comfortably in the international market without duplication of individual efforts. Establishing regulatory reciprocity will permit the sharing of established scientific issues in one country to be held with equal validity in another. The FDA refers to this effort as *global harmonization*. Already in 1996 countries in the European Community have agreed upon common standards and methodologies.

FDA: CONSUMER ADVOCATE

The FDA acts as a consumer advocate to protect the public health. Congress charges the FDA with the regulatory oversight of commercially distributed products available for interstate commerce. One of its responsibilities is to ensure that commercial products are properly manufactured. Commercially marketed products are monitored to guard against hidden defects through programs like postmarketing surveillance.

In the area of health care, one major responsibility is to reliably establish the risk-benefit ratio for new drugs and devices based upon the regulatory mandate as detailed in the Code of Federal Regulations 21§860.7(c): *valid scientific evidence*. The FDA collects information about the clinical benefits (efficacy parameters), the anticipated adverse events (safety parameters), and the unanticipated adverse events (e.g., medical device reporting as part of postmarket surveillance) of various medical products. The FDA disseminates that information to the public and the medical profession. The Federal Food, Drug and Cosmetic Act[1] mandates certain regulatory authority to the Secretary of Health and Human Services and consequently to the Commissioner of the FDA.

Within the Federal Food, Drug and Cosmetic Act (henceforth, the Act) are sections dealing with violations of interstate commerce such as the adulteration or misbranding (or mislabeling) of foods, drugs, devices, and cosmetics. *Misbranding* refers to misleading labeling or advertising that fails to reveal material facts about the use or consequences resulting from the use prescribed in the labeling or advertising.[2] The exact statutory definitions, penalties, or remedies for these prohibited acts are not the subject of this chapter. However, the interested reader would be served by reviewing the relevant sections in the Act. The Act goes on to describe the regulatory requirements of producers of drugs and devices to register with the FDA and obey certain manufacturing and marketing requirements. All reporting requirements are by law to the Secretary of Health and Human Services but in practice to the FDA.

THE ROLE OF THE CENTER FOR DEVICES AND RADIOLOGICAL HEALTH

Within the FDA, the Center for Devices and Radiological Health (CDRH) administers programs to protect the public health in the fields of devices and radiological health. These programs protect the public health by ensuring quality in manufacture, distribution, advertising, and proper labeling of devices. One aspect of labeling identifies the specific risk-benefit issues outlined by specifying the important safety and effectiveness issues. For medical devices, important labeling information about safety and effectiveness is principally obtained by conducting well-controlled clinical studies.

Labeling also depends upon the claims made for the intended use of the device by the sponsor.* The

Sponsor is the term applied to a person, individual, partnership, corporation or association, academic institution, or basically any legal entity. A sponsor is a person or entity that initiates but does not actually conduct the investigation. An *entity* is a group other than an individual which uses one or more of its employees to conduct a clinical study that it has initiated.

Act mandates labeling of medical devices so that commercially available devices are not misbranded. *Labeling* refers not only to a display of written, printed, or graphic material on the immediate container of any commercial product, but other relevant written or printed material accompanying the product as well.[3] A device is misbranded if the labeling or advertising is misleading.[4] Labeling relates directly to the prohibited act of misbranding previously mentioned.

The CDRH serves several regulatory roles. One important mission is to detect hidden defects in medical devices through postmarketing surveillance. Postmarketing surveillance and reporting requirements of the CDRH are meant to uncover any manufacturing problems, hidden defects, or other problems that might cause a device to be misbranded or a health hazard. Postmarketing surveillance and device reporting requirements overcome some of the restrictions imposed by limited but statistically significant clinical trials. In large-scale manufacturing, it is possible to expose the more esoteric safety issues and to monitor for consistent quality of production by adhering to regulatory requirements called *good manufacturing practices*. In its other role as monitor for clinical studies, the scientific review process focuses on assisting in device development, ensuring an appropriate level of performance for a device, and assessing clinical outcomes. Other areas in CDRH focus on other aspects of commercial production and marketing.

Through its congressional mandate to administer the investigational device exemption (IDE) and the premarket application (PMA) processes, the Office of Device Evaluation within the CDRH participates with the sponsors in monitoring controlled clinical studies. The six divisions within the Office of Device Evaluation oversee the controlled clinical studies that generate the information necessary to properly address labeling issues for the specific intended use of a given device. By concentrating on safety and effectiveness through controlled clinical studies, procedural outcomes and risk-benefit issues can be assessed. This provides the information necessary for labeling of the device, physician training guidelines, and informed consent. A major mission of the Division of Ophthalmic Devices in the Office of Device Evaluation at CDRH is to evaluate the submissions for ophthalmic devices to determine safety and effectiveness issues for the intended use.

DEFINITION OF LABELING

The term *label* has a specific meaning in the regulatory arena. According to Section 201(k) of the Act: "label means a display of written, printed, or graphic matter upon the immediate container of any article; and a requirement made by or under authority of this Act that any word, statement, or other information appear on the label shall not be considered to be complied with unless such word, statement, or other information also appears on the outside container or wrapper." Additionally in Section 201(m), "labeling means all labels and other written, printed, or graphic matter (1) upon any article or any of its containers or wrappers, or (2) accompanying such article." The last statement refers to the familiar product inserts for drugs. However, for new devices, product labeling takes the form of a "Summary of Safety and Effectiveness Document" which chronicles the information and conclusions gained from the clinical studies.

The aspect of labeling that clinicians are most familiar with is the product insert, which details the risks and benefits of the product for its intended use. The risk-benefit statement applies only to the intended use for which the product was studied. Prescribing a different dosing schedule or using the product to treat a disease or condition for which it (the product) was not tested constitutes an off-label use. The controversy surrounding off-label use arises not from the FDA's prohibition of it, but rather from the fact that in off-label use the risks and benefits are officially unknown. It is the mandate of the FDA to ensure that the issues of safety and effectiveness be known for the devices it regulates. However, the FDA concedes that off-label use of a drug or device by a physician involves the practice of medicine and falls within the scope of his or her medical license.

MEDICAL DEVICES: DEFINITION IN THE CODE OF FEDERAL REGULATIONS

A description of the scope and diverse range of products that are medical devices will give an appreciation of the dimensions of this task. The Act defines a medical device as "any instrument, apparatus, implement, machine, contrivance implant, *in vitro* reagent or other similar or related article, including any component, part or accessory that is:

- recognized in the official National Formulary, or the United States Pharmacopeia or any supplement to them,
- intended for use in the diagnosis of disease or other conditions, or in the cure, mitigation, treatment, or prevention of disease in man or other animals, or
- intended to affect the structure or any function of the body of man or other animals, and which does not achieve its primary intended purposes through chemical action within or on the body of man or other animals and which is not dependent upon being metabolized for the achievement of any of its principal intended purposes."[5]
- Generally speaking, the range of devices that CDRH regulates includes any medical product that does not have a pharmacologic or biologic mode of action.

THE FEDERAL CHARGE FOR SAFETY AND EFFECTIVENESS

The federal charge cited in Title 21 of the Code of Federal Regulation (CFR) § 860.7 for devices refers to reliance on "valid scientific evidence" to determine whether there is "reasonable assurance that a device is safe and effective for its intended use and condition of use"[6] when "accompanied by adequate directions for use and warnings against unsafe use that will provide clinically significant results."[7] The federal charge for safety is that the "probable benefits to health . . . for its intended use . . . when accompanied by adequate directions and warnings against unsafe use, outweigh any probable risks."[8] The federal charge for effectiveness is that in "a significant portion of the target population, the use of the device for its intended uses and conditions of use . . . will provide clinically significant results (efficacy)."[9]

THE MEDICAL DEVICES AMENDMENTS OF 1976

The Medical Devices Amendments of 1976 were enacted to provide a framework for the regulation of medical devices. The rapid technological developments affecting the medical devices market necessitated separating the regulation of medical devices from its former association with drugs. The Medical Device Amendments of May 28, 1976, directed the FDA to initially classify all then contemporary devices in commercial distribution into classes that reflect the level of regulation that will provide a "reasonable assurance of safety and effectiveness."[10] Advisory Panels were convened by mandate of the Act. Depending upon the device's potential to cause harm, the Panel assigned devices to three classes that imposed graded regulatory oversight. All medical devices commercially marketed before 1976 were grandfathered in order to avoid any disruption in market availability. Even today, any device may be subject to reclassification based upon new information regarding a currently marketed and labeled device or secondary to establishing a performance standard necessary for downgrading to Class II, for example (see "The Classification of Medical Devices").

THE OPHTHALMIC ADVISORY PANEL

As discussed above, the Medical Device Amendments of May 28, 1976, required certain changes in the regulation of medical devices. Written into the Act was the requirement to establish panels of experts to evaluate the safety and effectiveness of the devices regulated by the FDA. The Panels are a diversified conglomerate of experts from clinical and administrative medicine, engineering, biological and physical sciences, other related professions, and even representatives from the regulated industry.[11] The Ophthalmic Advisory Panel's first task was to classify all of the devices that were commercially marketed prior to May 28, 1976. A grace period built into this regulation allowed devices in the pipeline to proceed under previous regulation, while existing devices were grandfathered. The regulatory vehicle referred to from this section of the Act, known as 510(k), represents the grandfathering allowance. All new devices that presented significant risk of harm must proceed down the more rigorous regulatory pathway via the IDE/PMA.

The Division of Ophthalmic Devices works closely with the Panel members to achieve proper labeling and classification for devices. The members of the Panel are special government employees while working on Panel matters. The Ophthalmic

Advisory Panel usually meets for public session four times per year. The meeting's agenda is announced in the Federal Register. The meetings, which are open to the public, range from device classification, guidance document discussion, and presentation of premarket applications for Panel decision on commercial marketing to FDA business important to the Panel's work. Transcripts of the meeting can be obtained through the Freedom of Information(FOI) Act by contacting the FOI focal point at:

Division of Ophthalmic Devices HFZ-460
9200 Corporate Blvd.
Rockville, Maryland 20850.

THE CLASSIFICATION OF MEDICAL DEVICES

The classification of a medical device for commercial distribution in the United States will determine the regulatory vehicle chosen and the manufacturing requirements necessary to provide the labeling that reflects a "reasonable assurance of the safety and effectiveness of the device."[12] Because of the diversity and scope of medical devices, the federal charge to the FDA concerning all devices requires an equally broad charge, a reasonable assurance of safety and effectiveness. Briefly, to be complete but not comprehensive, Section 513 of the Act establishes the following device classifications:

- Class I devices require the least regulation and are subject to "General Controls." These controls include manufacturing location (site) registration, device listing, premarket notification usually,* and adherence to "Good Manufacturing Practices (GMP)."
- Class II devices are subject to General Controls as well as "Special Controls" that provide a reasonable assurance of safety and effectiveness. Special Controls may include, but are not limited to, performance standards or criteria set by an FDA guidance document, controlled clinical studies, patient registries, and postmarket surveillance studies. Performance standards[13] provide reasonable assurance of safety and effectiveness through established provisions of

*Many ophthalmic Class I devices are exempt from premarket notification.

manufacture and testing; provision for the recognized performance characteristics in conformity with established standards for similar devices; restriction of the sale, distribution, and use by a qualified practitioner licensed by law; and required form and content of labeling for the proper installation, maintenance, and operation for the intended use of the device.[14] These criteria suggest a group of devices that are in a mature product cycle about which much is known, facilitating establishment of such standards.

- Class III devices for ophthalmic purposes are so classified because they present an unreasonable risk of injury[15] or visual impairment. All new devices for human use introduced into interstate commerce for commercial distribution after May 28, 1976, are assigned to Class III unless substantial equivalence to a predicate device is shown or petitioned for classification into Class I or Class II.[16] Basically, a Class III device is a device or technology about which insufficient information exists to address the charge of reasonable assurance of safety and effectiveness, precluding sufficient labeling information. The charge of the sponsor is to submit the device to testing under the auspices of the FDA in order to gather information sufficient to eventually downgrade the device by specifying individual Performance Standards, Special Controls, and General Controls, all mentioned above for Class II devices. Interestingly, establishment of Performance Standards is the mechanism by which a group of similar Class III devices marketed for the same intended use can be reclassified as Class II.[17] Obviously, the pioneering sponsor of the first-of-a-kind device has a larger burden to bear than those who follow with a similar device.

REGULATION OF CLINICAL STUDIES

To perform any clinical study to gather scientific evidence about the performance of a medical device in the domestic patient population requires an IDE. Section 520(g) of the Act gives the FDA authority to regulate investigational devices. A FDA-approved IDE allows a device to be shipped lawfully for the purpose of conducting a clinical study. The primary regulations regarding clinical studies of investigational devices cite the Code of Federal Regulations, Title 21: Part 812: Procedures for the Conduct of Clinical Studies with Devices; Part 50: General Elements of Informed Consent; and Part 56: Procedures and Responsibilities for Institutional Review boards (IRBs).

SAFETY, EFFECTIVENESS, AND LABELING

New Class III devices require the highest level of regulatory control because of the relative lack of information for labeling and for judging safety and effectiveness. Two sequential regulatory vehicles are needed to commercially market a new Class III device. The regulatory vehicle known as the *premarket application (PMA)* is a legal order to commercially market a device. The PMA process, complete with preclinical and clinical data derived from a clinical study under an *investigational device exemption (IDE)*, defines the safety and effectiveness of the device for its intended use; this satisfies some of the regulatory requirements for commercial marketing of a Class III device. Other requirements are related to the inspections of the sponsor's manufacturing facilities and records prior to receiving the PMA approval letter. Following commercial marketing, the device and the manufacturer are subject to the regulatory requirements and postmarket surveillance that had been waived during the clinical study under the IDE regulations.

FDA APPROVAL ORDER AND RISK

An FDA approval order (letter) for a premarket application (PMA) legally permits the introduction of a medical product, a device for our purposes here, into interstate commerce. The reason that FDA-approval of the device itself is not a correct statement is that the FDA approves the premarket application (PMA) and not the named device per se. In fact, it is specifically prohibited to advertise that the FDA endorses or approves a device.

A legally marketed device that has been through the regulatory process does not imply that the device is without risk. FDA approval of the PMA indicates a reasonable assurance of safety and effectiveness for the intended use; this is clearly not the same as stating that there is no risk. The device classification system evolved based upon the inherent risk to human health. At all device classification levels, the system works because issues of safety and effectiveness are defined and addressed with adequate labeling in order to assess risk. With any classification, inevitably problems will surface that illustrate shortcomings in the system. This topic will be revisited with a discussion of the microkeratome and LASIK.

IDE REGULATIONS

In order to be legally distributed for commercial use, medical devices must be properly labeled for intended use. The central issue with new Class III devices is that they have not been shown to be safe and effective to draft the appropriate labeling. To distribute such an improperly labeled medical device would violate the Act. Other provisions of the Act would also be in violation. To remedy this situation, Congress proposed the IDE as a regulatory vehicle. The 1976 Medical Devices Amendments to the Act provide exemptions for investigational devices from certain required provisions of the Act. Consistent with protection of the public health and ethical standards, an IDE encourages the discovery and development of useful devices, provides optimum freedom for investigators, and, most important, protects the safety of the investigational subject.

IDE regulations for devices are different than for drugs because of the diversity of the products, the variety of the study designs, and the conventional lack of a study control. A fast-changing technology also requires a more flexible approach to the IDE process for many devices. The stage in the life cycle of a product also affects the regulatory vehicle and the time to market. A very new technology will take the longest time to run the regulatory gauntlet, while a more mature technology may find the process less formidable. The former probably requires a full IDE and PMA, while the latter, for a mature commercial device, may need only a 510(k) without any complicated clinical study.

Recognition that time to market is an obstacle to patient care has prompted certain alternatives to the conventional regulatory approach such as the IDE/PMA expedited review process. In general,

Class III devices like refractive lasers pose significant risks to the patient (i.e., the patient may get hurt). The expedited review process is not applicable here. An FDA-approved IDE, with IRB oversight and informed consent protection for the study subject, eventuating in a PMA submission, is the conventional regulatory approach for new Class III devices at this time.

THE CONTROLLED CLINICAL STUDY

The controlled clinical study is the application of the scientific method to clinical investigation while not exploiting patients or exposing them to unnecessary risks or safety hazards. Controlled clinical studies are the key to the labeling that supplies reliable information on device performance, instructions on proper use, and expected clinical outcomes when used for the labeled indications. Defining the safety and effectiveness parameters often remains theoretical for the intended use of a device until the clinical study is analyzed because biological systems are unpredictable. The controlled clinical study defines the safety and effectiveness issues so that the physician can evaluate new technology on its demonstrated scientific merits. The value of the process is that a given device can be expected to perform reliably and predictably, without hidden defects. A properly licensed and experienced practitioner can use a commercially marketed and labeled device for its intended use to treat appropriate patients with reasonable assurance of safety and efficacy and achieve a predictable clinical outcome.

THE PURPOSE OF LABELING

Using a device has much in common with writing a medication prescription. A physician would not prescribe a medication with which he or she was not thoroughly familiar. From a regulatory perspective, using a device is no different from putting a professional signature on a prescription pad for a drug prescription. The labeling that is being discussed is no different from what appears in the *Physicians' Desk Reference* (PDR), except that it applies to a device or diagnostic tool and is not bound in a tome along with countless others labels.

The reason the FDA insists on physician training for a particular device can be argued from several perspectives. The most intellectually satisfying approach is that in order to obtain predictable results and properly manage the issues of safety and effectiveness, the physician must understand and replicate exactly the methodology used in the clinical study. As a special control, the FDA can insist that a device be marketed as "restricted" because additional measures are needed to provide reasonable assurance of safety and effectiveness.

In order to operate a newly marketed Class III device properly for its intended use, as labeled, one has to be familiar with the methodology that was used to generate the labeling from the controlled clinical study. The only way a physician can obtain this instruction is through the auspices of the clinical study investigators with the permission of the company that sponsored the IDE study and the antecedent investigational device. This information is strictly confidential, not to be divulged by the FDA, and proprietary to the company. In order to use the device *per protocol*, the physician must be familiar with all aspects of the controlled clinical study to achieve reproducible results (the scientific gold standard). One question stands as the cornerstone of all well-conducted, scientific studies: Are the results reproducible? That is the scientific challenge; the intended benefit derived by conducting the controlled clinical study; and the driving force behind properly training the treating physician in the precise methodology of the study.

REFRACTIVE DEVICES AND PHASE I AND II STUDIES

A device goes through developmental improvement and refinement in Phase I and Phase II of the clinical trial. Phase I clinical trials are usually very limited in size. Phase I, or a feasibility study, often determines if there is any value in expanding to a Phase II study for the purpose of defining the safety issues in a somewhat larger patient population. For excimer laser refractive surgery, Phase I studies were abandoned since a lack of adequate fixation was an important issue for safety and effectiveness. For corneal inlays and refractive intraocular lenses (IOLs), Phase I studies are necessary for safety reasons associated with any implant. Intrastromal

corneal inlays and refractive IOLs raise issues of biocompatibility, long-term tissue interactions, and toxicity. The relative reversibility of these intrastromal corneal implants, and even of some refractive IOLs, is an important safety factor in their favor.

REFRACTIVE DEVICES AND PHASE III STUDIES: THE EVOLVING REGULATORY PROCESS

By the time of Phase III studies, the marketable device is ready for a controlled clinical study with a statistically significant sample size to define safety and effectiveness issues. For refractive lasers, all of which are Class III devices,* the recommended, significant sample size was a holdover from the former years of IOL studies, where sample size was an established number. Since the regulatory requirement is "valid scientific evidence" based upon well-controlled studies analyzed using appropriate statistical methods,[18] the actual sample size to meet this standard may not be 700 cases as previously established. The sponsor's burden is to provide valid arguments to support the position that the sample size should be driven by valid statistical methodology rather than an established precedent. What is not contestable is the issue of accountability. The Ophthalmic Advisory Panel has made it quite clear that evaluating the results of the clinical studies requires sterling accountability of the cohort.

Another factor that will help to move this process along, in addition to justifying sample size, is following certain long-term safety and effectiveness issues through postmarket surveillance. The Ophthalmic Advisory Panel has suggested this. Postmarket surveillance is one of the special controls referred to for Class II devices. This is further evidence that refractive laser devices are a maturing technology. A dual effect is achieved through a shortened study duration and the simultaneous improvement in accountability that necessarily follows.

The last technique to move the process along is to allow more liberal inclusion criteria for the fellow eye. Finding patients with bilateral inclusion criteria for simple myopic protocols is a challenge. Since the

---

*Do not confuse device classification of lasers with federal classification of lasers as devices that emit radiation: 21CFR§1040.10.

fellow eye does not contribute to scientific evidence on primary efficacy parameters but can contribute to the safety parameters, anticipating enrollment of the fellow eye in a separate astigmatic protocol will facilitate enrollment. Since the simple myopic protocol is usually the first study to make it to the PMA stage, anything that facilitates enrollment will shorten the time until a PMA is submitted. These factors reflect the improved comfort with the safety and effectiveness of a maturing and evolving device, technology, and refractive procedure. When at least four similar devices have been through the PMA process,[19] it only remains for a sponsor to eventually define appropriate performance standards,[20] meet other criteria mentioned previously, and apply to the advisory Panel to reclassify those refractive laser devices for whom the performance standard applies into Class II. Once this is accomplished, it may be possible, although not assured, to travel the less arduous 510(k) pathway of substantial equivalence to the market. Every regulatory submission is unique; what is constant is the acceptance by FDA staffers of reasonable explanations and justifications for choosing various methodologies. These are merely suggestions and do not rule out the possibility that another, more streamlined mechanism might exist to facilitate the regulatory process.

SIGNIFICANT VERSUS NONSIGNIFICANT RISK CLINICAL STUDIES

The choice of a regulatory vehicle that is selected to evaluate the safety and effectiveness of a device is determined by several considerations. The class of the device, the marketing claims of the device manufacturer, and the determination of significant risk should factor in choosing the most appropriate regulatory vehicle. The main choices for Class II and III devices are 510(k) for substantial equivalence or an IDE and PMA when issues of safety and effectiveness remain ill-defined. Device classification has already been reviewed. The determination of significant risk of the investigational device in question is a sometimes confusing requirement. The determination of significant risk (SR) or nonsignificant risk (NSR) is of great consequence. All clinical studies to gather scientific evidence about the performance of a medical device in the domestic patient population require an IDE. Any clinical study that involves

human subjects requires oversight by an IRB. The sponsor has to justify to the IRB whether the study is an SR or an NSR. If the IRB disagrees or has questions, it may defer to the FDA for an SR/NSR determination. Either way, certain protections are afforded the clinical study subject by the federal regulations concerning IRBs. If a clinical study is considered an NSR and the IRB approves the submitted protocol, the investigator has in essence an IDE which, because the study is NSR, allows the clinical investigation to commence without the need to notify the FDA. Should the sponsor then wish to market the device at the conclusion of the NSR study, the appropriate regulatory requirements would need to be filed with the FDA, as is required for any device to be marketed for commercial purposes. However, if the study is determined to be SR, the sponsor must submit the IDE protocol to the FDA for approval prior to initiating the clinical study.

FOREIGN STUDIES

A discussion of what constitutes a valid clinical study is incomplete without reference to the regulatory requirements that permit the inclusion of nondomestic sites in a controlled clinical study. Two situations exist: either the sponsor has a FDA-approved IDE or the sponsor does not have a FDA-approved IDE. Although the former situation is preferred, either way the submitted data in support of a PMA from a foreign site(s) should comply with all of the provisions of 21 CFR § 812: IDE regulations. In addition, the FDA will accept the PMA submission if the clinical study began after November 19, 1986; if the data collected are valid; and if the investigators have conducted the study in accordance with the "Declaration of Helsinki" as a minimum requirement to protect the study subjects. Should the sponsor wish to use nondomestic data exclusively to support a PMA, the data must be shown to be applicable to the domestic population; the studies must be conducted by clinical investigators of recognized ability and expertise; the data must be considered valid without the need for an on-site inspection, but this option is not precluded; and it is recommended that a presubmission meeting with the FDA be arranged to negotiate these matters.[21]

SUBSTANTIAL EQUIVALENCE: THE 510(k) ROUTE

If no claims of superiority to a predicate device (a device that is already legally marketed in the United States) for the same intended use are made, the marketing claims of the manufacturer then allow Class I and II, and even some Class III, devices to enter the regulatory process via Section 510(k) of the Act. In premarket notification (510(k) application), the sponsor must demonstrate that the device is substantially equivalent (SE) to a legally marketed predicate device for the same intended use: a me-too device. The purpose of determining SE is that the issues of safety and effectiveness should be the same for the predicate and proposed devices, allowing proper labeling for the intended use. The issue of safety is dealt with by the labeling, often avoiding the need to conduct a controlled clinical study. The 510(k) process provides for an accelerated regulatory pathway to commercial marketing. The device need not perform better, and can even perform worse, than the predicate device. If the performance and safety are properly defined by the labeling, the intent of the regulation has been fulfilled. As far as devices are concerned, the role of the FDA is to provide proper dissemination of valid scientific information so that informed choices can be made. The FDA is not in the business of making value judgments about the devices themselves, so long as the labeling adequately reflects the safety and effectiveness and the public health is not compromised.

The 510(k) provision is a special provision of the Medical Device Amendments of 1976. It allows the FDA to grandfather most preamendment devices in commercial distribution before enforcement of the 1976 amendments, including commercially available Class III devices. The reasoning is that if a device was available prior to the Medical Device Amendments of 1976, its very position in the marketplace establishes its safety and effectiveness. For example, the commercially available preamendment microkeratome, initially classified as Class I, serves as the predicate for the microkeratome presently used for LASIK (laser in situ keratomileusis). LASIK raises new issues of safety and effectiveness for the new intended use compared to the excimer laser for superficial PRK and the microkeratome for its preamendment indications. The regulatory

dilemma is that sufficient scientific information is currently unavailable about LASIK for proper labeling of the microkeratome and refractive laser for this new use. Once the labeling issues have been defined and analyzed, the indications for intended use of the device can then be expanded through the simple process of supplementing the existing PMA. This is the mechanism by which the performance of the procedure with such devices would no longer be considered off-label.

OFF-LABEL USE

Safety and effectiveness data for a given indication are not strictly applicable when an off-label use is contemplated. Therefore, such off-label use of a device may be in violation of the Act (misbranding). However, the FDA's policy on the off-label use of various devices has been historically to view it as a practice of medicine issue and not an FDA concern. As has been pointed out, the objective of device classification is to define risk. The practice of medicine using technologically advanced medical devices will always conflict with the FDA's mandate that requires risk to be specified through proper labeling.

For example, the unknown risk and the lack of valid scientific evidence about LASIK have prompted the FDA to reconsider how to handle this issue. At domestic sites that are performing LASIK without an FDA-approved IDE, the FDA is requesting the investigators to submit clinical study protocols, file with IRBs, and observe informed consent regulations. The associated regulatory requirements placed on these sponsor-investigators are the associated prohibitions on promotion and other practices detailed in 21CFR§812.7. Briefly, financial charges to the clinical study subjects are restricted, the study cannot be unreasonably prolonged, and advertising cannot imply any claims for safety or effectiveness.

An alternative is to define LASIK not as two procedures (an initial lamellar keratectomy and an independent photorefractive procedure), but rather as one continuous procedure. Under these circumstances, the device with the greater risk (the Class III refractive laser) may determine the class of any associated devices used for the procedure. This approach has precedence with respirators, condoms, and defibrillators, in which the identical device was classified differently depending on its intended use. In this manner, the regulatory relationship of corneal lamellar keratectomy procedures and the microkeratome remains unaffected. The same would not be true if the microkeratome were to be considered for reclassification. This example epitomizes the controversy surrounding a contemporary regulatory impasse. The resolution of this difficult regulatory and public health issue probably depends on the completion of controlled clinical studies on LASIK to supply sufficient information for appropriate labeling as a new indication for refractive lasers.

EFFICACY PARAMETERS OF REFRACTIVE LASERS

Efficacy implies a clinical benefit, while *effectiveness* refers to whether the device does what it is supposed to do. Device effectiveness for Class III refractive lasers would be best measured by recording differences in corneal power before and after laser treatment. The reason is that refractive lasers claim to alter the shape of the cornea, with the caveat "after healing occurs." The best method of demonstrating this would be to measure the altered corneal curve that results from the laser treatment after healing has been completed. Since certain assumptions about corneal topography are no longer valid after photorefractive keratectomy (PRK), standard keratometry is no longer an accurate measure of corneal power. Unfortunately, lacking another effectiveness parameter, we must settle for an efficacy parameter based upon a subjective manifest refraction: deviation from the intended target correction (DIC). Like any surrogate endpoint, the DIC substitutes as the primary refractive efficacy parameter for device effectiveness. Substitution of an efficacy parameter for the more appropriate effectiveness parameter is reflected in the labeling.

Only in simple myopia does the magnitude of the refraction correlate with a certain level of uncorrected visual acuity. Given certain limitations, uncorrected visual acuity is the best single measure of overall efficacy, either visual or refractive, since this is the clinical benefit sought by the patient. This is especially important for astigmatic treatments since refractive simplifications, like spherical equivalence, hide any uncorrected residual astigmatism. Additionally, vector analysis of residual astigmatic data diverts attention from the important issue of clinical benefit to the patient. If astigmatic treatment is successful, the refractive and visual efficacy results should be reduced to results comparable to or even better than those anticipated for simple myopic PRK studies.

The difficulty in analyzing inadequately treated compound myopic astigmatism after PRK arises because of the lack of correlation between the residual refractive error and the uncorrected visual acuity. If the astigmatic treatment is not completely successful in eliminating the astigmatic component of the refractive error (astigmatism of less than 1.0 D), determining the overall success of a clinical study statistically is complicated, since uncorrected visual acuity and residual refractive error are not linked, as in simple myopic PRK.

To achieve excellent results in eliminating compound myopic astigmatism, one should verify that the refractive and keratometric axes are coincident before attempting to treat astigmatism with refractive laser devices. If the axes are different, choosing which axis to correctly apply the astigmatic treatment is problematic. Successful astigmatic treatment hinges on a reliable manifest refraction and meticulous attention to detail in expertly applying the laser treatment to the bona fide astigmatic axis on the cornea. Unless the astigmatic component in astigmatic PRK is reduced below ± 1.00 D, statistical analysis of the resulting refractive and visual efficacy data merely diverts attention from the issue of clinical benefit to the patient. Failure to eliminate astigmatism when treating astigmatic PRK will not be compensated for by fancy mathematical arguments to the contrary. Patient satisfaction will be the yardstick by which success in astigmatic treatment is measured.

The treatment of such conditions as higher myopia, presbyopia, and hyperopia presents different issues. The problems of higher myopia involve answering the following questions:

1. What are the acceptable uncorrected visual acuity endpoints?
2. What level of safety parameters is acceptable?
3. How safe are retreatments?

Presbyopia and hyperopia present completely different problems in the design of the refractive treatment pattern. Some of the safety issues will be the same as in PRK, but the efficacy criteria remain to be defined by the success of the treatments. At issue will certainly be achieving stable and predictable refractive outcomes. Considering that presbyopia and possibly myopia are progressive conditions, it may be unreasonable to expect a permanent solution to a dynamic biologic refractive system over the long run.

SAFETY AND EFFICACY PARAMETERS AND REFRACTIVE LASERS

Just as refractive laser technology and the PRK procedure have evolved over time, the focus of safety and effectiveness has changed. Initially, demonstrating device performance and simply achieving visual recovery were pleasant surprises to the early investigators. Then, as the device was used, safety concerns surfaced involving laser beam calibration, beam homogeneity, corneal haze, loss of best spectacle corrected visual acuity, decentration, irregular astigmatism, central islands, induced astigmatism, and patient visual symptoms. Many of these safety issues have not been totally eliminated. However, our tolerance of them and their significance has definitely diminished through improvements in laser beam homogeneity, delivery, procedural improvements, and physician experience. Patient visual symptoms remain a significant safety concern, but their impact must be reconciled with the patient's tolerance of this limitation. With improvements in device, procedure, and technical expertise, these safety issues have surrendered prominence to other concerns. With the increase in the size of the ablation zone, corneal ulcers were expected to dominate safety but didn't. Meanwhile, increasing effectiveness has continuously achieved higher levels of uncorrected visual acuity and refractive accuracy. Hopefully, this process will continue to evolve and improve for the benefit of the patient.

REFRACTIVE LASERS IN THE UNITED STATES

The first refractive lasers to become commercially available in the United States were for the limited intended use of correcting simple myopia. To expand the indications for use to astigmatism or hyperopia, the sponsors have needed only to submit supplements to the PMAs documenting the scientific validity of the new indications.[22] A whole new PMA process has fortunately not been necessary. It should be emphasized, though, that previous limitations of commercial availability to one company's refractive laser with restrictions in labeled use created significant public health concerns. One presently marketed excimer laser is not capable of astigmatic treatment without the use of an ablatable mask. The other commercially-marketed excimer laser is capable of astigmatic treatment by either the sequential or simultaneous technique, but this capability has been locked out. The physician's desire to completely treat a patient's full refractive condition has resulted in creative approaches such as LASIK and combining PRK with astigmatic keratotomy.

The issues of safety and public health are basic to the FDA's mission. The use of the presently marketed excimer lasers for indications not in the PMA order (off-label use) raises other public health concerns. The crux of the matter is that the device is not properly labeled when used off-label and is therefore misbranded. The additional issue of advertising off-label uses is equally problematic for the FDA. Also of concern is the combination of PRK with sequential, astigmatic keratotomy to get around the astigmatic limitation with the laser as presently labeled. Another concern is the multiple treatment passes for the treatment of high myopia, since the laser is locked out over -7.00 D, or the overtreatment of myopes with -1.00 D, resulting in hyperopic overcorrection. The issue of LASIK need not be recounted here. In the author's opinion, expanding the FDA-approved indications for the excimer laser will be in the best interest of public health. The additional issue of advertising off-label uses will evaporate with the expanded, approved indications. The only regulatory remedy for these issues is to rewrite the refractive laser guidance document, facilitate the PMA and IDE process through options previously discussed, apply for performance standards[23] to reclassify refractive lasers at an appropriate time, and train physicians properly so that iatrogenic complications do not cast a pall over this emerging technology before it is able to stand on its own.

REFERENCES

1. Refers to title [21], United States Code: The Federal Food, Drug and Cosmetic Act of July 1993 (The Act, July 1993). For sale by the Superintendent of Documents, U.S. Government Printing Office, Washington, DC 20402.
2. [Sec. 201(n)] The Act, July 1993.
3. [Sec. 201(m)(k)(m)].
4. [Sec. 201(n)].
5. [Sec. 201(h)(1)(2)(3)].
6. Part 21, *Code of Federal Regulations* (CFR)§870.7 (c)(2).
7. 21CFR§870.7(e)(1).
8. 21CFR§870.7(d)(1).
9. 21CFR§870.7(e)(1).
10. [Sec. 513.(a)(1)(A)(I)].
11. [Sec. 513(b)(2)].
12. [Sec. 513(a)(1)(A)(B)(C)].
13. [Sec. 514(a)(b)].
14. [Sec. 514(2)(A)(B)(C)].
15. [Sec. 513(a)(1)(C)(ii)(II)].
16. See Reclassification [Sec(513)(f)(1)].
17. [Sec. 514(b)(1)].
18. 21CFR§870.7(f)(2).
19. [Sec. 520(h)(4)(B)].
20. [Sec. 514(a)(b)].
21. 21CFR§814.15.
22. 21CFR§814.39(a)(1).
23. [Sec. 514(a)(b)].

Index